Rights-Based Approaches
to Public Health

Elvira Beracochea, MD, MPH, has more than 25 years of experience as a physician, public health and international development expert, human rights advocate, epidemiologist, health policy advisor, researcher, health systems and hospital manager, consultant, professor, and coach. She has worked in more than 30 countries in Latin America, Africa, Asia, Eastern Europe, and the South Pacific. She is committed to help realize the right to health and the right to development. In 2005, she founded MIDEGO, an organization with an urgent rights-based mission: to accelerate the achievement of the Millennium Development Goals (MDGs). She has developed "Health for All NOW," a continuous innovation process to help achieve the MDGs and empower health professionals. In addition, she teaches Epidemiology at George Mason University.

Corey Weinstein, MD, CCHP, has been in the practice of medicine in California for 40 years. He began visiting prisoners in 1971 doing medical rights and advocacy. In 1980, he founded a group called Prisoner Health Advocates.

He is the immediate past chair of the International Human Rights Committee (IHRC) of the American Public Health Association (APHA) and was on the task force that wrote the 2003 *APHA Standards for Health Services in Correctional Institutions.* As a member of the IHRC, he works with the World Health Organization Health in Prison Project and the World Federation of Public Health Organizations advocating for prisoner rights.

Dr. Weinstein is a founder of California Prison Focus (CPF), a 20-year-old community-based human rights organization that works with prisoners in California's high-security prisons.

Dabney P. Evans, MPH, is executive director of the Emory University Institute of Human Rights. She is a senior associate faculty in the Hubert Department of Global Health at the Rollins School of Public Health at Emory University. Evans teaches courses in Interdisciplinary Perspectives in Human Rights and Health and Human Rights.

Evans serves on the Medical Education in Cooperation With Cuba (MEDICC), a nongovernmental organization whose aim is improving health care quality and accessibility in the United States, Cuba, and throughout the world. She is the current chair of the International Human Rights Committee of the American Public Health Association. She serves on the advisory boards of the Center for Trauma and Torture Survivors, the Refuge Media Project, and the Hubert H. Humphrey Fellowship. Evans is faculty advisor to two student groups: Physicians for Human Rights (PHR) based in the Emory University Medical School and Human Rights Action (HuRA) based in the Rollins School of Public Health. In 2007, she was the recipient of the Martin Luther King Jr. Community Service Award.

Rights-Based Approaches to Public Health

ELVIRA BERACOCHEA, MD, MPH
COREY WEINSTEIN, MD, CCHP
DABNEY P. EVANS, MPH

Editors

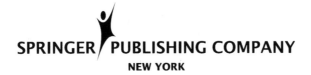

SPRINGER PUBLISHING COMPANY
NEW YORK

Springer Publishing Company, LLC
11 West 42nd Street
New York, NY 10036
www.springerpub.com

Acquisitions Editor: Jennifer Perillo
Senior Production Editor: Diane Davis
Cover Design: David Levy
Composition: Absolute Service, Inc., Gil Rafanan, Project Manager

ISBN: 978-0-8261-0569-1
E-book ISBN: 978-0-8261-0570-7

10 11 12 13/ 5 4 3 2 1

The author and the publisher of this work have made every effort to use sources believed to be reliable to provide information that is accurate and compatible with the standards generally accepted at the time of publication. Because medical science is continually advancing, our knowledge base continues to expand. Therefore, as new information becomes available, changes in procedures become necessary. We recommend that the reader always consult current research and specific institutional policies before performing any clinical procedure. The author and publisher shall not be liable for any special, consequential, or exemplary damages resulting, in whole or in part, from the readers' use of, or reliance on, the information contained in this book. The publisher has no responsibility for the persistence or accuracy of URLs for external or third-party Internet Web sites referred to in this publication and does not guarantee that any content on such Web sites is, or will remain, accurate or appropriate.

Library of Congress Cataloging-in-Publication Data

Rights-based approaches to public health / Elvira Beracochea, Corey Weinstein, Dabney P. Evans, editors.
    p. ; cm.
  Includes bibliographical references and index.
  ISBN 978-0-8261-0569-1 — ISBN 978-0-8261-0570-7 (e-book)
 1. Health care reform. 2. Right to health care. 3. Public health—Social aspects. I. Beracochea, Elvira. II. Weinstein, Corey. III. Evans, Dabney P.
  [DNLM: 1. Health Care Reform—methods. 2. Evidence-Based Practice. 3. Human Rights. 4. Internationality. 5. Organizational Case Studies. 6. Public Health. WA 530.1]
  RA394.R555 2011
  362.1'0425—dc22

                                    2010040005

Special discounts on bulk quantities of our books are available to corporations, professional associations, pharmaceutical companies, health care organizations, and other qualifying groups.

If you are interested in a custom book, including chapters from more than one of our titles, we can provide that service as well.

For details, please contact:
Special Sales Department, Springer Publishing Company, LLC
11 West 42nd Street, 15th Floor, New York, NY 10036-8002
Phone: 877-687-7476 or 212-431-4370; Fax: 212-941-7842
Email: sales@springerpub.com

Printed in the United States of America by Gasch Printing.

To the students of public health
who will be shaping these
new approaches to our work.
You are the ones who will deepen
our understanding of how to work
collaboratively with our communities
and institutions and empower them
to help create a better future.

Contents

Contributors

Charles Allen III, MSPH, is the Advisor to the Mayor & Director, Office of Coastal and Environmental Affairs, City of New Orleans.

Neil Arya, BASc, MD, CCFP, is a Family Physician and Director of Global Health at the University of Western Ontario. He is an Adjunct Professor of Environment and Resource Studies and of Health Studies at the University of Waterloo and Assistant Clinical Professor part time at McMaster University.

Laurel Baldwin-Ragaven, AB, MD CM, is a family physician, bioethics scholar and human rights advocate. She is the Medical and Executive Director of the Malta House of Care, a non-profit mobile medical van providing free primary health care services to the uninsured in Hartford, Connecticut.

Dhrubajyoti (Dru) Bhattacharya, JD, MPH, LLM, is an Assistant Professor of Health Policy in the Department of Preventive Medicine and Epidemiology, Loyola University Chicago Stritch School of Medicine, Director of the M.P.H. track in Health Policy and Law, and also serves as a Visiting Professor of Law at Loyola University Chicago School of Law.

Kathy Boudin, MA, EdD, is the Director of The Criminal Justice Initiative: Supporting Children, Families and Communities, located in The Columbia University School of Social Work where she is also an adjunct professor. She also works for The Center for Comprehensive Care at St. Lukes-Roosevelt Hospital with the Coming Home Program, addressing health needs for people with a history of incarceration.

Nichola Cadge, MPH, RGN, works in the Department of International Development.

Ujwal Chhetry, MA, received his Masters of Arts degree in Sustainable International Development from Brandeis University. In 2009, he was awarded Bridgewood Feldwater Fellowship to do a study on Rights Based Approach to HIV/AIDS in India. He is currently working as a Program Assistant in MIDEGO, Inc.

Khagendra Dahal, MBBS, MD, is currently the second year resident in Internal Medicine at St. Elizabeth's Medical Center, Boston, Massachusetts.

Don C. Des Jarlais, PhD, is Director of Research for the Baron Edmond de Rothschild Chemical Dependency Institute at Beth Israel Medical Center, Professor of Epidemiology and Population Health of Albert Einstein College of Medicine, a Senior Research Fellow with the National Development and Research Institutes, Inc., and a Guest Investigator at Rockefeller University in New York.

Ariel Frisancho is a health coordinator of CARE Peru.

Lance Gable, JD, MPH, is an assistant professor of law at Wayne State University Law School and a scholar at the Centers for Law and the Public's Health, a Collaborative at Georgetown and Johns Hopkins Universities.

Helene D. Gayle is president and chief executive officer of CARE USA, a leading international humanitarian organization with programs to end poverty in nearly 70 countries.

Jocelyn E. Getgen, JD, MPH, is the Program Director at Virtue Foundation.

Jay Goulden is program director for CARE Peru.

Jennifer Kasper, MD, MPH, FAAP, is on the faculty of the Division of Global Health in the Department of Pediatrics at Massachusetts General Hospital and an Instructor at Harvard Medical School. She is a former President and current Chair of the International Volunteer Committee of Doctors for Global Health.

George Kent is a professor in the Department of Political Science at the University of Hawai'i.

Alexandra Kirby, MA, is a consultant for the Global Drugs Policy program of the Open Society Institute.

Judy Kitts, MA, is a Negotiations Analyst for the Ministry of Aboriginal Relations and Reconciliation with the government of British Columbia.

Amanda M. Klasing, MA, JD, is a Fellow in the Women's Rights Division at Human Rights Watch, and was formerly the RFK Social Justice Fellow at RFK Center for Justice and Human Rights.

David Lee, MD, is Director of Technical Strategy and Quality at the Center for Pharmaceutical Management, Management Sciences for Health, Arlington, Virginia.

Leslie London, MD, MB, ChB, is a senior specialist in public health at the University of Cape Town, South Africa. He is the director of the School of Public Health and Family Medicine and the head of its Health and Human Rights Programme.

Kasia Malinowska-Sempruch, MSW, is a director of the Global Drugs Policy program at the Open Society Institute.

Benjamin Mason Meier, JD, LLM, PhD, is an Assistant Professor of Global Health Policy at the University of North Carolina at Chapel Hill and a Scholar at the O'Neill Institute for National and Global Health Law at Georgetown University.

Padmini (Mini) Murthy, MD, MPH, MS MPhil, CHES, is Assistant Professor, Department of Health Policy and Management and Global Health Program Director at New York Medical College School of Public Health. She is also Assistant Professor in the Department of Family and Community Medicine. Dr. Murthy is the NGO co-representative of the Medical Women's International Association to the United Nations.

David P. Novello, JD, is the principal in the Law Offices of David Novello, LLC in Washington, D.C. He has practiced environmental law in government and private practice for 25 years, and has taught at the Georgetown University Law School and the University of Maryland School of Law.

Mehlika Ozden Hoodbhoy, MA, was a consultant to HealthRight International.

Roshni D. Persaud, JD, MPH, is an attorney in the Office of Legal Affairs of the New York City Health and Hospitals Corporation and serves an Adjunct Assistant Professor for Hofstra University's Department of Health Professions and Family Studies, where she teaches Health Law and Ethics.

Andrew D. Pinto, MD, CCFP, MSc, is a family physician at St. Michael's Hospital in Toronto and is completing a fellowship in public health.

Mila Rosenthal, PhD, is the executive director of HealthRight International, a global health and human right organization working to build lasting access to health for excluded communities around the world and at home in the United States.

Leonard Rubenstein, JD, is at the Center for Public Health and Human Rights at the Johns Hopkins Bloomberg School of Public Health.

Anja Rudiger, PhD, is director of the Human Right to Health Program at the National Economic and Social Rights Initiative (NESRI).

Margaret L. Satterthwaite, MA, JD, is Associate Professor of Clinical Law and a Faculty Director of the Center for Human Rights and Global Justice at New York University School of Law.

Monika Sawhney, PhD, is currently working as an Assistant Professor of Global Health at Mercer University, Macon, Georgia. At Mercer, she is setting up an undergraduate program in Global Health.

Salaam Semaan, MPH, DrPH, is Deputy Associate Director for Science, National Center for HIV/AIDS, Viral Hepatitis, STD, and TB Prevention, Centers for Disease Control and Prevention (CDC), Atlanta, Georgia.

Clyde Lanford (Lanny) Smith, MD, MPH, DTM&H, FACP, is an Associate Professor of Clinical Medicine and Clinical Family & Social Medicine in the Residency Programs in Primary Care and Social Internal Medicine, Montefiore Medical Center, Albert Einstein College of Medicine (AECOM) and serves as Global Health Advisor at AECOM.

Tanya Telfair Sharpe, (EIS 2000) PhD, MS, is the Deputy Director for the Office of Health Equity of CDC's National Center for HIV/AIDS, Hepatitis, STDs, and TB Prevention where she works to achieve health equity for ethnic/racial and gender minorities.

Vandana Tripathi, MPH, was the Director of Programs of HealthRight International and is currently enrolled in a PhD program in the Department of Population, Family, and Reproductive Health at the Johns Hopkins University Bloomberg School of Public Health.

Emily Waller, MPH, is the Program Manager of the Program on International Health and Human Rights in the Department of Global Health and Population at the Harvard School of Public Health.

Ann Yoachim, MPH, is the Program Manager of the Institute on Water Resources Law and Policy and an Adjunct Instructor in the School of Public Health and Tropical Medicine, Tulane University.

Anthony B. Zwi, MB BCh, DOH, DTM&H, MSc, PhD, FFPHM, AFPHM, is Professor of Global Health at the School of Public Health and Community Medicine at the University of New South Wales, Sydney, Australia.

Foreword

How I wish this important book were available in 2002 when I began my 6 years as UN Special Rapporteur on the right to the highest attainable standard of health!

In the early years, when talking with health professionals, I sometimes felt like I was speaking a foreign language. Human rights are enshrined in the World Health Organization Constitution, Declaration of Alma-Ata, Ottawa Charter for Health Promotion, and other important documents agreed to by the health community, but I soon found that the language of human rights did not enjoy widespread currency among health professions.

Of course, there is much common ground between the health and human rights communities: Both groups wish to establish effective, integrated, responsive health systems accessible to all; both stress the importance of not only access to health care but also access to water, sanitation, health information, and education; both understand that good health is not the sole responsibility of a health department, but a wide range of public and private actors; both prioritize the struggle against discrimination and disadvantage; both stress cultural respect; and so on. And yet, despite the inspiring and pioneering work of Jonathan Mann and his colleagues at the Harvard School of Public Health and the Francois-Xavier Bagnoud Center for Health and Human Rights, I found little awareness of the manifest common ground between health and human rights—which is why this book would have helped so much as I assumed my mandate in 2002.

This wide-ranging collection explores how public health professionals have begun to utilize rights-based approaches in their work, the challenges they have faced, and the lessons they have learned. Although written with practitioners in mind, the discussion will also be of interest to scholars. With an orientation toward the United States, it will also engage health and human rights professionals in many other countries.

In 2002, the UN Commission on Human Rights adopted a resolution establishing a new human rights monitoring mechanism: a Special Rapporteur on the right to the highest attainable standard of health. Although the commission had been establishing such mechanisms in relation to civil and political rights for some decades, it was not until the late 1990s that it turned its attention to economic, social, and cultural rights. The Government of Brazil, supported by other developing countries, drove the initiative to establish a new mechanism on the right to the highest attainable standard of health. Developed countries, on the other hand, were circumspect. Indeed, two—United States and Australia—voted against the resolution establishing this new mandate.

The Rapporteur's task may be very briefly summarized as requiring the mandate holder to help states better promote and protect the right to the highest attainable standard of health (sometimes shortened to "the right to health").

After lengthy consultations, I set out my broad approach to the mandate. In brief, I identified three main objectives: to raise the profile of the right to health as a fundamental human right; to clarify the contours and content of the right to health; and to find practical ways of operationalizing the right to health. Of course, these objectives could only be realized with the advice and assistance of a wide range of allies. Moreover, I identified two interrelated themes that would recur throughout my reports: (a) poverty and the right to health, and (b) discrimination and the right to health.

There are striking similarities between, on the one hand, these three objectives (especially the first and third) and twin themes and, on the other hand, the issues running through this book.

Like other Rapporteurs, my output had three official forms: thematic reports, country reports, and "communications," that is, letters of complaint to governments. Over 6 years, I wrote some 30 right-to-health reports. All are in the public domain.[1] The thematic reports look at issues such as sexual and reproductive rights, access to medicines (including the duties of states and pharmaceutical companies), mental disability, water and sanitation, maternal mortality, the skills drain, the health-related Millennium Development Goals, and indicators and benchmarks. One thematic report published *Human Rights Guidelines for Pharmaceutical Companies in relation to Access to Medicines*. The country reports are on Mozambique, Peru, Romania, Uganda, Lebanon/Israel (following the war

---

[1]All available at: http://www.essex.ac.uk/human_rights_centre/research/rth/index.aspx

of mid-2006), Sweden, and India. A report on Colombia/Ecuador (the aerial spraying of glyphosate along their common border) is forthcoming. An additional country report looks at donors' human rights responsibilities of international and cooperation in health by exploring Sweden's role in relation to (a) Uganda's health sector and (b) the health-related activities of the World Bank and International Monetary Fund. Under the rubric of country reports, I also reported on the World Trade Organization, Guantanamo Bay, and the pharmaceutical company GlaxoSmithKline. All of these country reports were preceded by visits to the place or institution in question, except Guantanamo Bay where the Bush Administration imposed unacceptable conditions on the visit: Specifically, the authorities refused to allow private interviews with the detainees. All the thematic and country reports were presented, in writing and orally, to either the UN General Assembly or Human Rights Council/Commission, where they were discussed.

Clearly, a number of these right-to-health reports resonate with specific chapters in this book, such as those on medicines, water, conflict, and the Millennium Development Goals.

It is not possible here to review my methods of work, although it should be emphasized that my colleagues and I consulted very widely before preparing either thematic or country reports. These consultations were not only with government officials, public officials, civil society groups, and academics. They also included listening to the most disadvantaged, such as internally displaced people living in the conflict zone of northern Uganda, the inhabitants of remote villages in Peru's *sierra*, and the bombed-out inhabitants of south Beirut and southern Lebanon.

When reviewing these reports, it is possible to identify some trends and phases in my approach to the mandate that bear on some of the discussions in the chapters of this book.

Promulgated by the UN Committee on Economic, Social and Cultural Rights in 2000, General Comment 14 represents a critically important stage in the evolution of our understanding of the right to the highest attainable standard of health. The General Comment shaped much of my work, just as it shapes much of the discussion in this book. However, as its name suggests, the General Comment provides a *general* analysis of the right to health. Building on this analysis, my reports endeavor to make the right to health more specific and accessible. Thus, some reports take the analysis provided by General Comment 14 and apply it to specific elements of the right to health, such as access to medicines. Others apply the General Comment to specific right-to-health issues, such as the skills drain, and specific groups of people, such as those with mental disabilities. Also, country reports apply the comment's general analysis to the right to health in specific jurisdictions.

This specific application of General Comment 14 permitted the development and refinement of the analysis set out in general terms in the comment. For example, the comment briefly underscores the crucial importance of accountability, whereas most of my reports consider and apply this vital human rights concept, sometimes in considerable detail. Although the comment devotes two important paragraphs to indicators and benchmarks, I had the opportunity to prepare three reports on this issue, the last of which sets out a methodology for a human rights-based approach to health indicators. Like some of the chapters in this book, this process of applying General Comment 14 to specific contexts helps to refine the analytical framework for "unpacking" the right to health.

The application and refinement of this analytical framework was necessary but not sufficient. Experience showed that some health workers were understandably uncomfortable with the legal and abstract nature of the framework. For many health workers, the framework remained divorced from the realities of public health and medicine.

This led to closer cooperation with health workers and a revised approach typified, for example, by the reports on Peru, Uganda, Sweden, and India. The Ugandan report focuses on a single issue: neglected diseases, that is, those diseases mainly afflicting the poorest people in the poorest communities. The framework set out in General Comment 14, and subsequently refined, informs the Ugandan report, but the report endeavors to be more operational in its discussion about, for example, incentives to encourage health professionals to work in Uganda's underserved areas; participation in Uganda's village health teams; the burden placed on the Ugandan authorities by the uncoordinated health interventions of the international community; the need to enhance research and development for neglected diseases; the importance of an *integrated* health system; accountability and an enhanced role for the Ugandan Human Rights Commission; and so on. As in my earlier reports, the framework's elements are still there —access, participation, accountability and others—but they are applied in a more practical, operational manner. My report on Peru, by the way, benefited greatly from collaboration with CARE Peru (and others), as discussed in chapter 15.

Around this time there were other shifts in emphasis in my approach to the mandate. For example, I began to give more emphasis to the common ground between medicine, public health, and the right to health; the indispensable role of health workers in the delivery of the right to health; and how the right to health can help health workers deliver their professional objectives. All these arguments are found in the earliest reports but, as the mandate unfolded, they began to have greater prominence. If they are to succeed, however, such arguments cannot rely on excessively legal phrases and abstract analysis that risk alienating many health workers whose primary interest is the formulation and practical implementation of health policies, programs, and projects. At the same time, the empowering, transformative message of human rights must not be sacrificed.

Discussions with health workers revealed another problem. The thematic reports were focusing on specific issues, specific groups of people, and so on. Moreover, some of the country visits were now single issue, such as Uganda (neglected diseases) and India (maternal mortality). Although this focused approach brings major advantages, it has a serious drawback: it can lead to a fractured consideration of the right to the highest attainable standard of health, making it more difficult to look at larger, systemic issues on which the right to health depends. This focused approach was the mandate's equivalent of narrow vertical health interventions that, without care, can undermine the wider health system.

This was one of the factors that led to my examination of health systems from the right-to-health perspective. Also, at last the international community was beginning to recognize that many health systems were failing and collapsing. After years of neglect, the clarion cry was to strengthen health systems. For these and other reasons, the UN Human Rights Council passed a resolution in 2006 asking me to prepare a report on health systems and the right to health, a topic that is addressed in an early chapter in this volume.

Like all the contributions to this book, my UN reports not only confirm that health and human rights occupy much common ground, they also show how health and human rights complement and reinforce each other.

Obviously, the realization of the right to the highest attainable standard of health depends on health professionals enhancing public health and delivering medical care. Of course, the right to health cannot be realized without health professionals! Equally, the classic, traditional objectives of the various health professions can benefit from the new, dynamic discipline of human rights. Human rights can help to reinforce existing, good health programs, and they can sometimes help to identify new, equitable health policies. They can help to ensure that health policies and programs are equitable, effective, evidence-based, robust, participatory, inclusive, and meaningful to those living in poverty. The supportive role of human rights extends to the provision of medical care, as well as public health. Also, provided it is done in an appropriate manner, framing a pressing health concern as a human rights issue can enhance its legitimacy and importance. In short, health professionals can use human rights to help them achieve their professional objectives.

This highlights one of the great strengths of this book: It is a place for public health practitioners to share and explore their experiences through the human rights "lens." In this way, it provides a snapshot of where the public health community stands in relation to human rights. The case studies give us applied examples of how human rights are being used in contemporary public health.

At root, those working in health and human rights are both animated by a similar concern: the well-being of individuals and populations. This book will be an invaluable asset to both communities as they work to achieve their common goals.

Paul Hunt
UN Special Rapporteur on the right to the highest attainable standard of health
(2002–2008)

Rights-Based Approaches
to Public Health

PART I

Introduction

CHAPTER 1

Introduction: Why Do Rights-Based Approaches to Health Matter?

Elvira Beracochea, Dabney P. Evans, and Corey Weinstein

INTRODUCTION

In late 2000, I (Dabney Evans) found myself in a dusty carpet mill outside the city of Kathmandu, in the small Himalayan country of Nepal. Although it was a clear winter day, the carpet mill was poorly lit; carpet and dust particles obscured my view. On the floor of one of the massive carpet looms sat a young woman, a Tibetan refugee. As I looked closer, I saw that an infant was strapped to her chest in a sling.

As a public health professional, I knew that the educational level and age of a child's mother is significantly related to infant birth outcomes (such as birth weight and gestational age). What would the future hold for that baby and her young mother? From a human rights perspective, several issues clamored for my attention. The young woman was a refugee . . . was she able to complete an education before leaving her home country? What kind of traumas might she have faced on her journey? What was her political status now and did she have access to any support services? She had secured a job in the carpet factory . . . but were the working conditions fair? Could she take breaks to eat, use the restroom, or nurse her child? Was she being paid a fair wage? And finally, what about her health and that of her infant?

This scenario underlines the interdependence of rights and the ways in which they may impact one another. Yes, the woman had a right to work, but perhaps working in the carpet factory was impinging on her right to receive education or negatively impacting the health of her child.

Preventable deaths are what brought me (Elvira Beracochea) to work to realize everyone's right to health. Too many times, I have seen infants die from preventable diarrhea and dehydration, patients with TB whose health centers have run out of medicine, and young mothers in shock because of postpartum hemorrhage who arrive at a health center too late to do anything.

As a doctor, I have worked to reduce preventable deaths in developing countries for more than 25 years. In spite of all our medical knowledge and technology, diarrhea and dehydration, pneumonia, measles, polio, malaria, TB, AIDS, and treatable pregnancy complications still kill people unnecessarily. We know how to prevent and treat these conditions, we have the resources to do it, and we know where people at risk of dying are (in Haiti, sub-Saharan Africa, and India, mostly). How can we prioritize the health needs of those that need health care the most?

The answer is by going beyond needs and ensuring the *right to health* to everyone on this planet. In a rights-based approach (RBA) to public health, everyone has the right to access current medical knowledge about prevention and treatment. As a public health professional, I believe I have the responsibility to protect and help realize the right to health because I have the knowledge to do so and the good fortune to live in a country where I can advocate equal access to resources. Implementing such an approach requires a commitment to not pass on to the next generation of public health professionals the same burden of disease our generation inherited. The next generation will have to fight antibiotic resistance, AIDS and emerging infectious diseases, cancer, diabetes, and cardiovascular conditions; they should not have to fight diarrhea, infant pneumonia, polio, measles, malaria, TB, or lack of appropriate obstetric care. It is time we prevent these deaths on a global scale.

My aim for this book is to help more public health professionals use RBAs to prevent unnecessary deaths and help the next generation of public health professionals learn from our success and mistakes. Thus, they will have a head start on realizing the right to health for all.

I (Corey Weinstein) have traveled many lonely roads in the past 40 years going from prison to prison as a human rights advocate. I've watched with horror as the United States has become what Dr. Andrew Coyle calls "the nation that loves prisons," and the world's biggest jailer. My organization's slogan is "uplifting prisoners' rights to preserve human rights."

Throughout my career, I have seen many prisoners suffer needlessly. Louie was our investigator in D Block at Pelican Bay State Prison; he documented every time the guards brutalized a prisoner during a cell extraction. He got his information through the air vent and drain pipe phone system. He was killed by deliberate medical neglect. Charisse took on the medical department at her prison in Chowchilla. She fought successfully for better care while she was being poisoned with iron overload through medical mistreatment of her sickle cell disease. She declined to retire to the locked nursing unit for intravenous therapy and ultimately gave her life to the struggle. Preston was killed by guard gunfire for engaging in a weaponless standup fistfight set up by staff in a small concrete exercise yard they called *Little Vietnam.*

Two critical issues brought human rights into the foreground of our work: the medical neglect of and discrimination against prisoners with HIV that caused needless tragedy and suffering; and the burgeoning use of long-term solitary confinement on a massive scale that fractured the minds of women and men so confined. The resulting despair and violence increased the suffering inside. These are matters that go beyond the narrow confines of court-adjudicated civil rights or medical neglect. Beginning in the mid-1990s, organizations working with prisoners began to appeal to the United Nations under the human rights treaties implemented during the Clinton administration.

In the midst of the devastation of mass incarceration, we used a new paradigm that appealed to the best in society and connected us to others from various sectors and across national boundaries. In a human rights framework, RBAs codify and deepen the strategies of radical community organizing from the 1960s and 1970s. Deep within the essence of RBAs is the knowledge that ordinary people have the capacity to manage their own lives and society quite well using knowledge and resources that we have developed and that must be shared freely. That is the dream that finds partial realization in the work of each of the authors in this book.

PUBLIC HEALTH AND HUMAN RIGHTS

Although public health practitioners have always identified strongly with the ideals of social justice, it was not until the past decade that health and human rights truly entered the foreground of public health debates. The groundbreaking work of Jonathan Mann (see for example Mann et al., 1994) presented the stigma and discrimination faced by people living with HIV and AIDS as not only a health issue but also a human rights issue.

Since that time, the subdiscipline has grown tremendously—including the launch of an international journal on health and human rights, numerous texts, international conferences on the topic, and the appointment of the United Nations Special Rapporteur on the right to health.

Even though research and practical work related to health and human rights has grown exponentially, those engaged in this work still face tremendous challenges and growing pains. Although the legal definition of the right to health has gained great clarity based on various international documents, which will be discussed in this chapter and throughout the book, the methods for effective program planning, implementation and evaluation have remained challenging for those in the field. The gap remains between international human rights law ("paper") and public health professionals, who largely see themselves as "people people" as opposed to "paper people."

As public health scholars Easley, Marks, and Morgan (2001) put it,

> the challenge facing public health professionals wishing to be more engaged in human rights is to go beyond the emotional attachment to social justice and human rights and acquire the knowledge of the field and the skills necessary to put human rights into health practice (p. 1924).

Despite the challenges in interpreting and applying international human rights law and the right to health, some health professionals have undertaken novel approaches in an attempt to test the efficacy of RBAs to public health. After all, RBAs must be proved to positively impact both health and human rights if we can expect their methods to be adopted more broadly in the public health community. The purpose of this text is to explore how public health professionals have begun to use RBAs in their work, the challenges they have faced, and the lessons they have learned.

WHAT DO WE MEAN BY "RIGHTS-BASED APPROACHES"?

One of the great strengths of the concept of human rights is that the language of rights is available to all. It is evocative and often emotional when anyone makes a claim about their rights. Just imagine your sentiments whenever you hear someone proclaim, "My rights are being violated!" The early pioneers of human rights might have only imagined a day when the concept of human rights was so widespread that individuals might make such statements.

However, the overly liberal use of rights language may be inappropriate and may distort the concept of human rights. Occasionally people will lay claim to "the right to (fill in the blank)" without any basis in international human rights law. It is for this reason that an explicit definition of "rights-based" must be agreed on. Throughout this text, the term *rights-based* implies *an explicit connection to normative documents in the field of international human rights.* Such documents include *hard law* (such as international human rights treaties) and *soft law* (such as reports and general comments developed within the international and/or regional human rights realm). We will discuss some of the seminal documents related to the right to health over the following pages.

INTERNATIONAL HUMAN RIGHTS DOCUMENTS AND THE RIGHT TO HEALTH

Key international documents that discuss and define the right to health include, but are not limited to, Article 25 of the Universal Declaration of Human Rights (UDHR); Article 12 of the International Covenant on Economic, Social and Cultural Rights (ICESCR); General Comment 14; Reports of the United Nations Special Rapporteur on the Right to Health; and the Office of the United Nations High Commissioner on Human Rights/World Health Organization Fact Sheet. A more in-depth discussion of the evolution of these documents is provided in chapter 2; here we will summarize the key passages related to the right to health within each document.

The Universal Declaration of Human Rights

The UDHR[1] was adopted by the General Assembly of the United Nations on December 10, 1948. Article 25 states the following with regard to health:

1. Everyone has the right to a standard of living adequate for the health and well-being of himself and of his family, including food, clothing, housing and medical care and necessary social services, and the right to security in the event of unemployment, sickness, disability, widowhood, old age or other lack of livelihood in circumstances beyond his control.
2. Motherhood and childhood are entitled to special care and assistance. All children, whether born in or out of wedlock, shall enjoy the same social protection.

The International Covenant on Economic, Social and Cultural Rights

The ICESCR[2] is a treaty adopted by the United Nations General Assembly on December 16, 1966, and in force since January 3, 1976. Article 12 states:

1. The States Parties to the present Covenant recognize the right of everyone to the enjoyment of the highest attainable standard of physical and mental health.
2. The steps to be taken by the States Parties to the present Covenant to achieve the full realization of this right shall include those necessary for:
   (a) The provision for the reduction of the stillbirth-rate and of infant mortality and for the healthy development of the child;
   (b) The improvement of all aspects of environmental and industrial hygiene;
   (c) The prevention, treatment and control of epidemic, endemic, occupational and other diseases;
   (d) The creation of conditions which would assure to all medical service and medical attention in the event of sickness.

General Comment 14 on the Right to the Highest Attainable Standard of Physical and Mental Health

General Comment 14[3] offers an authoritative interpretation of the meaning of the right to health as defined in Article 12 of the ICESCR. It also links the right to health to other rights and other international rights documents:

1. Health is a fundamental human right indispensable for the exercise of other human rights. Every human being is entitled to the enjoyment of the highest attainable standard of health conducive to living a life in dignity. The realization of the right to health may be pursued through numerous, complementary approaches, such as the formulation of health policies, or the implementation of health programmes developed by the World Health Organization (WHO), or the adoption of specific legal instruments. Moreover, the right to health includes certain components which are legally enforceable.
2. The human right to health is recognized in numerous international instruments. . . . The right to health is recognized, inter alia, in article 5 (e) (iv) of the International Convention on the Elimination of All Forms of Racial Discrimination of 1965, in articles 11.1 (f) and 12 of the Convention on the Elimination of All Forms of Discrimination against Women of 1979 and in article 24 of the Convention on the Rights of the Child of 1989. Several regional human rights instruments also recognize the right to health, such as the European Social Charter of 1961 as revised (art. 11), the African Charter on Human and Peoples' Rights of 1981 (art. 16) and the Additional Protocol to the American Convention on Human Rights in the Area of Economic,

Social and Cultural Rights of 1988 (art. 10). Similarly, the right to health has been proclaimed by the Commission on Human Rights, as well as in the Vienna Declaration and Programme of Action of 1993 and other international instruments.

3. The right to health is closely related to and dependent upon the realization of other human rights, as contained in the International Bill of Rights, including the rights to food, housing, work, education, human dignity, life, non-discrimination, equality, the prohibition against torture, privacy, access to information, and the freedoms of association, assembly and movement. These and other rights and freedoms address integral components of the right to health.

Reports of the United Nations Special Rapporteur on the Right to Health

Special Rapporteurs are independent experts appointed by the United Nations Commission on Human Rights (now the Human Rights Council) to examine and report on a situation or a specific human rights theme. In 2002, the first Special Rapporteur on the right to health was appointed by the United Nations. This person reports to United Nations annually on the status of the right to health around the world.[4]

In addition to his contributions in more clearly defining the right to health under international human rights law, the United Nations Special Rapporteur on the right to health has also significantly contributed to RBAs through his work relating to monitoring and evaluating the right to health using indicators.[5] As in public health evaluations, the importance of various methods and techniques is useful. Indicators must measure process as well as short and long-term outcome and may include qualitative and quantitative indicators.

Office of the United Nations High Commissioner on Human Rights/World Health Organization Fact Sheet

This document[6] outlines the way in which the right to health relates to vulnerable groups. In general, the human rights paradigm is particularly concerned with groups whose members may be particularly vulnerable to human rights violations (such as racial minorities, women, children, refugees, persons with disabilities) as evidenced by numerous treaties, which define the rights of those groups. This focus complements the population focus of most public health work. These documents, ratified or not, serve as guides to advocate, promote, and negotiate for increased fulfillment of the right to health.

A more in-depth discussion of international documents and their impact on health will be provided in chapter 6 by George Kent.

COMMON ELEMENTS OF RIGHTS-BASED APPROACHES

RBAs consider the social, political, historical, and economic contexts that frame the ways in which health is produced, experienced, and understood (Yamin, 2008).

Based on a call for the development of common methods in RBAs, *The Human Rights Based Approach Statement of Common Understanding*[7] was developed under the auspices of the United Nations Development Programme. It states that human rights principles should guide all phases of programming and in all sectors (including health) engaging in development work. These principles may guide public health work more generally through the incorporation of an RBA. The basic human rights principles discussed in the *Common Understanding* include the following:

- Human rights are universal and inalienable. All people in the world are entitled to them. They cannot voluntarily be given up, nor can others take them away. As stated in Article 1 of the UDHR, "All human beings are born free and equal in dignity and rights."
- Human rights are indivisible. Whether of a civil, cultural, economic, political, or social nature, they are all inherent to the dignity of every person. Consequently, they all have equal status as rights, and cannot be ranked in a hierarchical order.
- Human rights are interdependent and interrelated. The realization of one right often depends, wholly or in part, upon the realization of others. For instance, realization of the right to health may depend, in certain circumstances, on realization of the right to education or information.
- All individuals are equal as human beings and by virtue of the inherent dignity of each person. All human beings are entitled to their human rights without discrimination of any kind, such as race, color, sex, ethnicity, age, language, religion, political or other opinion, national or social origin, disability, property, birth, or other status as explained by the human rights treaty bodies.
- Every person and all peoples are entitled to active, free, and meaningful participation in, contribution to, and enjoyment of civil, economic, social, cultural, and political development in which human rights and fundamental freedoms can be realized.
- States and other duty bearers are answerable for the observance of human rights. In this regard, they have to comply with the legal norms and standards enshrined in human rights instruments. Where they fail to do so, aggrieved rights holders are entitled to

institute proceedings for appropriate redress before a competent court or other adjudicator in accordance with the rules and procedures provided by law.

One retrospective analysis (Rand & Watson, 2008) suggested that rights-based projects include the following eight elements:

- A thorough analysis of underlying causes of poverty, including power, gender, and risk;
- Community-centered development, including sustainable capacity and decision-making ability;
- Duty bearers who are engaged, strengthened, and accountable;
- Advocacy for sustainable change;
- Alliance building;
- Engagement at multiple levels;
- A focus on marginalized and discriminated groups; and
- A presentation of the issues as rights issues relative to international standards.

Each of these elements should, at a minimum, be considered when developing a project and incorporated to the extent appropriate.

RIGHTS-BASED APPROACHES VERSUS NEEDS-BASED APPROACHES

Some professionals have shifted from a *needs-based approach* (NBA) to an *RBA*, giving people the ability to claim what is rightfully theirs as opposed to simply receiving aid. The NBA is commonly used and allows public health professionals to prioritize the health problems of a group or community and subjugate the needs of the individual to the needs of the majority. This is a classic example of *utilitarianism*, the ethical theory that holds that actions should be evaluated based on whether they benefit the greatest good for the greatest number. This conflicts with a key tenet of human rights: rights are universal. Therefore, everyone has the right to health; no one has more right than another. One challenge with RBAs, then, is to balance the rights of individuals with the rights of communities and especially vulnerable populations.

The NBA can also be used as an excuse for poor public health performance. Accounting for poor performance is easier when needs exceed resources. We know that resources are never enough; there is always a way to spend all that we have and more. We also know that spending more

FIGURE 1.1 Checklist for Assessing Rights-Based Approaches in Public Health

Human Right Principle	Yes or No?
Are issues presented as rights issues relative to international standards as opposed to need based issues?	
Action: If no, identify explicitly the sources of international standards that relate to the issue at hand.	
Is the approach based on a thorough analysis of underlying causes of vulnerability and poverty including power, gender, and risk?	
Action: If no, examine factors which may influence vulnerability, specifically poverty, and other demographic variables foe the population under consideration.	
Is the approach centered on community development including sustainable capacity and decision making ability?	
Action: If no, how might the program incorporate participatory approaches for community engagement?	
Are duty bearers engaged strengthened and accountable?	
Action: If no, how can stakeholders be included in program processes?	
Do advocacy efforts advocate for sustainable change?	
Action: If no, how might sustainability be incorporated?	
Are alliances being built among all stakeholders?	
Action: If no, consider listing all potential stakeholder and inviting their participatory engagement.	
Is there engagement at multiple levels in the health system?	
Action: If no, consider if such exclusions are necessary and relevant.	
Do programs focus on marginalized and discriminated groups?	
Action: If no, examine the vulnerable groups that may potentially be impacted and devise a plan to address these impacts.	

money on health does not necessary lead to better health. There is evidence that citizens of more affluent countries, such as the United States, do not enjoy better health outcomes than other countries. In a rights-based public health system, health would not be something only the rich can afford and in which charity is used to meet the health needs of poor, minority, or marginalized groups. In a rights-based public health system, the government has to fulfill *everyone's* right to health through evidence-based and effective services at national, state, and local levels. A well-implemented rights-based program or service calls for ensuring that everyone's rights are considered and everyone's responsibilities are accounted for. Partnerships between local governments and civil society organizations and stronger advocacy for the rights of the poor and sick are essential.

Because limited resources prevent many public health programs from meeting the needs of all, many public health professionals dismiss RBAs as too idealistic or impractical; in the end, rights become part of the public health rhetoric and their value as a public health approach is weakened.

Accountability is another key component of RBAs to public health. In clinical settings, health professionals are accountable for helping their patients. In contrast, most public health professionals are not used to accounting for their own duties and taking responsibility for the resources entrusted to them. In addition, communities are not organized to claim their rights and demand accountability from government at various levels. Public health professionals need to use the information they collect to account for progress toward meeting the rights of all citizens in their area of responsibility.

In this new way of delivering public health services, public health professionals monitor the health rights of the communities they serve, then create and manage efficient programs to reach the needs of every individual and family.

We suggest that you consider the questions and actions in the checklist for assessing rights-based approaches in public health (Figure 1.1) to assess how well rights are being protected and served in your area of public health. This simple assessment tool will help you take the first steps toward moving from a needs-based to rights-based public health system.

RIGHT HOLDERS, DUTY BEARERS, AND NON-STATE ACTORS

Fundamentally, human rights describe the relationship between individuals (or groups) and the State. This relationship forms the core of most human rights doctrine because nation states have, in recent history, become the most powerful entities in the world. Individuals and groups are often referred to as *rights holders* because the rights discussed in the human rights paradigm are predominantly described in terms of the individual. These rights adhere to individuals because we are human and we are inherently born in dignity.

States are known as *duty bearers* because they assume responsibility to promote and protect human rights. In the past, these obligations have been categorized by the type of rights (civil and political, for example, as opposed to economic, social, and cultural). Another way of categorizing rights and their subsequent obligations is to describe them as either positive or negative. A *positive right* is a right to be subjected to an action of another person or group; a negative right is a right *not to be* subjected to an action of another person or group.

Presently, obligations of states are most commonly discussed in the following three ways: respect, protect, and fulfill. The obligation to *respect* is a pledge by the State to refrain from directly violating the right to health. The obligation to *protect* obliges the State to prevent other actors from violating the right to health. Finally, the obligation requires positive action on the part of the State toward the *fulfillment* of the right.[8]

In relation to public health, States are not anonymous entities. States are represented by politicians and lawmakers, as well as local public health staff. The role of rights-based public health workers is to work in close connection with State authorities to ensure that the right to health is fulfilled for everyone in the communities they serve and help account for the status of their health.

At a global level, the United Nations holds States accountable for their human rights obligations via the mechanisms defined in the various charter and treaty monitoring bodies of each organization. For example, the Human Rights Council is a charter body that holds a broad human rights mandate. Treaty monitoring bodies hold more specific mandates related to their area of law. For instance, the Committee Against Torture specifically examines State behavior with regard to the obligations set forth within the Convention Against Torture. Additionally, under the auspices of the United Nations High Commissioner for Human Rights, several UN country teams have implemented RBAs in their work. They integrate human rights in country level analysis and planning, the development of theme groups on rights-related topics, support for human rights advisors in country and existing human rights mechanisms, advocacy and awareness raising, and the integration of human rights activities into postconflict, peace-building, and humanitarian operations (United Nations Development Group, n.d.).

The final players within the field of human rights are *non-State actors*. Non-State actors may include any private individual or groups such as transnational or multinational corporations (referred to as TNCs and MNCs, respectively) as well as nongovernmental organizations (NGOs) and civil society organizations (CSOs). Mediators between the two, particularly when the rights-holder cannot advocate for his or her own rights, are sometimes referred to as *right claimers*. This is the case of a parent claiming the rights of his child, or an organization claiming the rights of rape victims to receive AIDS treatment.

Non-State actors may play a positive role by advocating for those whose rights are not being protected. Likewise, some non-State actors may negatively impact rights by directly or indirectly violating human rights. Although MNCs are often categorized as the "bad guys" and NGOs as the "good guys," it is important to note that the potential positive or negative impact of non-State actors is not cut and dry. The obligations of non-State actors are not clearly defined under auspices of the current human rights regime; the role and potential responsibilities of non-State actors is currently evolving.

Within this framework, public health professionals are in a unique position. When working directly for federal, state, or local government agencies, they may themselves be State actors and assume the corresponding responsibilities. If they work within NGOs and CSOs, they are non-State actors. As individuals, they assume certain rights and responsibilities. It is therefore important for all public health professionals to reflect on the role they are in and the corresponding rights and responsibilities that follow in order to act appropriately.

Rights holders can also be duty-bearers when it comes to ensuring health. For example, communities have the right to health and the duty to participate in the delivery of health services. When using an RBA, all duty-bearers demonstrate responsibility and accountability at various levels. Take child immunization programs for instance. Parents and guardians have the right to ask the government to provide vaccines. However, they also have the responsibility to bring their children for immunization at the right time. The responsibility and accountability for a child's immunization is shared by all duty-bearers at various levels in the health system: the nurse that efficiently provides the vaccine, the public health professional that manages and oversees the immunization program, all the way up to the local and national government authorities that approved the budget and purchased the vaccines and syringes. They all have a duty to protect the right to health of that child.

EFFICACY OF RIGHTS-BASED APPROACHES TO HEALTH

Several organizations, including United Nations International Children's Emergency Fund (UNICEF), Cooperative for Assistance and Relief Everywhere (CARE), and Save the Children, have begun implementing RBAs into their work, along with evaluations of project efficacy (Rand & Watson, 2008;

UK Interagency Group on Rights-Based Approaches, 2007). When compared to nonrights-based projects, "rights-based projects show a greater range and depth of positive impacts, and these are more likely to be sustained over time" (UK Interagency Group on Rights-Based Approaches, p. 34). Rights-based projects are also seen to address underlying structural causes of poverty and disadvantage as well as working in partnership with various stakeholders to address social problems. Overall results of RBAs include:

- Asset accumulation, such as improved access to maternal and neo-natal health services, increased protection against HIV/AIDS, and increased gender equity; in addition, the quality and retention of assets gained also showed improvement in combination with the use of RBAs;
- Reduction of vulnerability by treating vulnerability as a structural issue itself rather than as a symptom of other social ills;
- Improved linkages between citizen and state resulting in reduced social exclusion and vulnerability; in addition, increased willingness and ability of actors to fulfill their obligations as well as accountability;
- Improved access to justice and increased social and political capital;
- Diversification of livelihood security;
- Increased knowledge and skills through capacity building; and
- Improved protection against social discrimination on the basis of gender or other vulnerabilities as well as improved protection from social exploitation (UK Interagency Group on Rights-Based Approaches, 2007).

Participants in a retrospective analysis of projects using RBAs identified the following nine categories of impact:

- Changes to policy and practice;
- Impact at multiple levels;
- Affirmation of human dignity;
- Change in power dynamics;
- Strengthened mechanisms for civil society claims on rights and duty holder accountability;
- Increased peace and personal security;
- Opened political culture;
- Greater responsiveness, responsibility, and accountability among duty holders; and
- Fundamental and sustainable change (Rand & Watson, 2008).

How to measure the impact of RBAs within each of these categories is still under development and may likely be the focus of the next wave of research.

CONCLUSION

In the chapters ahead, you will see various attempts at dealing with the RBA versus NBA dilemma, particularly in difficult situations such as prisons, high-conflict areas, and developing countries. You will learn what works and what has not worked yet. The fact that an RBA has not been adopted at global scale is not an indication that the approach is not feasible, but that we have not figured out a way to respect each other's rights and account for our own responsibilities yet. As you read this book, we suggest you reflect on your own rights and responsibilities to your fellow citizens. We hope it inspires you to think of other ways to further a rights-based agenda.

REFERENCES

Easley, C. E., Marks, S. P., & Morgan, R. E. (2001). The challenge and place of international human rights in public health. *American Journal of Public Health, 91*(12), 1922–1925.

Mann, J., Gostin, L., Gruskin, S., Brennan, T., Lazzarini, Z., & Fineberg, H. (1994). Health and human rights. *Health and Human Rights, 1*(1),6–93.

Rand, J., & Watson, G. (2008). *Rights-based approaches: Learning project.* Oxfam America and CARE USA. Retrieved November 24, 2009, from http://www .hrea.org/erc/Library/display_doc.php?url=http%3A%2F%2Fwww.oxfam. org.uk%2Fresources%2Fdownloads%2FRights-based%2520Approaches%2F English%2FRights_Based_App_Book.pdf&external=N

UK Interagency Group on Rights-Based Approaches. (2007). *The impact of rights-based approaches to development: Evaluating/learning process Bangladesh, Malawi, and Peru.* Retrieved November 24, 2009, from www.crin.org/docs/ INter_Agency_rba.pdf

United Nations Development Group. (n.d.) *UN country teams: Working together on human rights.* Retrieved December 21, 2009, from http:// www.undg.org/docs/7655/UN%20country%20teams%20working%20 together.doc

Yamin, A. E. (2008). Will we take suffering seriously?: Reflections of what it means to apply a human rights framework to health and why we should care. *Health and Human Rights, 10*(1), 45–63.

NOTES

[1]For more on the obligations to respect, protect, and fulfill, see UN ICESCR General Comment 12 on the right to adequate food (http://daccessdds.un.org/doc/UNDOC/GEN/G99/420/12/PDF/G9942012.pdf?OpenElement) and UN ICESCR General Comment 14 on the right to the highest attainable standard of health (http://daccessdds.un.org/doc/UNDOC/GEN/G00/439/34/PDF/G0043934.pdf?OpenElement)

[2]Office of the United Nations High Commissioner for Human Rights. Retrieved from http://www2.ohchr.org/english/law/cescr.htm

[3]United Nations. Retrieved from http://www.unhchr.ch/tbs/doc.nsf/%28symbol%29/E.C.12.2000.4.En

[4]Office of the United Nations High Commissioner for Human Rights. Retrieved from http://www2.ohchr.org/english/issues/health/right/

[5]Official Documents System of the United Nations. Retrieved from http://daccess-dds-ny.un.org/doc/UNDOC/GEN/G06/114/69/PDF/G0611469.pdf?OpenElement

[6]Office of the United Nations High Commissioner for Human Rights, & World Health Organization. Retrieved from http://www.ohchr.org/Documents/Publications/Factsheet31.pdf

[7]United Nations International Children's Emergency Fund. Retrieved from http://www.unicef.org/sowc04/files/AnnexB.pdf

[8]For more on the obligations to respect, protect, and fulfill, see UN ICESCR General Comment 12 on the right to adequate food (http://daccessdds.un.org/doc/UNDOC/GEN/G99/420/12/PDF/G9942012.pdf?OpenElement) and UN ICESCR General Comment 14 on the right to the highest attainable standard of health (http://daccessdds.un.org/doc/UNDOC/GEN/G00/439/34/PDF/G0043934.pdf?OpenElement)

CHAPTER 2

Rights-Based Approaches to Public Health Systems

Benjamin Mason Meier, Lance Gable, Jocelyn E. Getgen, and Leslie London

INTRODUCTION

A rights-based approach to public health systems focuses on underlying determinants of health – the economic, political, and social systems that determine health status and have far greater impact on health than the provision of medicine. With an understanding that health vulnerability is societally structured, public health systems can be seen to protect and promote the health of entire societies, employing multidisciplinary interventions to address the underlying causes of health and disease. By employing the language of human rights in health-related issues such as equity, discrimination, and social marginalization, public health advocates can achieve tangible health policy gains. However, it is necessary that public health scholars first gain a deeper understanding of the language of human rights and how these legal obligations can be applied in alleviating underlying determinants of health at the societal level through public health systems.

International human rights offer a powerful policy discourse to address underlying determinants of health through public health systems, creating government obligations to fulfill the "conditions in which people can be healthy" (Institute of Medicine, 1988, p. 7). By framing health disparities as a "rights violation," public health advocates benefit from international legal standards by which to frame government responsibilities and evaluate government policies, shifting the analysis of health reform from quality of care to social justice (Parmet, 2009). Applying the legal language of human rights to health policy debates, public health advocates can create a rights-based approach to disease prevention and health promotion through population-based public health systems (Hunt & Backman, 2009).

This chapter reviews the terms of the human rights debate, assesses the evolution of human rights for the public's health, and applies the normative frameworks of the right to health to reform the public health systems necessary to address underlying determinants of health through national and global health policy.

EVOLUTION OF HUMAN RIGHTS TO ADDRESS UNDERLYING DETERMINANTS OF HEALTH

Health rights have evolved to meet societal threats to health. If the right to health is to be viewed as historically situated and subject to normative evolution, it is important to understand the circumstances that have led policymakers to embrace changing conceptions of health in international law. Through advances in health threats, theories, and technologies, the means to achieve health have changed in fundamental ways not envisioned by the original framers of the right to health. At the population level, the field of public health, an outgrowth of the U.S. public health campaigns of the early part of the 20th century, has taken on international importance in health policy debates.

Reflecting this changing health landscape, international legal frameworks under a right to health have evolved from a right to medical interventions to a right to all those underlying conditions that structure health, including such disparate underlying determinants of health as resource distribution, gender, violence and armed conflict, and other "socially related concerns." This part chronicles the policy dynamics of the right to health at three seminal moments in its history, including (a) the expansive aspirational language of the 1948 Universal Declaration of Human Rights (UDHR), (b) the weakened legal obligations of the 1966 International Covenant on Economic, Social and Cultural Rights (ICESCR), and (c) the reclaimed public health standards of the 1978 Declaration of Alma-Ata, which would be codified by the United Nations in 2000 to address underlying determinants of health in General Comment 14 to the ICESCR.

With the United Nations seeking to rebuild a world ravaged by war and to address the deprivations that occurred during the Depression and War that followed, the 1948 UDHR includes a right to health that moves beyond medical care, providing for a right to "*a standard of living adequate for the health* [italics added] and well-being of himself and of his family, including food, clothing, housing and *medical care* [italics added] and necessary social services" (UDHR, 1948, art. 25). In preparing this right to a standard of living adequate for health, derived from drafts of the American Law Institute, there was widespread international agreement that the human right to health included both the fulfillment of medical care and the realization of underlying determinants of health – including within this right public health regulations for food safety and nutrition, sanitary housing, disease prevention, and comprehensive social security (Eide, 1993). In operating through public health systems, it was clear that government responsibility for the attainment of health included obligations to provide the security and material environment necessary for the fulfillment of healthy conditions.

But with states subsequently avoiding the right to health at the height of the Cold War, the United Nations General Assembly summarily weakened proposals for a right to health in the 1966 ICESCR, eliminating the definition of complete health and reference to "social well-being" from the right and replacing it with the ambiguous "highest attainable standard of health" (ICESCR, 1966, art. 12). Furthering this ambiguity in the content of the right, the General Assembly removed from the right any specific mention of underlying determinants of health—nutrition, housing, sanitation, recreation, economic and working conditions—leaving in its place the vagueness of government responsibility for "environmental and industrial hygiene" (ICESCR, art. 12).

As ideas about health changed in the late 1960s, however, so too did support for human rights to address underlying determinants of health through public health systems. Although human rights discourses on health had veered away from a focus on public health and toward curative medicine during the post-War enthusiasm for scientific advancement, public health systems had showed far greater promise in preventing disease and promoting health, shifting public health discourse back toward underlying determinants of health through "primary health care" – that is, health care in addition to the underlying social, political, and economic determinants of health (Rosen, 1974). With health framed as a widespread social imperative rather than a limited medical challenge, human rights would be seen as instrumental to the realization of public health systems.

In 1978, as the ICESCR was coming into law, the World Health Organization (WHO) and the United Nations International Children's Emergency Fund (UNICEF) held an international conference to revitalize public health systems from a human rights perspective. This international conference, with representatives from 134 state governments, would adopt a Declaration on Primary Health Care, a document that has come to be known as the Declaration of Alma-Ata (WHO, 1978). Returning to the rights-based emphasis on underlying determinants of health in the Constitution of the WHO, the Declaration of Alma-Ata began with the statement that:

> health—which is a state of complete physical, mental and social well-being, and not merely the absence of disease or infirmity—is a fundamental human right [that] requires the action of many other social and economic sectors in addition to the health sector. (WHO, 1978, pmbl.)

To address underlying determinants of health under the Declaration of Alma-Ata, representatives laid out seven specific governmental obligations for essential aspects of "primary health care," including such underlying determinants as education concerning prevailing health problems and the methods of preventing and controlling them; promotion of food supply and proper nutrition; an adequate supply of safe water and basic sanitation; maternal and child health care, including family planning; immunization against the major infectious diseases; prevention and control of locally endemic diseases; appropriate treatment of common diseases and injuries; and the provision of essential medicines (WHO, 1978). Although WHO's focus on underlying determinants of health would wane in the ensuing years, the United Nations would reengage human rights for the public's health as it became clear that the right to health necessitated a contemporary reinterpretation if it were to frame rights-based public health systems (Meier, 2010).

CURRENT RIGHTS-BASED FRAMEWORKS FOR PUBLIC HEALTH SYSTEMS

The United Nations Committee on Economic, Social and Cultural Rights (CESCR) has taken the lead in developing a modernized right to health commensurate with an understanding of public health systems. General Comment 14, promulgated by the CESCR in 2000, interpreted the ICESCR to find that the right to health:

> is not confined to the right to health care. On the contrary, the drafting history and the express wording of article 12.2 acknowledge that *the right to health embraces a wide range of socio-economic factors that promote conditions in which people can lead a healthy life, and extends to the underlying determinants of health* [italics added], such as food and nutrition, housing, access to safe and potable water and adequate sanitation, *safe and healthy working conditions, and a healthy environment* [italics added]. (¶ 4)

Thus, the CESCR finds the right to health to be an inclusive right, not restricted to medical care and treatment, but encompassing a broader array of underlying factors that impact health. At a minimum, these underlying determinants of health include access to safe and potable water, adequate sanitation, adequate supply of safe food, nutrition and housing, healthy occupational and environmental conditions, access to health-related education and information (including on sexual and reproductive health), and participation in health-related decision making at community, national, and international levels (CESCR, 2000).

The right to health, according to General Comment 14, entitles individuals "to a system of health protection which provides equality of opportunity for people to enjoy the highest attainable level of health" (CESCR, 2000, ¶ 8). In realizing this right, a state must consider four key measures when assessing its compliance across the facilities, goods, services, and programs that comprise its public health system:

- *Availability*—the state must ensure that a "sufficient quantity" exists of resources integral to health, including sanitation, safe and potable drinking water, functional health services, trained health care professionals, adequate treatment facilities, and access to essential medicines.
- *Accessibility*—the state must remove barriers to access to health facilities, goods, and services, whether these barriers are imposed through economic, geographic, physical, or informational means.
- *Acceptability*—the state's health facilities, goods, and services must be satisfactory, according to cultural traditions and standards of medical ethics.
- *Quality*—the state's health facilities, goods, and services must maintain a level of quality consistent with medical and scientific standards (CESCR, 2000).

In meeting the substance of these commitments under the right to health, states assume three types of obligations:

- *Respect*—avoid interference with the right to health through its actions or omissions
- *Protect*—constrain the actions of third parties that may undermine the right to health.
- *Fulfill*—take affirmative steps to achieve the right to health (CESCR, 2000).

Through these overlapping frameworks, General Comment 14 recognizes the interconnectedness of governmental and nongovernmental actors in creating a robust public health system that can adequately support the necessary range of economic, political, and social determinants of health. To carry out these obligations, states must adopt a "national strategy" to realize the right to health and support a public health system that adequately maintains underlying determinants of health. Furthering this strategy, states must promulgate the necessarily legal infrastructure to support these measures and develop an implementation plan with appropriate "transparency" and "accountability" (CESCR, 2000, ¶¶ 53–56).

Although the right to health remains subject to "progressive realization"—affording states time to construct health systems in accordance with the "maximum available" national resources—General Comment 14 nevertheless imposes significant parameters on the application of the right to health through public health systems (Freedman, 2009). As states each develop national plans, benchmarks, and indicators, investigations have begun to determine whether measurable progress has been made toward realizing the right to health (Backman et al., 2008).

Further elucidating the content and application of General Comment 14, several analytical reports by the United Nations Special Rapporteur on the Enjoyment of the Highest Attainable Standard of Physical and Mental Health have examined the relationship of health systems to the right to health, recognizing that "a strong health system is an essential element of a healthy and equitable society" (UN Report of the Special Rapporteur, 2008, p. 12). Drawing on WHO's identification of six building blocks for a health system (health services; health workforce; health information systems; medical products, vaccines, and technology; health financing; and leadership, governance, and stewardship [WHO, 2007]), the Special Rapporteur has analyzed the interface between these building blocks and the right to health, concluding with a series of legal reforms to strengthen public health systems through national health policy (UN Report of the Special Rapporteur, 2008).

APPLICATION OF A RIGHTS-BASED APPROACH TO PUBLIC HEALTH SYSTEM REFORM

In examining the national experience, it has become clear that a rights-based approach to public health system development and reform means much more than simply ratifying international treaties. To address the multiple levels between the international human right to health and national public health system reform, this part aims to clarify through comparative case studies the evidence for rights-based approaches to advancing public health systems and to outline through international legal standards the basis for rights-based health reform in the United States. (A more extended discussion of a rights-based approach to U.S. health care reform is discussed in chapter 4.)

Comparative Analysis of Rights-Based Health System Reforms

Analyzing these data across rights-based health system reforms, three themes emerge: (a) the place of social determinants within a rights-based approach; (b) equity as an explicit goal of a rights-based public health system; and (c) how a human rights approach addresses vulnerability.

Social Determinants of Health and a Rights-Based Approach

Although General Comment 14 clearly recognizes that the right to health encompasses underlying determinants of health, taking direct account of socioeconomic determinants in a rights-based framework is not always explicit. For example, in the United Kingdom, recent policy concerns for reducing avoidable health inequalities have led to attempts to include selected social and economic factors within resource allocation formulae to take better account of the impacts of social determinants on health inequalities (Smith, 2008). However, such exploratory work is not recognized as asserting a rights-based agenda in the British context. Similarly, research with parliamentarians in Southern and Eastern Africa has illustrated that members of health portfolio committees frequently identified key socioeconomic determinants outside of the health sector—such as food security, social grants, and education (which are elements of the right to health)—as important challenges for their work, but did not identify them within a rights paradigm (London et al., 2009). Bringing the lens of discrete legal obligations to these determinants of health will help to sharpen state accountability in ways that have not yet emerged.

Equity as an Explicit Goal of a Rights-Based Public Health System

Unlike earlier conceptions of equity as one of several important but competing public health considerations for public health system reform, there is increasing recognition that health equity is, of itself, the critical goal of a rights-based system rather than a goal instrumental to the achievement of a public good (Evans et al., 2001). The WHO Commission on Social

Determinants of Health (2008) has provided much of the evidence that inequalities in income, social situation, and power are the key obstacles to reducing health inequalities and are more important than investments in health care alone, finding that health systems that make equity an explicit goal are more likely to achieve overall reductions in morbidity and mortality. As seen under the Brazilian Unified Health System (Sistema Único de Saúde), an equity-based system can offer new ways of working at the primary health care level and establishing new forms of accountability, successfully reducing mortality and morbidity (Cornwall & Shankland, 2008). Under counterfactual conditions—where neoliberal health care reforms subordinated equity to considerations of efficiency, requiring cutbacks in state expenditure and reductions of public services—ideologically driven decisions for public health systems have generally been profoundly negative in equity of coverage and access to services (De Vos et al., 2006). Despite the recent moderation of these detrimental health care reforms, human rights principles provide a sustained framework for moving toward equity in the creation of effective public health systems to address underlying determinants of health.

A Human Rights Approach and Vulnerability

Finally, because human rights are inherently focused on substantive equality, rights-based approaches would give preference to the needs of vulnerable groups. Complementing efforts to afford greater protections for vulnerable groups, a rights-based approach recognizes and strengthens the agency of vulnerable groups to take action to change the conditions of their vulnerability (London, 2007). The engagement by civil society actors with the state could help to advance rights-based programming through collective agency and engagement in public health policy reform (Yamin, 2000). Through such engagement, vulnerable groups would find a voice in the policy process, breaking with the idea of health service users as either passive recipients or as empowered clients, but rather as rights-holding citizens engaging with a state that is obligated to establish mechanisms for citizen participation.

U.S. Rights-Based Health System Reforms

Applying such rights-based approaches to health policy reform in the United States, public health systems can address underlying determinants of health—including gender, race, and age—through human rights frameworks to inform public health policies and improve health outcomes (Yamin, 2005). International human rights treaties, such as the

Convention on the Elimination of All Forms of Discrimination against Women (CEDAW), the Convention on the Elimination of All Forms of Racial Discrimination (CERD), and the Convention on the Rights of the Child (CRC), provide these frameworks to establish rights-based policies for U.S. public health system reform.

To address gender as an underlying determinant of health, systemic reform efforts must combat gender inequality and discrimination. Rights-based U.S. health care reform strategists thus incorporate human rights norms enumerated in the CEDAW and its interpretive documents. The CEDAW establishes a state obligation to take "all appropriate measures, including legislation, to ensure the full development and advancement of women, . . . human rights and fundamental freedoms on a basis of equality with men" (CEDAW, 1979, art. 3). Despite U.S. reluctance to ratify the CEDAW, local NGOs and governments have applied rights-based frameworks to improve women's health outcomes, including a San Francisco ordinance based on CEDAW principles, which resulted in the dramatic expansion of intervention and prevention services to women-survivors of intimate partner violence and sexual assault (Murase, 2005).

Similarly, to address race as an underlying determinant of health, the CERD enumerates legally binding obligations to employ a rights-based framework for combating racial inequity in health. Indeed, CERD obligates the U.S. government to take affirmative steps to:

> eliminate racial discrimination in all its forms and to guarantee the right of everyone . . . to equality before the law, notably in the enjoyment of . . . the rights to public health, medical care, social security and social services. (CERD, 1966, art. 5)

Rights-based health system reform efforts must work toward eliminating racial discrimination at structural and programmatic levels as well as racial disparities in health outcomes. As an example of attempts to do so, NGOs have evaluated the reproductive health of minority women in the United States in light of government obligations under the CERD, focusing on issues of maternal mortality, sexually transmissible infections and unintended pregnancies where women of color are adversely affected (Center for Reproductive Rights, 2007).

Finally, to address age as an underlying determinant of health, the CRC offers a human rights framework to formulate rights-based approaches for the improvement of children's health. Human rights norms prioritize the protection of children, the provision of child health services, and children's participation in improving their health outcomes (Waterston & Goldhagen, 2007). To that end, the CRC specifically focuses on state obligations to diminish infant and child mortality, develop primary health care, combat disease and malnutrition, ensure appropriate prenatal and postnatal health education and care for mothers, and develop preventive health care, guidance for parents, and family planning education and services (CRC, 1989).

Although the United States has not ratified the CRC, strategists such as the Campaign for U.S. Ratification of the Convention on the Rights of the Child have incorporated its norms into domestic health care reform efforts by advocating for public health systems to address issues of child survival, development, protection, and participation (Todres, Wocjik, & Revaz, 2006). Following the lead of other state and local governments, the city of Chicago has incorporated the CRC's norms in a resolution to "advance policies and practices that are in harmony with the principles of the Convention on the Rights of the Child in all city agencies and organizations that address issues directly affecting the City's children" (Campaign for a New Domestic Human Rights Agenda, 2009).

CONCLUSION

Framing health inequities as a "rights violation" offers international standards by which to frame government responsibilities and evaluate conduct. By applying human rights standards as a substantive and decision-making framework, human rights can be applied to create a rights-based approach to underlying determinants of health through public health systems.

REFERENCES

Backman, G., Hunt P., Kholsa R., Jaramilla-Strouss C., Mikuria Fikre B., Rumble C., et al. (2008). Health systems and the right to health: An assessment of 194 countries. *Lancet, 372,* 2047–2085.

Campaign for a New Domestic Human Rights Agenda. (2009). *State and local human rights agencies: Recommendations for advancing opportunity and equality through an international human rights framework.* Retrieved September 6, 2010, from http://www.ushrnetwork.org/sites/default/files/State_and_Local_Human_Rights_Agencies_Report.pdf

Center for Reproductive Rights. (2007). *Supplementary information about the United States, Scheduled for review during the CERD Committee's 72nd session.* Retrieved September 6, 2010, from http://reproductiverights.org/sites/crr.civicactions.net/files/documents/CERD%20Shadow%20Letter%20Final_07_08_0.pdf

Convention on the Elimination of All Forms of Discrimination Against Women. (1979). New York: United Nations.

Convention on the Elimination of All Forms of Racial Discrimination. (1966). New York: United Nations.

Convention on the Rights of the Child. (1989). New York: United Nations.

Cornwall, A., & Shankland, A. (2008). Engaging citizens: Lessons from building Brazil's national health system. *Social Science & Medicine, 66*(10), 2173–2184.

De Vos, P., De Ceukelaire, W., Van der Stuyft., P. (2006). Colombia and Cuba: contrasting models in Latin America's health sector reform. *Tropical Medicine and International Health, 11*(10), 1604–1612.

Eide, A. (1993). Article 25. In A. Eide, G. Alfredsson, G. Melander, L. A. Rehof, A. Rosas (Eds.), *The universal declaration of human rights: A commentary.* Scandinavian University Press: Oslo, Norway.

Evans, T., Whitehead, M., Diderichsen, F., Bhuyia, A., & Wirth, M. (Eds.). (2001). *Challenging inequalities in health. From Ethics to Action.* New York: Oxford University Press.

Hunt, P., & Backman, G. (2009). Health systems and the right to the highest attainable standard of health. *Health and Human Rights, 10*, 81–92.

Institute of Medicine. (1988). *The future of public health.* Washington, DC: Institute of Medicine.

International Covenant on Economic, Social and Cultural Rights. (1966). New York: United Nations.

London, L. (2007). 'Issues of equity are also issues of rights': Lessons from experiences in Southern Africa. *BMC Public Health, 7:* 14.

London, L. Mbombo, N., Thomas, J., Loewenson, R., Mulumba, M., & Mukono, A. (2009). Parliamentary committee experiences on promoting the right to health in east and southern Africa. *EQUINET Discussion Paper 74.* Harare: EQUINET.

Meier, B. M. (2010). Global health governance and the contentious politics of human rights: Mainstreaming the right to health for public health advancement. *Stanford Journal of International Law, 46*, 1–50.

Murase, E. M. (2005). *CEDAW Implementation Locally: Lessons from San Francisco.* Retrieved September 6, 2010, from http://www.iwpr.org/PDF/05_Proceedings/Murase_Emily.pdf

Parmet, W. E. (2009). *Populations, public health, and the law.* Washington, DC: Georgetown University Press.

Public Interest Projects. (2009). *Chicago city council passed resolution supporting the Convention on the Rights for the Child.* Retrieved July 30, 2010, from http://www.ushumanrightsfund.org/news/chicago-city-council-passed-resolution-supporting-

Rosen, G. (1974). *From medical police to social medicine: Essays on the history of health care.* New York: Science History Publications.

Smith, P. C. (2008). Resource allocation and purchasing in the health sector: The English experience. *Bull World Health Organ, 86*(11), 884–888.

Todres, J., Wocjik, M. E., & Revaz, C. R. (Eds.). (2006). *The U.N. convention on the rights of the child: An analysis of treaty provisions and implications of U.S. ratification.* Ardsley, NY: Transnational Publishers.

UN Committee on Economic, Social and Cultural Rights. (2000). The Right to the Highest Attainable Standard of Health, CESCR General Comment 14. 22d Sess., Agenda Item 3, U.N. Doc. E/C.12/2000/4.

UN Report of the Special Rapporteur on the right of everyone to the enjoyment of the highest attainable standard of physical and mental health. (2008). Human Rights Council, 7th session, Agenda item 3, at 12, UN doc. A/HRC/7/11, 31 January 2008.

Universal Declaration of Human Rights. (1948). New York: United Nations.

Waterston, T., & Goldhagen, J. (2007). Why children's rights are central to international child health. *Archives of Disease in Childhood, 92,* 176–180.

World Health Organization. (1978). *Primary health care: Report of the International Conference on Primary Health Care.* Geneva: World Health Organization.

World Health Organization. (2007). *Everybody's business: Strengthening health systems to improve health outcomes.* Geneva: World Health Organization.

World Health Organization. (2008). *Closing the gap in a generation: Health equity through action on the social determinants of health. Final Report of the Commission on Social Determinants of Health.* Geneva: World Health Organization.

Yamin, A. E. (2000). Protecting and promoting the right to health in Latin America: selected experiences from the field. *Health and Human Rights, 5*(1), 116–148.

Yamin, A. E. (2005). The right to health under international law and its relevance to the United States. *American Journal of Public Health, 95,* 1156–1161.

CHAPTER 3

Rights-Based Approaches and Health Disparities in the United States

Roshni D. Persaud

INTRODUCTION

The financial expenditures with respect to the U.S. health care system are an ever-increasing drain on the federal budget, the economy, and employers.[1] It is reported that the United States spends more on health care costs than any other nation in the world.[2] In 2007, health care expenditures spiraled up to an astounding $2.2 trillion for the fiscal year.[3]

Despite the astronomical amount of money spent by the United States, health disparities among various demographic groups continue to persevere.[4] More specifically, low-income Americans and racial and ethnic minorities experience a disproportionately higher prevalence of disease, fewer treatment options, and reduced access to care.[5] For example:

- Infant mortality rates are 2.5 times higher for African Americans,[6] and 1.5 times higher for American Indians, than for Caucasians[7];
- The mortality rate for heart disease for African Americans is higher than for Caucasians[8];
- A total of 50% of all AIDS cases are among minorities who account for 25% of the U.S. population[9];
- The prevalence of diabetes is 70% higher among African Americans and twice as high among Hispanics compared to Caucasians[10];

- Asian Americans and Pacific Islanders have the highest rate of tuberculosis of any racial or ethnic group[11];
- Cervical cancer is nearly 5 times more likely among Vietnamese American women than Caucasian women[12];
- Women are not as likely as men to get lifesaving pharmaceuticals for heart attacks[13]; and
- More women than men need cardiac bypass surgery or suffer a heart attack after an angioplasty.[14]

With an increase in the unemployment rate, these disparities will theoretically continue to increase.[15]

This chapter will begin by defining health disparities.

HEALTH DISPARITIES DEFINED

Generally, government entities and public health experts examine the "health" of a population, through various epidemiological statistics such as infant mortality and life expectancy.[16]

Infant mortality is regarded as a critical indicator in the overall health and welfare of a nation because it is correlated with factors such as maternal health, quality and access to medical care, socioeconomic conditions, public health practices, and the financing of health care services.[17] Currently, the United States fares poorly with regard to infant mortality and life expectancy as compared to other industrialized countries.[18] More specifically, the U.S. infant mortality rate is 6.69 deaths per 1,000 live births, which is higher than most of the world's industrialized nations.[19] The Centers for Disease Control and Prevention (CDC) asserts that the elevated rates of infant mortality in the United States are "due in large part to disparities which continue to exist among various racial and ethnic groups in this country, particularly African-Americans."[20]

Additionally, U.S. life expectancy, which is 78.11 years, lags 49th in the world, and falls far behind other wealthy nations such as Japan, France, Germany, and the United Kingdom.[21] Moreover, the U.S. record with regard to access to health care and public health services is weak.[22] In fact, the World Health Organization (WHO) ranked the performance of the U.S. health care system 37th among all nations because of disparities by race and income.[23]

The term *health disparity* has various meanings in differing environments and is a notion used almost exclusively within the United States.[24] In 1999, the National Institutes of Health (NIH) convened an NIH-wide working group that was given the responsibility of creating a strategic plan for reducing health disparities.[25] It was that group that devised the first NIH definition of "health disparities."[26] The definition states that:

> Health disparities are differences in the incidence, prevalence, mortality, and burden of diseases and other adverse health conditions that exist among specific population groups in the United States.[27]

In the year 2000, the Minority Health and Health Disparities Research and Education Act, (U.S. Public Law 106–525) provided a legal definition of health disparities, which states in relevant part that a population will be considered a health disparity population if:

> there is a significant disparity in the overall rate of disease incidence, prevalence, morbidity, mortality, or survival rates in the population as compared to the health status of the general population.[28]

One should be cognizant of the fact that, a broad spectrum of populations is affected by health disparities; the most noteworthy "include racial and ethnic minorities, residents of rural areas, women, children, the elderly, and persons with disabilities."[29]

For purposes of this chapter, "health disparities" will be used to describe both the disparities in health status, which are "differences in health conditions and in health outcomes"; and disparities in health care, which are, "differences in the preventive, diagnostic and treatment services offered to people with similar health conditions."[30] Moreover, the varied factors that contribute to health disparities will be explored in this chapter.

VARIABLES THAT CONTRIBUTE TO HEALTH DISPARITIES

The factors that contribute to health disparities within the United States are multifactorial.[31] The Institute of Medicine (IOM) reports that characteristics related to the patient, the health care system, and the clinical encounter all may impact racial and ethnic health disparities in a detrimental manner.[32]

Patient Variables

Patient variables are the characteristics of a patient that may influence health disparities.[33] For example, when a patient delays seeking medical care, elects not to follow a prescribed treatment regimen offered by the health care professional, or refuses medical attention altogether, this can have a harmful impact on their health.

Other patient variables that have been correlated with health disparities include socioeconomic status (SES), which is generally "measured by wealth, poverty, education, literacy and occupation."[34] One particular research study determined that lower SES was a chief contributor to increased cancer mortality risk among racial/ethnic minorities, thus signifying an interaction between SES and race/ethnicity.[35]

Language barriers are also implicated in creating health disparities. For example, it has been shown that when a patient is unable to properly communicate with the health care provider, it can potentially result in a decrease of "medication compliance, self-management of chronic disease, and overall health outcomes."[36]

Poor health literacy also contributes toward health disparities.[37] The Agency for Healthcare Research and Quality reports that only 12% of the 228 million adults in the United States have the necessary skills to access and use health information to make proper health care decisions.[38]

Mistrust of health care providers may also preclude certain populations from seeking medical care and may serve as another element that contributes to health disparities.

Health Care Systems Variables

Health care systems variables can pose various challenges for patients and may contribute to increased disparities in health.[39] More specifically, navigating the health care system for a patient can be quite complex and thus, reduce the chance that a patient will receive quality care.[40] Additionally, the way a health care institution is structured, the financial system, and the geographic location also serve as potential barriers. For example, if a patient of lower SES lives a far distance from the hospital or does not have sufficient money for transportation costs to the hospital, he or she may not obtain much needed care. Moreover, lack of diversity within the health care system, lack of minority health care providers, lack of cultural sensitivity, and unavailability of language services are other relevant factors that may contribute to health disparities.

Clinical Encounter Variables

Clinical encounter variables are the characteristics of an individual provider that may influence health disparities.[41] Some physicians and health care providers may have certain stereotypes or biases that may be detrimental to various patient populations. Researchers for one study found that physicians rated African American patients as "less intelligent, less educated, more likely to abuse drugs and alcohol, more likely to fail to comply with medical advice, more likely to lack social support, and less likely to participate in cardiac rehabilitation than white patients."[42] Such biases can have negative implications in the care and provision of health care services provided to patients.

LACK OF HEALTH INSURANCE COVERAGE AND ITS IMPACT ON HEALTH DISPARITIES

According to the 2009 National Health Care Disparities Report, "all population groups should receive equally high quality of care."[43] Moreover, accessing a health care system and receiving suitable health care in time for the services to be effective are essential factors in guaranteeing positive health outcomes.[44] Unfortunately, the sobering disparity with respect to rates of insurance and access to health care for racial and ethnic minorities, as well as low-income populations in the United States remains an issue of grave concern.[45] In 2008, the U.S. census reported that 46.3 million people were without health insurance coverage[46] and around 90 million Americans lacked health insurance at some point during the year."[47] Racial and ethnic populations within the United States lack insurance coverage at an even higher rate than Caucasians.[48] This translates to racial and ethnic minorities with reduced access to health care and as a logical consequence—an elevated level of morbidity and mortality.

Recent research efforts have documented a significant correlation between individual access to health care and individual health.[49] Most notably, a Harvard Medical study determined that the lack of health insurance coverage may account for up to 44,789 deaths a year in the United States and provides evidence for the aforementioned assertion.[50] Moreover, the 2009 National Health Care Disparities Report found that uninsured people tend to get "the worst care."[51] Individuals without health insurance are also less likely to seek much needed medical care and are less likely to obtain prescriptions for chronic medical conditions. Thus, they are unable to receive suitable health care in time for the services to be effective and the negative health outcomes could be devastating.

Studies suggest that the provision or expansion of health insurance coverage alone would not eliminate disparities in health care. One expert cautions that expanding insurance coverage would not be meaningful in terms of people accessing care if the health coverage is not sufficient to cover the crux of a patient's medical bills.[52] For example, medical care would not be affordable or an option if people have to pay large deductibles or a large share of their entire medical bill.[53] A consistent sentiment held by health care researchers is "health insurance can only make people healthier if they can access care."[54] Moreover, the literature suggests that the lack of insurance does not fully account for all the differences in health care related to race, ethnicity, and SES, and it has been proposed "that even if an individual had health insurance coverage it would greatly reduce but not completely eliminate disparities in care."[55] It should also be noted that the 2009 National Health Care Disparities Report determined that "even when people are of the same socio-economic status and have the same type of health insurance coverage, and when co-morbidities, stage of presentation and other confounding variables are controlled for, members of racial and ethnic minority groups in the United States typically receive lower-quality health care than do their Caucasian counterparts."[56]

HEALTH CARE REFORM AND ITS IMPACT ON HEALTH DISPARITIES

Currently, the U.S. health care system is supported by a combination of social and private insurance, with mainly private providers dominating the market.[57] Although approximately three fifths of the population (around 150 million people) benefit from employer-sponsored health insurance, 46.3 million people remain uninsured.[58] According to the 2009 National Healthcare Disparities Report, Americans without health care coverage are much less likely than those with private insurance to obtain recommended care, especially preventive services.[59] The report further delineates that although some racial differences in lack of insurance have tapered in the past 10 years, disparities related to ethnicity, income, and education continue to persist.[60]

In March 2010, wide-sweeping national health care reform was effectuated when President Barack Obama signed the Patient Protection and Affordable Care Act and the Health Care and Education Reconciliation Act into law.[61] Although racial and ethnic health disparities are not a primary focus of this health reform law, the legislation does address several issues that impact health care disparities within the United States.

For example, in an April 2010 press release, Kathleen Sebelius, secretary of the Department of Health and Human Services, acknowledged that "minorities were less likely to have insurance and less likely to get the treatments they needed."[62] She stated that in the reformed system, it is expected that "an increasing number of Americans will be able to obtain medical care, regardless of their race or ethnicity and the quality of care will improve."[63]

The law is expected to insure approximately 32 million of the 46 million individuals who are currently uninsured, more than half of whom are people of color.[64] It will also require that most U.S. citizens and legal residents obtain health coverage.[65] Those without coverage will have to pay a tax penalty, however, exceptions will be granted for certain groups. Additionally, the law will create state-managed "American Health Benefit Exchanges," which will enable individuals who meet certain criteria to buy health coverage.[66]

The law also endeavors to expand Medicaid eligibility to all non-Medicare eligible individuals younger than 65 years of age, which includes children, pregnant women, parents, and adults without dependent children with specified income levels.[67] This will be beneficial for certain populations who are considered "disparity populations" namely, women and children. States will also be afforded the option to create a Basic Health Plan for uninsured individuals with incomes between 133 and 200% of the federal poverty level (FPL) who would otherwise be eligible to receive premium subsidies in the Exchange.[68]

A national high-risk pool to provide health insurance for individuals with preexisting medical conditions will also be created for a temporary period.[69] Moreover, U.S. citizens and legal immigrants who have a preexisting medical condition and who have been uninsured for a minimum of 6 months will be able to enroll in the high-risk pool and receive subsidized premiums.[70] Furthermore, effective 6 months following enactment, preexisting condition exclusions for children will be barred.[71] It is anticipated that the legislation will permit various populations who have been previously unable to obtain health insurance because of preexisting conditions to get much needed care, thereby reducing morbidity and mortality rates. The populations that stand to benefit include racial and ethnic populations with chronic disease and people of lower SES with chronic diseases.

Individual and group health plans will not be able to place lifetime limits on the dollar value of coverage and insurers will also be precluded from terminating coverage (except in cases of fraud).[72] Theoretically, for example, a young child diagnosed with a type of cancer that can be extremely expensive will not be dropped from coverage if his or her aggregated medical bills accrued over a lifetime exceed a certain dollar amount.

The law also mandates improved collection and reporting of information pertinent to race, ethnicity, gender, primary language, disability status, and for underserved rural and frontier populations.[73] Moreover, the law mandates the compilation of access and treatment data for people with disabilities.[74] Effective 2 years following enactment of the law, the secretary for the Department of Health and Human Services will be vested with the responsibility of analyzing the aggregate data that monitor trends in health disparities.[75]

According to the 2009 National Healthcare Disparities Report the most prevailing disparity was the lack of preventive care.[76] For example, a large number of minorities had worsening disparities in the percentage of adults older than 50 years old who received proper screening for colon cancer.[77] Furthermore, African Americans and Hispanics had elevated mortality rates from the disease.[78] The reform bill earmarks money for prevention and public health programs,[79] which should allow Americans increased access to free preventive services that will hopefully thwart diseases and thus preclude more costly treatment.[80] The new legislation will also create a grant program to support the delivery of evidence-based and community-based prevention and wellness services targeted at improving prevention activities. It will also support programs targeted at reducing chronic disease rates and addressing health disparities that occur especially in rural and frontier areas.[81]

The bill expands programs aimed at increasing the number of medical professionals and will also seek to diversify the health care workforce.[82] As a logical consequence, minority populations would have greater accessibility to health care workers. Plus, some minority populations may be more willing to obtain services from a diverse group of health professionals that would be culturally sensitive and "in tune" with their needs.[83]

IS THE "RIGHT TO HEALTH" GUARANTEED UNDER U.S. LAW?

The definition of "health" has taken on many forms in the past few decades and for many is an elusive notion.[84] Moreover, the "right to health" is an even more difficult concept to articulate or describe.[85] The "health" of a person may be defined narrowly, to refer to a state in which an individual is not afflicted with a disease or experience pain.[86] The WHO on the other hand defines "health" broadly in the following manner: "Health is a state of complete physical, mental and social well-being, and not merely the absence of disease or infirmity."[87] The distinction between these definitions is important because the narrow definition is somewhat limited in scope whereas the broad definition of health seems to implicate a wide range of factors that contribute toward leading a "healthy" life. Taking this into consideration, the "right" to health under the broad definition could theoretically include a "general, unlimited right to health; a right to health care or medical care; a right to a basic package of medical needs; a right to health care coverage or insurance; or other variations."[88]

United States Federal Constitution

The Federal Constitution of the United States confers no right to health or medical care.[89] It should be noted, however, that the preamble to the U.S. Constitution does specify a state duty to promote the public good,[90] but the explicit text leaves the discharge of this obligation to the discretion of the legislature.[91] The Constitution also provides Congress with the authority to support the establishment of federal health programs and also authorize regulations to enhance the delivery of health care and promote the public's health.[92] Despite the fact that the police power resides with the states, constitutional authority for numerous federal health activities stem from the constitutional requirement that Congress provide for the general welfare.[93]

More specifically, the Federal Constitution contains language that permits Congress to tax and spend in order to provide for the common defense and general welfare of the United States.[94] This specific power permits the federal government to allocate financial resources in the provision of services and has been described as encouraging states and the public to engage in activities that achieve commendable goals, such as the implementation of the international human right to health.[95] Another significant power of the federal government is the regulation of interstate commerce.[96] Under this clause, Congress possesses the apparent authority to initiate health care reform, establish national health boards and payment systems, and regulate health insurance.[97] Currently, there are two health insurance programs, which are sponsored by the government; Medicare, which provides coverage for the elderly population, and Medicaid, which provides coverage for the "deserving poor."[98]

State Law

On a state level, policy makers and public health officials are able to enact and implement various policies and laws through a legal mechanism known as the *police power.*"[99] The police power generally refers to the inherent authority of a state to make all laws necessary and proper to preserve or promote public health, public safety, and the public welfare.[100] The police powers of a government are quite broad and take many forms.[101] For example, health care professionals are required to obtain a professional license from a local government agency.[102] Health care facilities are also required to abide by various accreditation standards.[103] Restaurants and other types of food establishments are closely monitored and regulated by state government.[104] Despite repeated challenges, the breadth and depth of the state police power in the regulation of the public health has been continually affirmed by the U.S. Supreme Court.[105]

Would a Constitutional Right to Health Care Have a Positive Effect on Health Disparities?

One question to consider in this discussion is whether an explicit constitutional right to health care would make a difference in accessing health care or impacting health outcomes.[106] Some have taken the position that the empirical data and comparative law demonstrate that a constitutional right to health care would not have an impact with respect to health care or health outcomes.[107] More specifically, research did not find a correlation between a constitutional right to health or health care and the government's promise to provide universal coverage.[108] Moreover, the research also determined that there is no association between the constitutional right to health and/or medical care and the two health outcome indicators: infant mortality and life expectancy.[109] One example that clearly illustrates this example is Japan. Japan has the most favorable infant mortality and life expectancy rates, yet it does not provide a constitutional right to health or medical care.[110]

It is important to note that despite the fact that more than two thirds of the constitutions from abroad contain some sort of statement with respect to health and health care,[111] many of these constitutional statements have been described as "aspirational."[112] As a practical matter, these constitutional clauses do not confer people with specific legal rights.[113] Additionally, these constitutional statements have been described as mere recommendations that various governments adopt to demonstrate their commitment toward the goal of promoting a healthy society.[114]

INTERNATIONAL TREATIES AND RATIFICATION BY THE UNITED STATES

Official adoption of the international human rights to health, particularly with respect to ratification of relevant international and regional treaties, has been limited by the United States.[115] However, in the past decade, human rights discourse has emerged as a powerful tool in many parts of the world for achieving the conditions necessary for the attainment of good health.[116]

The problem of defining and implementing a right to health has been characterized by one author as threefold: (a) indeterminacy (how to categorize it),[117] (b) justiciability (how to enforce it),[118] and (c) progressive realization (how to raise the standard over time).[119] Review of the most salient international treatises containing statements allocating the right to health clearly demonstrates the issue at point. For example, international documents as far back as 1946 acknowledge health (and consequently the prevention and treatment of disease) as a human right.[120] It is reported, however, that not a single document moves past the aspirational plane to impose tangible obligations on government.[121]

In the following subsection of this chapter, you will be presented with an array of international treaties and documents (which have been introduced in previous chapters) that expound about the human right to health and/or medical care; unfortunately, many of these documents simply provide suggestions for enforceability procedures. Some documents even lack the most basic scheme for domestic enforcement. Consequently, these documents are largely disregarded by the United States and several foreign governments.[122] Moreover, it has been documented that a host of these documents "may offer moral direction for policymaking to international organizations like the WHO," however, these documents provide "no protection for individuals seeking access to health care."[123]

The aforementioned assertion, however, is subject to debate given recent legal developments in jurisdictions outside of the United States. It has been proposed that although various international treatises provide limited enforceability in ensuring the right to health or health care, there is developing jurisprudence in jurisdictions such as South Africa and United Kingdom, which in fact illustrate judicial enforcement of certain health and health care-related rights.[124] Most notable is the South African case, *Treatment Action Campaign v. Minister of Health*, which held that HIV-positive pregnant women have the right to obtain treatment in public hospitals and clinics to prevent mother-to-child transmission of the HIV virus.[125] Moreover, in another case, the European Court of Human Rights held that the deportation of an individual suffering from AIDS to his or her native country would constitute "cruel, inhumane, or degrading treatment" because of the fact that his or her native country could not provide proper medical treatment, and this precipitating factor would ultimately result in an earlier demise[126].

To date, the United States has failed to ratify any of the United Nation's treaties and instruments recognizing the international human right to health with the exception of the International Convention on the Elimination of all Forms of Racial Discrimination (ICERD), and the International Covenant on Civil and Political Rights (ICCPR), which contains other health-related rights.[127] Furthermore, the United States has not ratified any regional treaties recognizing the international human right to health.[128] Therefore, as a practical matter, the United States is not required as a state party to implement the international human right to health.[129]

The following subsections will provide a brief synopsis of some of the most salient treaties and declarations that address the right to health and health care. The following listing and review is not meant to be exhaustive but will serve rather as an introduction.

Universal Declaration of Human Rights

The United States is a member of WHO, which is an specialized international public health agency within the United Nations.[130] The organization's primary responsibility lies in providing a leadership role with respect to issues germane to global health, establishing norms and standards, molding health research, supplying evidence-based policy alternatives, providing technical support to countries, and tracking and analyzing health trends.[131]

The constitution of the WHO declares that "the enjoyment of the highest attainable standard of health is one of the fundamental rights of every human being without distinction of race, religion, political belief, economic or social condition."[132] Moreover, "health is a state of complete physical, mental and social well-being and not merely the absence of disease or infirmity."[133]

In 1948, the United States agreed to abide by the obligations set forth by the Universal Declaration of Human Rights (UDHR). With respect to the right to health and health care, Article 25 states in relevant part that:

> everyone has the right to a standard of living adequate for the health and well-being of himself and of his family, including food, clothing, housing and medical care and necessary social services . . .[134] [Additionally,] Motherhood and childhood are entitled to special care and assistance. All children, whether born in or out of wedlock, shall enjoy the same social protection.[135]

Over time, WHO has provided clarification of this definition, which ultimately cumulated in a "right to primary health in accordance with the ability of the state and the international community to provide it."[136] As a declaration, however, the UDHR does not impose specific obligations on state parties. This declaration is important because it envisions a spectrum of variables that affect the general health of a human being and it further provides protection for women and children, both who suffer from disparities in health and health care within the United States.

The International Covenant on Civil and Political Rights

The ICCPR was ratified by the United States on June 8, 1992, and although it does not contain a specific provision safeguarding the right to health; it does incorporate several enumerated rights that are directly or indirectly associated to a person's enjoyment of his or her right to health.[137] The respective provisions of the ICCPR, which could arguably be linked to the right to health include the following: the right to not be subjected to torture or to cruel, inhuman or degrading treatment or punishment (Article 7); the right to not be subjected without free consent to medical or scientific experimentation (Article 7); and the right to not be held in slavery or servitude or to be required to perform forced or compulsory labor (Article 8).[138]

In 1992, the United States ratified the ICCPR, with five reservations, five understandings, and four declarations.[139] Some have noted that with so many reservations, its implementation has little domestic effect.[140] The U.S. declaration stating that "the provisions of Article 1 through 27 of the Covenant are not self-executing" is noteworthy and illustrative of the aforementioned assertion. Generally, when a treaty or covenant is "not self-executing," and in the instance where Congress has failed to take an active part in implementing the agreement with legislation, no private right cause of action is created by ratification.[141] Thus, the ICCPR on the surface appears to be binding on the United States as a matter of international law; however, it does not form a part of the domestic law of the nation. It is interesting to note that in the United States pursuant to 45 CFR Part 46, Section 46.116, "no investigator may involve a human being as a subject in research . . . unless the investigator has obtained the legally effective informed consent of the subject."[142] The aforementioned regulation is important because of past research abuses that took place in the United States with respect to various minority populations.

The Tuskegee study serves as one such example. In 1932, the Public Health Service, working in conjunction with the Tuskegee Institute, commenced a study to record the natural history of syphilis in hopes of justifying treatment programs for blacks.[143] The research study was called the "Tuskegee Study of Untreated Syphilis in the Negro Male."[144] At the commencement of the study, 600 African American men were enrolled, 399 with syphilis, 201 did not have the disease.[145] Sadly, the study was conducted without the benefit of the patients' informed consent.[146] Essentially, researchers told the men they were being treated for "bad blood," a local term used to describe several ailments, inclusive of syphilis, anemia, and fatigue.[147] Unfortunately, the men did not receive the proper treatment needed to cure their illness, even when a standard treatment became available for syphilis.[148] In exchange for taking part in the study, the men received free medical exams, free meals, and burial insurance.[149] The study that was originally projected to last 6 months was actually permitted to persist for 40 years.[150]

International Convention on the Elimination of all Forms of Racial Discrimination

The United States ratified the ICERD in October 1994, and the convention entered into force for the United States on November 20, 1994.[151] According to Article 5 of ICERD:

> States Parties undertake to prohibit and to eliminate racial discrimination in all its forms and to guarantee the right of everyone, without distinction as to race, color, or national or ethnic origin, to equality before the law, notably in the enjoyment of the following rights: Economic, social and cultural rights, in particular, the right to public health, medical care, social security and social services.[152]

Because of the U.S. ratification of ICERD, it is obligated to comply with and implement the provisions of ICERD just as it would any other domestic law or international treaty, subject to the U.S. reservations that were entered when it ratified ICERD.[153] Moreover, the U.S. Constitution Article 6 clause 2 clearly delineates that treaties are "the law of the land."[154] As a consequence, the United States has agreed to be legally bound by ICERD's mandate "to protect and promote equality and non-discrimination" in the enjoyment of the human right to health.[155] This treaty is relevant because it obligates countries to eradicate discrimination both domestically and internationally.[156]

When the United States ratified ICERD, it agreed to submit reports to the Committee on the Elimination of Racial Discrimination, (the UN body charged with assessing state compliance with the convention).[157] It is reported, however, that the recent U.S. April 2007 report:

> fails to thoroughly discuss how racial discrimination prevents the enjoyment of the right to health and environmental health for people of color in the United States, nor does the report accept state responsibility for respecting, protecting, and fulfilling equal access to these rights.[158]

The report, titled "Unequal Health Outcomes in the United States," asserts that racial discrimination in health care access and treatment is a human rights violation that warrants serious attention from both the ICERD Committee and policy makers in the United States.[159]

International Covenant on Economic, Social, and Cultural Rights

The International Covenant on Economic, Social and Cultural Rights (ICESCR)[160] Article 12 requires that state parties "recognize the right of everyone to the enjoyment of the highest attainable standard of physical and mental health."[161] Moreover, Article 10 (2) specifies that "special protection should be accorded to mothers during a reasonable period before and after childbirth. During such period working mothers should be accorded paid leave or leave with adequate social security benefits."[162]

This instrument also mandates specific state obligations with regard to the right to health, but does not define "health."[163] Article 12.2 sets forth some of the steps that must be implemented by states in achieving full realization of the aforementioned right and shall include those necessary for:

- "The provision for the reduction of the stillbirth rate and of infant mortality and for the healthy development of child" [164];
- "The improvement of all aspects of environmental and industrial hygiene"[165];
- "The prevention, treatment and control of epidemic, endemic, occupational and other diseases"[166]
- "The creation of conditions which would assure to all medical service and medical attention in the event of sickness."[167]

Usually, the right to health is closely associated with and dependent on the actualization of other human rights, including rights to equality and nondiscrimination.[168] Moreover, with respect to ICESCR, state parties undertake to guarantee that the right to health will be exercised without discrimination of any kind on the basis of gender and sex.[169]

The United States signed this document on October 5, 1977, but has failed to ratify it.[170] As a consequence, the United States is not obligated to adhere to the preceding provisions. If ratified and enforced by the United States, the infant mortality rate could potentially be reduced if the preceding clauses are complied with. In addition, as a general matter, working pregnant women who give birth to a child are not provided with paid leave in the United States. Under the Family and Medical Leave Act (FMLA), certain employees may be eligible for up to 12 weeks of unpaid, job-protected leave per year.[171] FMLA also requires that the woman's group health benefits be maintained during the leave.[172] However, if a woman elects to be out of work for a longer time to rear her newborn, she would be without a job and without employer-sponsored insurance.

The Convention on the Elimination of All Forms of Discrimination Against Women

The Convention on the Elimination of All Forms of Discrimination Against Women (CEDAW) expressly addresses equality in health care on the following grounds.[173] Article 12 of CEDAW asserts that:

> States Parties shall take all appropriate measures to eliminate discrimination against women in the field of health care in order to ensure, on a basis of equality of men and women, access to health care services, including those related to family planning.[174]

Moreover, CEDAW specifies that "States Parties shall ensure that women receive appropriate services in connection with pregnancy, confinement and the post-natal period, granting free services where necessary, as well as adequate nutrition during pregnancy and lactation."[175]

The United States signed CEDAW on July 17, 1980, but has failed to ratify this document.[176] United States' ratification of the aforementioned provisions would serve to alleviate disparities experienced by women. For example, women of color fare worse than Caucasian women across a vast range of measures in almost every state, and in a few states these disparities were quite alarming.[177]

Convention on the Rights of the Child

The Convention on the Rights of the Child (CRC) provides significant detail with respect to children and the provision of health care.[178] For example, it indicates that parties must recognize "the right of the child to the enjoyment of the highest attainable standard of health and to facilities for the treatment of illness and rehabilitation of health."[179] The language further asserts that state parties shall "strive to ensure that no child is deprived of his or her right of access to such health care services."[180] Moreover, the treaty calls for extensive preventive and health education services, which include "pre-natal and post-natal health care for mothers." Additionally, state parties must take steps to eliminate "traditional practices prejudicial to the health of children."[181] Interestingly,

Article 23 sets forth health care and additional special services for disabled children.[182]

CRC has not been ratified by the United States; however, the United States has ratified the two following Optional Protocols: (a) the Optional Protocol to the CRC on the involvement of children in armed conflict was ratified on December 23, 2002 (with one declaration and five understandings); and (b) the Optional Protocol to the CRC on the sale of children, child prostitution, and child pornography was ratified on December 23, 2002 (with one declaration and six understandings).

Disparities experienced by children continue to persevere within the United States. According to the 2009 National Health Care Disparities Report, children who are members of racial and ethnic minority groups tend to face greater health risks.[183] As mentioned earlier, African American children and American Indian/Alaskan Native children had death rates about 1.5–2 times as high as Caucasian children in the year 2003.[184] Moreover, in 2005, African American infants were more than twice as likely as Caucasian infants to die during their first year.[185] Life expectancy at birth was 78.3 years for Caucasian children and 73.2 years for African American children, a troubling difference of about 5 years.[186] Ratification of the CRC could arguably be conducive in alleviating the health disparities experienced by children. For example, if prenatal care were provided to all women within the United States, the infant mortality rate could possibly be lowered because lack of prenatal services is strongly associated with infant mortality.

PROTECTIONS FOR INDIVIDUALS WHO ACCESS THE U.S. HEALTH CARE SYSTEM

An argument can be made for the proposition "that the United States has established a considerable legal infrastructure that effectively recognizes the human right to health for some groups under specified circumstances."[187] Although the United States has various disparity populations, it is plausible that without the following enumerated protections, these disparities could inevitably worsen.

The Employee Retirement Income Security Act of 1974

The Employee Retirement Income Security Act (ERISA) of 1974 is a federal law that delineates the minimum standards for most voluntarily established pension and health plans in private industry.[188] The law is intended to provide protection for individuals in these plans.[189] ERISA has numerous amendments that enhance the protections available to health benefit plan participants and beneficiaries.[190] Most notable is the Consolidated Omnibus Budget Reconciliation Act (COBRA), which provides certain workers and their families with the right to continue their health coverage for a limited time after certain events, such as the loss of a job.[191] Generally speaking, ERISA does not apply to group health plans created by or maintained by governmental entities, churches for their employees, or plans that are maintained solely to comply with applicable workers compensation, unemployment, or disability laws.[192] Moreover, ERISA does not apply to plans maintained outside the United States primarily for the benefit of nonresident aliens or unfunded excess benefit plans.[193]

The Emergency Medical Treatment and Active Labor Act

This Act has been described as "the only truly universal right to health care in the United States" and is often characterized as on of the building blocks of health care rights."[194] Emergency Medical Treatment and Active Labor Act (EMTALA) was enacted by Congress in 1986 to prevent the practice of "patient dumping," which is the turning away of poor or uninsured individuals who are in need of hospital care.[195] EMTALA's goal is to ensure public access to emergency medical services regardless of the individual's ability to pay.[196] The Social Security Act, Section 1867, sets forth specific obligations on Medicare-participating hospitals that offer emergency medical services to provide a medical screening examination (MSE) when a request is made for examination or treatment for an emergency medical condition (EMC), including active labor, regardless of an individual's ability to pay.[197] Hospitals are subsequently obligated to provide stabilizing medical treatment for patients with EMCs.[198] If the hospital is unable to stabilize a patient within its capability, or if the patient requests, an appropriate transfer should be implemented.[199]

The Health Insurance Portability and Accountability Act of 1996

The Office for Civil Rights enforces the Health Insurance Portability and Accountability Act (HIPAA) Privacy Rule and its implementing regulations, which protects the privacy of individually identifiable health information; the HIPAA Security Rule, which sets national standards for the security of electronically protected health information; and the confidentiality provisions of the Patient Safety Rule, which protect identifiable information being used to analyze patient safety events and improve patient safety.[200]

Patient Right to Make Informed Health Care Decisions

Under the Patient Self-Determination Act (PSDA) of 1990, every person has a right under state law (whether statutory or as recognized by the courts of the state) to make decisions relating to his or her medical care, including the right to accept or refuse medical or surgical treatment, and the right to formulate advanced directives.[201]

Title VI of the Civil Rights Act

Title VI of the Civil Rights Act (Title VI), and its implementing regulations, is the primary law related to eliminating racial and ethnic discrimination in health care delivery.[202] Title VI Section 601 provides: "No person in the United States, shall, on the grounds of race, color, or national origin, be excluded from participation in, be denied the benefits of, or be subject to discrimination under any program or activity receiving federal financial assistance."[203]

The term *discrimination* under Title VI applies to intentional acts or policies that unintentionally result in discrimination against racial and ethnic minorities."[204] One should be cautioned that this title has limited applicability because of the fact that it attaches only to recipients receiving federal funds[205] and regulatory agencies have also interpreted Title VI to exclude physicians in private practice.[206] Furthermore, the 2001 Supreme Court case *Alexander v. Sandoval* held that private individuals are precluded from bringing a lawsuit under the disparate impact regulations, thus rendering the federal government as the only enforcer when a violation of the law has been alleged by a racial and ethnic minority.[207] Despite these limitations, Title VI has the potential to positively affect the health care arena because a tremendous amount of federal money has been devoted to the health care enterprise during the past 4 decades.[208]

Americans With Disabilities Act

The Americans With Disabilities Act (ADA) took effect in July of 1992; however, the language of the Act has been the subject of ongoing judicial interpretation and definition because of its broad language.[209] Similar to Title VI, the ADA is not exactly a "health law"; however, its influence on health care for disabled individuals is viewed as remarkable because it expands access to care for this population. According to the ADA, a person suffering from a "disability" is an individual who has "1) a physical or mental impairment that substantially limits one or more major life activities, 2) a record of such an impairment, or 3) is regarded as having such an impairment."[210]

The regulations further delineate that a physical or mental impairment means: "Any physiological disorder, or condition, cosmetic disfigurement, or anatomical loss affecting one or more of the following body systems: neurological, musculoskeletal, special sense organs, respiratory (including speech organs), cardiovascular, reproductive, digestive, genito-urinary, hemic and lymphatic, skin, and endocrine."[211] Additionally, a mental impairment is considered for all intents and purposes as: "any mental or psychological disorder, such as mental retardation, organic brain syndrome, emotional or mental illness, and specific learning disabilities."[212] Diseases, infections, and chronic conditions such as HIV, cancer, diabetes, epilepsy, and emotional illness may be considered physical and mental impairments for purposes of the ADA.[213] However, for a person to qualify as suffering from a physical or mental disability pursuant to the ADA, these impairments must substantially limit one or more major life activities.[214] Examples of the aforementioned activities include walking, seeing, working, participating in community activities, caring for oneself, performing manual tasks, hearing, speaking, breathing, and learning.[215]

According to experts, the ADA's profound influence on health care for individuals with disability is noteworthy, in large part, because the law defines private physicians' offices and private hospitals as places of "public accommodation" without regard to whether they participate in federally assisted programs.[216] The Supreme Court's first case interpreting the ADA, *Bragdon v. Abbott*, demonstrates the statute's application and relevance to the disabled population.[217] In this matter, the dentist, Randon Bragdon, refused to fill a cavity of an HIV-infected woman by the name of Sydney Abbott in his office.[218] Abbott subsequently sued the dentist under Title III of the ADA, which prohibits disability discrimination by the operator of a place of public accommodation,[219] (a term that expressly includes the "professional office of a health care provider").[220] Although the dentist insisted that providing the requested services in his office would pose a "direct threat"[221] of HIV transmission to him, the district court rejected this argument and held in favor of Abbott.[222] A review of the court's analysis suggest that absent a "direct threat" or another type of defense—a refusal to provide dental treatment to a person based on the person's disability constitutes a violation of the ADA.[223]

The issue of when the direct threat defense may be used subsequently went to the Supreme Court, which addressed whether deference should be given to the individual judgment of a health care worker regarding the existence of a significant risk of transmission.[224] The Court ultimately held that the existence of significant risk and direct threat should be determined from the standpoint of the person who refuses to provide treatment, but it must be based on "objective medical or scientific information."[225] This case epitomizes an expansion of federal disability law because of the fact that prior to the enactment of the ADA, only recipients of federal funds were precluded from discriminating against individuals with disabilities.[226]

Laws Involving Reproductive Freedom

Generally speaking, reproductive rights encompass two critical principles: reproductive self-determination and access to reproductive health care, information, and services.[227] The following section will briefly outline the evolution of reproductive rights within the United States.

In the 1965 case, *Griswold v. Connecticut*, the Supreme Court struck down a state law that prohibited giving married people information, instruction, or medical advice on contraception.[228] Soon thereafter, in 1972, *Eisenstadt v. Baird*, the Supreme Court established the right of unmarried people to use contraceptives.[229]

The 1973 seminal case, *Roe v. Wade* held that a woman has a constitutional right of privacy, which also includes a woman's right to decide to have an abortion previability without undue interference from the government.[230] In this case, however, the Supreme Court also recognized a state interest in protecting potential life and attempted to delineate the extent in which states may regulate and even prohibit an abortion. Thus, the Court in Roe confirmed that the state has the power to restrict abortions after viability so long as the law contains exceptions for pregnancies that endanger the woman's life or health. Moreover, Roe recognized the state's legitimate interests in protecting the health of the woman and the life of the fetus from the commencement of pregnancy.

In the 1992 case, *Planned Parenthood of Southeastern Pennsylvania v. Casey*, the Supreme Court reaffirmed the "core" holdings of *Roe v. Wade*, which stated that women have a right to abortion prior to fetal viability, but states are permitted to restrict abortion access so long as these restrictions do not impose an "undue burden" on women seeking abortions. An abortion regulation constitutes an undue burden and is unconstitutional if its intended purpose or effect results in a substantial impediment in the path of a woman seeking an abortion of a nonviable fetus.[231] In addition, the court ruled that spousal consent pose an undue burden on the women.[232]

In the 2000 case, *Sternberg v. Carhart*, the Supreme Court concluded that the Nebraska statute making "partial-birth abortion" a crime was unconstitutional because it lacked any exception for preservation of health of the mother and because it imposed an undue burden on a woman's ability to choose a more common abortion procedure, thereby unduly burdening the right to choose abortion itself.[233]

It should be noted that the U.S. Supreme Court has recognized that, although a woman has a right to determine whether to terminate her pregnancy under the U.S. Constitution, the right is not absolute, and may be impeded in certain situations via governmental regulation.[234] It is documented that:

> the Supreme Court has sought to balance a woman's fundamental right to bodily autonomy with valid governmental interests in protecting its interests in the health of its citizens, in maintaining medical standards, and in protecting potential life in a variety of decisions.[235]

For example, on November 5, 2003, Congress passed the Partial-Birth Abortion Ban Act (PBABA) of 2003, which made it a federal crime to knowingly perform a partial-birth abortion.[236] At that time, Congress deliberately failed to include a health exception with respect to PBABA.[237] It is purported that this was done in full recognition of and in response to Stenberg.[238] The act did contain an exception allowing the performance of a partial-birth abortion to save the life of the mother, but not for the health of the mother.[239] After trial, the district court determined that the PBABA was unconstitutional on two separate grounds. First, the district court concluded Congress's finding regarding a medical consensus was unreasonable and thus the PBABA was unconstitutional because of its lack of health exception.[240] Second, the district court held that PBABA covered the most common late-term abortion procedure and thus imposed an undue burden on the right to an abortion.[241]

Consequently, the case was reviewed by the Supreme Court and in the 2007 case, *Gonzales v. Carhart*, the PBABA of 2003 was upheld as constitutional.[242] Several medical groups articulated concern that in supporting the PBABA, the Supreme Court essentially endorsed the substitution of congressional legislation for medical judgment. According to the American College of Obstetricians and Gynecologists' (ACOG) amicus brief opposing the PBABA, "the Act will chill doctors from providing a wide range of procedures used to perform induced abortions or to treat cases of miscarriage and will gravely endanger the health of women in this country."[243] For some, this is considered "a steady erosion of women's reproductive rights in this country."[244]

CONCLUSION

In the United States, various factors impact health disparities but the quality of health care can be enhanced for all patients with a comprehensive strategy that includes attending to the needs of health care providers and their patients, to the conditions of health care settings in which care takes place, to the broader policies and practices of health systems, and to state and federal policies that govern the operation of health systems.[245] It has also been illustrated that the utilization of public health legal partnerships can also enhance the public's health and this novel approach may very well make a sizeable impact in reducing health care disparities within the United States.

Moreover, the establishment and implementation of domestic law that reflect the language contained in international treatises ensuring the human right to health and health care is critical. The aforementioned proposed legislation should have some type of enforcement provisions that would increase the likelihood of adherence.

It is also important that those who work in the health care arena continue to be educated about the various social, medical, political, and legal determinants of health. Quintessentially, it is crucial that interdisciplinary teams inclusive of health care professionals, human rights advocates, attorneys, public health officials, nongovernmental organizations, local and foreign governments, academics, and health care institutions collaborate in effectuating the laudable goal of eradicating health and health care disparities within the United States and abroad.

NOTES

[1]New York State Bar Association. (2009). *Health law section summary report on health-care costs: Legal issues, barriers and solutions, 14*(2), 126.

[2]Department of Health and Human Services Report. Health Disparities: A Case for Closing the Gap. Retrieved January 20, 2010, from http://www.healthreform.gov/reports/healthdisparities/index.html

[3]Office of the Actuary, Centers for Medicare and Medicaid Services, National Health Expenditure. Projections for 2008. U.S. Department of Health and Human Services. Retrieved January 20, 2010, from http://www.cms.hhs.gov/NationalHealth ExpendData/03_NationalHealthAccountsProjected.asp#TopOfPage

[4]Department of Health and Human Services Report. Health Disparities: A Case for Closing the Gap. Retrieved January 20, 2010, from http://www.healthreform.gov/reports/healthdisparities/index.html

[5]Department of Health and Human Services Report. Health Disparities: A Case for Closing the Gap. Retrieved January 20, 2010, from http://www.healthreform.gov/reports/healthdisparities/index.html

[6]The United States Commission on Civil Rights. (1999) The health care challenge: Acknowledging disparity, confronting discrimination, and ensuring equality. Volume I: The role of governmental and private health care programs and initiatives. Retrieved from http://www.law.umaryland.edu/marshall/usccr/documents/cr12h34z.pdf [hereinafter U.S. Commission on Civil Rights]. Page 11.

[7]The United States Commission on Civil Rights. (1999) The health care challenge: Acknowledging disparity, confronting discrimination, and ensuring equality. Volume I: The role of governmental and private health care programs and initiatives. Retrieved from http://www.law.umaryland.edu/marshall/usccr/documents/cr12h34z.pdf [hereinafter U.S. Commission on Civil Rights]. Page 11

[8]The United States Commission on Civil Rights. (1999) The health care challenge: Acknowledging disparity, confronting discrimination, and ensuring equality. Volume I: The role of governmental and private health care programs and initiatives. Retrieved from http://www.law.umaryland.edu/marshall/usccr/documents/cr12h34z.pdf [hereinafter U.S. Commission on Civil Rights]. (147 deaths per 100,000 for Blacks compared to 105 deaths per 100,000 for Whites).

[9]The United States Commission on Civil Rights. (1999) The health care challenge: Acknowledging disparity, confronting discrimination, and ensuring equality. Volume I: The role of governmental and private health care programs and initiatives. Retrieved from http://www.law.umaryland.edu/marshall/usccr/documents/cr12h34z.pdf [hereinafter U.S. Commission on Civil Rights].

[10]The United States Commission on Civil Rights. (1999) The health care challenge: Acknowledging disparity, confronting discrimination, and ensuring equality. Volume I: The role of governmental and private health care programs and initiatives. Retrieved from http://www.law.umaryland.edu/marshall/usccr/documents/cr12h34z.pdf [hereinafter U.S. Commission on Civil Rights].

[11]The United States Commission on Civil Rights. (1999) The health care challenge: Acknowledging disparity, confronting discrimination, and ensuring equality. Volume I: The role of governmental and private health care programs and initiatives. Retrieved from http://www.law.umaryland.edu/marshall/usccr/documents/cr12h34z.pdf [hereinafter U.S. Commission on Civil Rights]. Page 31

[12]The United States Commission on Civil Rights. (1999) The health care challenge: Acknowledging disparity, confronting discrimination, and ensuring equality. Volume I: The role of governmental and private health care programs and initiatives. Retrieved from http://www.law.umaryland.edu/marshall/usccr/documents/cr12h34z.pdf [hereinafter U.S. Commission on Civil Rights].

[13]The United States Commission on Civil Rights. (1999) The health care challenge: Acknowledging disparity, confronting discrimination, and ensuring equality. Volume I: The role of governmental and private health care programs and initiatives. Retrieved from http://www.law.umaryland.edu/marshall/usccr/documents/cr12h34z.pdf [hereinafter U.S. Commission on Civil Rights]. Page 14–15.

[14]The United States Commission on Civil Rights. (1999) The health care challenge: Acknowledging disparity, confronting discrimination, and ensuring equality.

Volume I: The role of governmental and private health care programs and initiatives. Retrieved from http://www.law.umaryland.edu/marshall/usccr/documents/cr12h34z .pdf [hereinafter U.S. Commission on Civil Rights].

[15]Department of Health and Human Services Report. Health Disparities: A Case for Closing the Gap. Retrieved January 20, 2010, from http://www.healthreform.gov/ reports/healthdisparities/index.html

[16]Littell, A. (2002). Can a constitutional right to health guarantee universal health care coverage or improved health outcomes?: A survey of selected states. *Connecticut Law Review, 35,* 289.

[17]MacDorman, M. F., & Matthews, T. J. Retrieved April 4, 2010, from http://www.cdc .gov/nchs/data/databriefs/db09.pdf

[18]Centers for Disease Control and Prevention. Retrieved April 11, 2010, from http:// www.cdc.gov/nchs/fastats/deaths.htm

[19]MacDorman, M. F., & Matthews, T. J. Retrieved April 4, 2010, from http://www.cdc .gov/nchs/data/databriefs/db09.pdf

[20]Office of Minority Health and Health Disparities. Eliminate Disparities in Infant Mortality. Retrieved April 18, 2010, from http://www.cdc.gov/omhd/amh/factsheets/infant.htm

[21]Central Intelligence Agency. Retrieved from https://www.cia.gov/library/publications/ the-world-factbook/rankorder/2102rank.html

[22]Kinney, E. D. (2008). Recognition of the international human right to health and health care in the United States. *Rutgers Law Review, 60,* 354.

[23]Press Release, World Health Organization, & World Health Report 2000 (2001, February 21). Retrieved from http://www.who.int/whr/2000/en/press_release.htm

[24]Carter-Pokras, O., & Baquet, C. (2004). What is a health disparity? *Public Health Reports, 117,* 426–434. Retrieved from http://www.ncbi.nlm.nih.gov/pmc/articles/PMC1497467/ pdf/12500958.pdf

[25]Center to Reduce Cancer Health Disparities. Retrieved from http://crchd.cancer.gov/ disparities/defined.html

[26]Center to Reduce Cancer Health Disparities. Retrieved from http://crchd.cancer.gov/ disparities/defined.html

[27]Center to Reduce Cancer Health Disparities. Retrieved from http://crchd.cancer.gov/ disparities/defined.html

[28]United States Public Law 106–525. Retrieved from http://frwebgate.access.gpo.gov/ cgibin/getdoc.cgi?dbname=106_cong_public_laws&docid=f:publ525.106.pdf

[29]The Office of Minority Health. What Are Health Disparities? Retrieved April 15, 2010, from http://minorityhealth.hhs.gov/templates/content.aspx?ID=3559

[30]Centers for Prevention and Health Services: Issue Brief. (2009, February). Eliminating Racial and Ethnic Health Disparities; A Business Case Update for Employers National Business Group on Health. Retrieved from http://www.businessgrouphealth.org/ pdfs/Final%20Draft%20508.pdf

[31]Department of Health and Human Services. Institute of Medicine. Unequal Treatment: What Healthcare System Administrators Need to Know About Racial and Ethnic Disparities in HealthCare. March 2002. Retrieved from http://www.iom. edu/~/media/Files/Report%20Files/2003/Unequal-Treatment-Confronting-Racial-and-Ethnic-Disparities-in-Health-Care/DisparitiesAdmin8pg.ashx

[32]Institute of Medicine. (2002). Unequal treatment: What healthcare system administrators need to know about racial and ethnic disparities in health care. Retrieved from http://www.iom.edu/~/media/Files/Report%20Files/2003/Unequal-Treatment-Confronting-Racial-and-Ethnic-Disparities-in-Health-Care/DisparitiesAdmin8pg.ashx

[33]Institute of Medicine. (2002). Unequal treatment: What healthcare system administrators need to know about racial and ethnic disparities in health care. Retrieved from http://www.iom.edu/~/media/Files/Report%20Files/2003/Unequal-Treatment-Confronting-Racial-and-Ethnic-Disparities-in-Health-Care/DisparitiesAdmin8pg.ashx

[34]Centers for Prevention and Health Services: Issue Brief. (2009, February). Eliminating Racial and Ethnic Health Disparities; A Business Case Update for Employers National Business Group on Health. Retrieved from http://www.business grouphealth.org/pdfs/Final%20Draft%20508.pdf

[35]Byers, T. E., Wolf, H. J., Bauer, K. R., Bolick-Aldrich, S., Chen, V. W., Finch, J. L., et al. (2008). The impact of socioeconomic status on survival after cancer in the United States: Findings from the National Program of Cancer Registries' patterns of patient care study. *Cancer, 113*(3), 582–591.

[36]Reyes, C., Van de Putte, L., Falcon, A. P., et al. *Genes, culture, and medicines: Bridging gaps in treatment for Hispanic Americans.* Washington, DC: The National Alliance for Hispanic Health and The National Pharmaceutical Council; 2004. Retrieved April 15, 2010, from http://www.hispanichealth.org/pdf/hispanic_report04.pdf

[37]Centers for Prevention and Health Services: Issue Brief. (2009, February). Eliminating Racial and Ethnic Health Disparities; A Business Case Update for Employers National Business Group on Health. Retrieved from http://www.businessgrouphealth.org/pdfs/Final%20Draft%20508.pdf

[38]U.S. Department of Health and Human Services. *National healthcare disparities report.* Rockville, MD: Agency for Healthcare Research and Quality; 2007;94. AHRQ Publication No. 08-0041. Available at: http:// www.ahrq.gov/qual/qrdr07.htm

[39]Centers for Prevention and Health Services: Issue Brief. (2009, February). Eliminating Racial and Ethnic Health Disparities; A Business Case Update for Employers National Business Group on Health. Retrieved from http://www.businessgrouphealth.org/pdfs/Final%20Draft%20508.pdf

[40]Centers for Prevention and Health Services: Issue Brief. (2009, February). Eliminating Racial and Ethnic Health Disparities; A Business Case Update for Employers National Business Group on Health. Retrieved from http://www.businessgrouphealth.org/pdfs/Final%20Draft%20508.pdf

[41]Centers for Prevention and Health Services: Issue Brief. (2009, February). Eliminating Racial and Ethnic Health Disparities; A Business Case Update for Employers National Business Group on Health. Retrieved from http://www.businessgrouphealth.org/pdfs/Final%20Draft%20508.pdf

[42]U.S. Department of Health and Human Services. (2009). National Healthcare Disparities Report. Rockville, MD: Agency for Healthcare Research and Quality; AHRQ Publication No. 10-0004. Retrieved from http://www.ahrq.gov/qual/nhdr09/nhdr09.pdf

[43]U.S. Department of Health and Human Services. (2009). National Healthcare Disparities Report. Rockville, MD: Agency for Healthcare Research and Quality; AHRQ Publication No. 10-0004. Retrieved from http://www.ahrq.gov/qual/nhdr09/nhdr09.pdf

[44]U.S. Department of Health and Human Services. (2009). National Healthcare Disparities Report. Rockville, MD: Agency for Healthcare Research and Quality; AHRQ Publication No. 10-0004. Retrieved from http://www.ahrq.gov/qual/nhdr09/nhdr09.pdf

[45]Agency for Healthcare Research and Quality. National Healthcare Disparities Report, 2008. Retrieved from http://www.ahrq.gov/qual/nhdr08/nhdr08.pdf

[46]U.S. Census Bureau. Press Release. (2008). Income, Poverty, and Health Insurance Coverage in the United States: 2007. Available at http://www.census.gov/prod/2008pubs/p60-235.pdf

[47]Yacht, J. M. (2007, October 7). Time has come for universal health care in America. *Tampa Tribune*, at 2.

[48]Kaiser Commission on Medicaid and the Uninsured. (2006). The uninsured and their access to health care. Retrieved from http://www.kff.org/uninsured/upload/The-Uninsured-and-Their-Access-to-Health-Care-Oct-2004.pdf

[49]Wilper, A. P., Woolhandler, S., Lasser, K. E., McCormick, D., Bor, D. H., & Himmelstein, D. U. (2009). Health insurance and mortality in US Adults. *American Journal of Public Health*, (99)12.

[50]Wilper, A. P., Woolhandler, S., Lasser, K. E., McCormick, D., Bor, D. H., & Himmelstein, D. U. (2009). Health insurance and mortality in US Adults. *American Journal of Public Health*, (99)12.

[51]U.S. Department of Health and Human Services. (2009). National Healthcare Disparities Report. Rockville, MD: Agency for Healthcare Research and Quality; 2009;AHRQ Publication No. 10-0004. Retrieved from http://www.ahrq.gov/qual/nhdr09/nhdr09.pdf

[52]Abelson, R. (2009, September 17). Harvard Medical Study Links Lack of Insurance to 45,000 U.S. Deaths a Year. Retrieved from http://prescriptions.blogs.nytimes.com/2009/09/17/harvard-medical-study-links-lack-of-insurance-to-45000-us-deaths-a-year/

[53]Abelson, R. (2009, September 17). Harvard Medical Study Links Lack of Insurance to 45,000 U.S. Deaths a Year. Retrieved from http://prescriptions.blogs.nytimes.com/2009/09/17/harvard-medical-study-links-lack-of-insurance-to-45000-us-deaths-a-year/

[54]Abelson, R. (2009, September 17). Harvard Medical Study Links Lack of Insurance to 45,000 U.S. Deaths a Year. Retrieved from http://prescriptions.blogs.nytimes.com/2009/09/17/harvard-medical-study-links-lack-of-insurance-to-45000-us-deaths-a-year/

[55]Agency for Healthcare Research and Quality. Retrieved from http://www.ahrq.gov/qual/nhdr09/nhdr09.pdf

[56]Smedley, B. D. (2003). *Unequal treatment: Confronting racial and ethnic disparities in health care, 2003*. Washington, DC: Board of Health Sciences Policy, Institute of Medicine.

[57]Kinney, E. D. (2008). Recognition of the international human right to health and health care in the United States. *Rutgers Law Review*, 60(335).

[58]Littell, A. (2002). Can a constitutional right to health guarantee universal health care coverage or improved health outcomes?: A survey of selected states. *Connecticut Law Review*, 35, 289, 308.

[59]Department of Health and Human Services. Secretary Kathleen Sebelius Statement on New Health Care Quality, Disparity Reports. Press Release April 2010. Retrieved from http://www.hhs.gov/news/press/2010pres/04/20100413a.html

[60]Department of Health and Human Services. Secretary Kathleen Sebelius Statement on New Health Care Quality, Disparity Reports. Press Release April 2010. Retrieved from http://www.hhs.gov/news/press/2010pres/04/20100413a.html

[61]Patient Protection and Affordable Care Act (P.L. 111–148) and Health Care and Education Reconciliation Act (P.L. 111–152).

[62]Department of Health and Human Services. Secretary Kathleen Sebelius Statement on New Health Care Quality, Disparity Reports. Press Release April 2010. Retrieved from http://www.hhs.gov/news/press/2010pres/04/20100413a.html

[63]Department of Health and Human Services. Secretary Kathleen Sebelius Statement on New Health Care Quality, Disparity Reports. Press Release April 2010. Retrieved from http://www.hhs.gov/news/press/2010pres/04/20100413a.html

[64]Berry, B. (n.d.). Health Care Law Aims to Address Inequities in System. Kaiser Monthly Update On Health Disparities. *Shreveport Times*. Retrieved May 10, 2010, from http://www.kff.org/minorityhealth/report.cfm

[65]The Henry Kaiser Family Foundation. Focus on Health Reform: Summary of New Health Reform. Retrieved May 9, 2010 http://www.kff.org/healthreform/upload/8061.pdf

[66]The Henry Kaiser Family Foundation. Focus on Health Reform: Summary of New Health Reform. Retrieved May 9, 2010 http://www.kff.org/healthreform/upload/8061.pdf

[67]The Henry Kaiser Family Foundation. Focus on Health Reform: Summary of New Health Reform. Retrieved May 9, 2010 http://www.kff.org/healthreform/upload/8061.pdf

[68]The Henry Kaiser Family Foundation. Focus on Health Reform: Summary of New Health Reform. Retrieved May 9, 2010, from http://www.kff.org/healthreform/upload/8061.pdf

[69]The Henry Kaiser Family Foundation. Focus on Health Reform: Summary of New Health Reform. Retrieved May 9, 2010, from http://www.kff.org/healthreform/upload/8061.pdf

[70]The Henry Kaiser Family Foundation. Focus on Health Reform: Summary of New Health Reform. Retrieved May 9, 2010, from http://www.kff.org/healthreform/upload/8061.pdf

[71]The Henry Kaiser Family Foundation. Focus on Health Reform: Summary of New Health Reform. Retrieved May 9, 2010, from http://www.kff.org/healthreform/upload/8061.pdf

[72]The Henry Kaiser Family Foundation. Focus on Health Reform: Summary of New Health Reform. Retrieved May 9, 2010, from http://www.kff.org/healthreform/upload/8061.pdf

[73]The Henry Kaiser Family Foundation. Focus on Health Reform: Summary of New Health Reform. Retrieved May 9, 2010, from http://www.kff.org/healthreform/upload/8061.pdf

[74]The Henry Kaiser Family Foundation. Focus on Health Reform: Summary of New Health Reform. Retrieved May 9, 2010, from http://www.kff.org/healthreform/upload/8061.pdf

[75]The Henry Kaiser Family Foundation. Focus on Health Reform: Summary of New Health Reform. Retrieved May 9, 2010, from http://www.kff.org/healthreform/upload/8061.pdf

[76]Department of Health and Human Services. (2010, April). Secretary Kathleen Sebelius Statement on New Health Care Quality, Disparity Reports. Press Release. Retrieved from http://www.hhs.gov/news/press/2010pres/04/20100413a.html

[77]Department of Health and Human Services. (2010, April). Secretary Kathleen Sebelius Statement on New Health Care Quality, Disparity Reports. Press Release. Retrieved from http://www.hhs.gov/news/press/2010pres/04/20100413a.html

[78]Department of Health and Human Services. (2010, April). Secretary Kathleen Sebelius Statement on New Health Care Quality, Disparity Reports. Press Release. Retrieved from http://www.hhs.gov/news/press/2010pres/04/20100413a.html

[79]The Henry Kaiser Family Foundation. Focus on Health Reform: Summary of New Health Reform. Retrieved May 9, 2010, from http://www.kff.org/healthreform/upload/8061.pdf

[80]Department of Health and Human Services. (2010, April). Secretary Kathleen Sebelius Statement on New Health Care Quality, Disparity Reports. Press Release. Retrieved from http://www.hhs.gov/news/press/2010pres/04/20100413a.html

[81]The Henry Kaiser Family Foundation. Focus on Health Reform: Summary of New Health Reform. Retrieved May 9, 2010, from http://www.kff.org/healthreform/upload/8061.pdf

[82]Berry, B. (n.d.). Health Care Law Aims to Address Inequities in System. Kaiser Monthly Update On Health Disparities. *Shreveport Times*. Retrieved May 10, 2010, from http://www.kff.org/minorityhealth/report.cfm

[83]Berry, B. (n.d.). Health Care Law Aims to Address Inequities in System. Kaiser Monthly Update On Health Disparities. *Shreveport Times*. Retrieved May 10, 2010, from http://www.kff.org/minorityhealth/report.cfm

[84]Littell, A. (2002). Can a constitutional right to health guarantee universal health care coverage or improved health outcomes?: A survey of selected states. *Connecticut Law Review, 35*, 289.

[85]Littell, A. (2002). Can a constitutional right to health guarantee universal health care coverage or improved health outcomes?: A survey of selected states. *Connecticut Law Review, 35*, 289.

[86]Littell, A. (2002). Can a constitutional right to health guarantee universal health care coverage or improved health outcomes?: A survey of selected states. *Connecticut Law Review, 35*, 289.

[87]Preamble to the Constitution of the World Health Organization as adopted by the International Health Conference, New York, June 19 to July 22, 1946; signed on July 22, 1946 by the representatives of 61 States (Official Records of the World Health Organization, no. 2, p. 100) and entered into force on 7 April 1948. The definition has not been amended since 1948. Retrieved from http://www.who.int/suggestions/faq/en/index.html and http://www.who.int/governance/eb/who_constitution_en.pdf

[88]Littell, A. (2002). Can a constitutional right to health guarantee universal health care coverage or improved health outcomes?: A survey of selected states. *Connecticut Law Review, 35*, 289.

[89]The U.S. National Archives & Records Administration. The Constitution of the United States: A Transcription. Retrieved February 4, 2010, from http://www.archives.gov/exhibits/charters/print_friendly.html?page=constitution_transcript_content.html&title=The%20Constitution%20of%20the%20United%20States%3A%20A%20Transcription

[90]See U.S. Constitution pmbl. ("In Order to . . . promote the general Welfare . . ..''). Retrieved February 4, 2010, from http://www.archives.gov/exhibits/charters/print_friendly.html?page=constitution_transcript_content.html&title=The%20Constitution%20of%20the%20United%20States%3A%20A%20Transcription

[91]See U.S. Constitution art. I, § 8 (authorizing, but not requiring, Congress to tax and spend in order to "provide for the . . . general Welfare . . ..'').

[92]See U.S. Const. pmbl; U.S. Constitution art. I, § 8, cl. 1.

[93]U.S. Const. art. I, § 8 (authorizing, but not requiring, Congress to tax and spend in order to "provide for the . . . general Welfare . . ..").

[94]U.S. Const. art. I, § 8 (authorizing, but not requiring, Congress to tax and spend in order to "provide for the . . . general Welfare . . ..").

[95]Kinney, E. D. (2008). Recognition of the international human right to health and health care in the United States. *Rutgers Law Review, 60*(335).

[96]U.S. Const. art. 1, § 8, cl. 3.

[97]Kinney, E. D. (2008). Recognition of the international human right to health and health care in the United States. *Rutgers Law Review, 60*(335) citing. See Memorandum from Walter Dellinger and H. Jefferson Powell, Department of Justice, to Attorney General Janet Reno and Associate Attorney General Webster L. Hubbell (Oct. 29, 1993), Retrieved from http://www.usdoj.gov/olc/1stlady.htm

[98]Littell, A. (2002). Can a constitutional right to health guarantee universal health care coverage or improved health outcomes?: A survey of selected states. *Connecticut Law Review, 35,* 289, 308.

[99]Teitelbaum, J., & Wilensky, S. (2007). *Essentials of health policy and law* (p. 4). Boston: Jones & Bartlett Pub.

[100]See U.S. Const. pmbl; U.S. Const. art. 1, § 8, cl. 1.

[101]Teitelbaum, J., & Wilensky, S. (2007). *Essentials of health policy and law* (p. 144). Jones & Bartlett Pub.

[102]Teitelbaum, J., & Wilensky, S. (2007). *Essentials of health policy and law* (p. 144). Jones & Bartlett Pub.

[103]Teitelbaum, J., & Wilensky, S. (2007). *Essentials of health policy and law* (p. 144). Jones & Bartlett Pub.

[104]Teitelbaum, J., & Wilensky, S. (2007). *Essentials of health policy and law* (p. 144). Jones & Bartlett Pub.

[105]Kinney, E. D. (2008). Recognition of the international human right to health and health care in the United States. *Rutgers Law Review, 60,* 354.

[106]Sandhu, P. K. (2007). A legal right to health care: What can the United States learn from foreign models of health rights jurisprudence? *California Law Review, 95,* 1151, 1168.

[107]Sandhu, P. K. (2007). A legal right to health care: What can the United States learn from foreign models of health rights jurisprudence? *California Law Review, 95,* 1151, 1168.

[108]Kinney, E. D. (2008). Recognition of the international human right to health and health care in the United States. *Rutgers Law Review, 60*(335).

[109]Littell, A. (2002). Can a constitutional right to health guarantee universal health care coverage or improved health outcomes?: A survey of selected states. *Connecticut Law Review, 35,* 308–309 (finding no correlation between infant mortality or the presence of universal health coverage and a constitutional right to health in a survey of eleven countries).

[110]Littell, A. (2002). Can a constitutional right to health guarantee universal health care coverage or improved health outcomes?: A survey of selected states. *Connecticut Law Review, 35,* 308–309 (finding no correlation between infant mortality or the presence of universal health coverage and a constitutional right to health in a survey of eleven countries).

[111]Kinney, E. D., & Brian Alexander Clark, Provisions for Health and Health Care in the Constitutions of the Countries of the World. *Cornell International Law Journal, 37,* 285, 291.

[112]Sandhu, P. K. (2007). A legal right to health care: What can the United States learn from foreign models of health rights jurisprudence? *California Law Review, 95,* 1151, 1168.

[113]Sandhu, P. K. (2007). A legal right to health care: What can the United States learn from foreign models of health rights jurisprudence? *California Law Review, 95,* 1151, 1168 citing Sunstein, C. R. (2005). Why does the American Constitution lack social and economic guarantees? *Syracuse Law Review 56,* 1, 4.

[114]Littell, A. (2002). Can a constitutional right to health guarantee universal health care coverage or improved health outcomes?: A survey of selected states. *Connecticut Law Review, 35,* 289–293.

[115]Kinney, E. D. (2008). Recognition of the international human right to health and health care in the United States. *Rutgers Law Review, 60*(335, 345).

[116]Leary, V. A. (1994). The right to health in international human rights law. *Health and Human Rights, 1,* 24–56; Freeman, L. (1999). Reflection on emerging frameworks of health and human rights. In J. M. Mann, S. Gruskin, M. A. Grodin, & G. J. Annas (Eds.), *Health and human rights: A reader* (pp. 227–252). New York: Routledge; J. M. Mann et al. (1999). Health and human rights. In J. M. Mann, S. Gruskin, M. A. Grodin, & G. J. Annas (Eds.), *Health and human rights: A reader* (pp. 7–20). New York: Routledge.

[117]Kinney, E. D., & Clark, B. A. (2004). Provisions for health and health care in the constitutions of the countries of the world. *Cornell International Law Journal, 37* (285), 288–293.

[118]DiFlorio, C. V. (1992). Assessing universal access to health care: An analysis of legal principle and economic feasibility. *Dickinson Journal of International Law, 11, 139,* 142; Fidler, D. P. (1999). International law and global public health, *University of Kansas Law Review, 48,* 1, 40.

[119]Sandhu, P. K. (2007). A legal right to health care: What can the United States learn from foreign models of health rights jurisprudence? *California Law Review, 95,* 1151, 1168 citing George P. Smith II, G. P. (2005). Human rights and bioethics: formulating a universal right to health, health care, or health protections? *38 Vanderbilt Journal of Transnational Law, 38*(5), 1295, 1301.

[120]Jamar, S. D. (1994). The International Human Right to Health, *Southern University Law Review,* 22, 1, 19; see also Pulido, G. L. (2000). Immunity of volunteer health care providers in Texas: Bartering legal rights for free medical care, *Scholar, 2,* 323, 326.

[121]Sandhu, P. K. (2007). A legal right to health care: What can the United States learn from foreign models of health rights jurisprudence? *California Law Review, 95,* 1151, 1168.

[122]Littell, A. (2002). Can a constitutional right to health guarantee universal health care coverage or improved health outcomes?: A survey of selected states. *Connecticut Law Review, 35,* 289, 313.

[123]Sandhu, P. K. (2007). A legal right to health care: What can the United States learn from foreign models of health rights jurisprudence? *California Law Review, 95,* 1151, 1168 citing Friesen, T. (2001). The right to health care. *Health Law Journal, 9,* 205, 210., at 205.

[124]Minister of Health v. Treatment Action Campaign (TAC) (2002) 5 SA 721 (CC). Retrieved from http://www.escr-net.org/caselaw/caselaw_results.htm

[125]Treatment Action Campaign (TAC), Founding Affidavit (2001, August 21), filed in *Treatment Action Campaign v. Minister of Health,* No. 21182/2001 (High Court of South Africa, Transvaal Provincial Division). Retrieved from http://www.tac.org.za/ Documents/MTCTCourtCase/ccmfound.rtf The Pretoria High Court ruled in favor of TAC in December 2001 and ordered the Department of Health to produce a mother-to-child-transmission prevention plan. The South African government lodged an appeal against the decision, which was recently upheld by the Constitutional

Court of South Africa (No. CCT 8/02, July 5, 2002). Retrieved from http://www.tac
.org.za/Documents/MTCTCourtCase/ConCourtMOHVsTAC.txt The *Constitution of
South Africa* (1996) states "(1) Everyone has the right to have access to
a. health-care services, including reproductive health care; b. sufficient food and
water; [. . .](2) The State must take reasonable legislative and other measures, within
its available resources, to achieve the progressive realization of each of these rights.
(3) No one may be refused emergency medical treatment."

[126]See Case of D v. United Kingdom, 24 Eur. H.R. Rep. 423, 448, 454 (1997).

[127]Kinney, E. D. (2008). Recognition of the International Human Right to Health and
Health Care in the United States. *Rutgers Law Review, 60*(335).

[128]Kinney, E. D. (2001). The international human right to health: What does this mean
for our nation and world? *34 Indiana Law Review, 34,* 1457.

[129]Kinney, E. D. (2008). Recognition of the International Human Right to Health and
Health Care in the United States. *Rutgers Law Review, 60*(335).

[130]World Health Organization. About WHO. Retrieved April 25, 2010, from http://
www.who.int/about/en/

[131]World Health Organization. About WHO. Retrieved April 25, 2010, from http://
www.who.int/about/en/

[132]World Health Organization. (1992). W.H.O. Constitution. In *Basic documents of the
World Health Organization* (37th ed.); *see also* UN Doc. A/CONF. 32/8. Retrieved
from http://www.who.int/governance/eb/who_constitution_en.pdf

[133]World Health Organization. W.H.O. Constitution. In Basic *documents of the World
Health Organization* (37th ed. 1992); *see also* UN Doc. A/CONF. 32/8. Retrieved
from http://www.who.int/governance/eb/who_constitution_en.pdf

[134]1948 Universal Declaration of Human Rights. Article 25. Retrieved from http://
www.un.org/en/documents/udhr/

[135]1948 Universal Declaration of Human Rights. Article 25. Retrieved from http://
www.un.org/en/documents/udhr/

[136]Jamar, S. D. (1994). The international human right to health. *Southern University
Law Review,* 22(1), 46–47.

[137]World Health Organization. Regional Office for the Eastern Mediterranean. The
International Covenant on Civil and Political Rights Health and Human Rights.
Retrieved April 15, 2010, from http://www.who.int/hhr/Civil_political_rights.pdf

[138]World Health Organization. Regional Office for the Eastern Mediterranean. The
International Covenant on Civil and Political Rights Health and Human Rights.
Retrieved April 15, 2010, from http://www.who.int/hhr/Civil_political_rights.pdf

[139]United Nations Treaty Collection. Status of treaties. Retrieved April 6, 2010, from
http://treaties.un.org/Pages/ViewDetails.aspx?src=TREATY&mtdsg_no=IV-
4&chapter=4&lang=en#EndDec

[140]Black, A.; Hopkins, J. (Eds.). (2003). *The Eleanor Roosevelt papers.* Hyde Park, New
York: Eleanor Roosevelt National Historic Site. Retrieved April 5, 2010, from http://
www.gwu.edu/~erpapers/teachinger/glossary/cov-civilpol-rights.cfm

[141]Sei Fujii v. State 38 Cal.2d 718, 242 P.2d 617 (1952); see also Buell v. Mitchell 274
F.3d 337 (6th Cir., 2001).

[142]45 CFR 46 §46.116. There are other provisions with respect to this regulation that detail
the limited applicability and exceptions in obtaining informed consent for research.

[143]Centers for Disease Control. The Tuskegee Timeline. Retrieved from http://www
.cdc.gov/tuskegee/timeline.htm

[144]Centers for Disease Control. The Tuskegee Timeline. Retrieved from http://www
.cdc.gov/tuskegee/timeline.htm

[145]Centers for Disease Control. The Tuskegee Timeline. Retrieved from http://www
.cdc.gov/tuskegee/timeline.htm

[146]Centers for Disease Control. The Tuskegee Timeline. Retrieved from http://www
.cdc.gov/tuskegee/timeline.htm

[147]Centers for Disease Control. The Tuskegee Timeline. Retrieved from http://www
.cdc.gov/tuskegee/timeline.htm

[148]Centers for Disease Control. The Tuskegee Timeline. Retrieved from http://www
.cdc.gov/tuskegee/timeline.htm

[149]Centers for Disease Control. The Tuskegee Timeline. Retrieved from http://www
.cdc.gov/tuskegee/timeline.htm

[150]Centers for Disease Control. The Tuskegee Timeline. Retrieved from http://www
.cdc.gov/tuskegee/timeline.htm

[151]United Nations. International Convention on the Elimination of all Forms of Racial Discrimination. Retrieved from http://www.state.gov/documents/organization/100294.pdf

[152]United Nations. International Convention on the Elimination of all Forms of Racial Discrimination. Retrieved from http://www.state.gov/documents/organization/100294.pdf

[153]American Civil Liberties Foundation. Frequently Asked Questions. Convention on
the Elimination of All Forms of Racial Discrimination. Retrieved from http://www
.aclunc.org/issues/racial_justice/asset_upload_file567_6311.pdf

[154]American Civil Liberties Union. Frequently Asked Questions. Convention on the
Elimination of all Forms of Racial Discrimination. Retrieved from http://www
.aclunc.org/issues/racial_justice/asset_upload_file567_6311.pdf

[155]American Civil Liberties Union. Frequently Asked Questions. Convention on the
Elimination of all Forms of Racial Discrimination. Retrieved from http://www
.aclunc.org/issues/racial_justice/asset_upload_file567_6311.pdf

[156]American Civil Liberties Foundation. Frequently Asked Questions. Convention on
the Elimination of All Forms of Racial Discrimination. Retrieved from http://www
.aclunc.org/issues/racial_justice/asset_upload_file567_6311.pdf

[157]CERD Working Group on Health and Environmental Health. (2008, January). A
Report to the U.N. Committee on the Elimination of Racial Discrimination.
Unequal Health Outcomes in the United States: Racial and ethnic disparities in
health care treatment and access, the role of social and environmental determinants of health, and the responsibility of the state. Retrieved from http://www
.prrac.org/pdf/CERDhealthEnvironmentReport.pdf

[158]CERD Working Group on Health and Environmental Health. (2008, January). A
Report to the U.N. Committee on the Elimination of Racial Discrimination.
Unequal Health Outcomes in the United States: Racial and ethnic disparities in
health care treatment and access, the role of social and environmental determinants of health, and the responsibility of the state. Retrieved from http://www
.prrac.org/pdf/CERDhealthEnvironmentReport.pdf

[159]CERD Working Group on Health and Environmental Health. (2008, January). A
Report to the U.N. Committee on the Elimination of Racial Discrimination.
Unequal Health Outcomes in the United States: Racial and ethnic disparities in
health care treatment and access, the role of social and environmental determinants of health, and the responsibility of the state. Retrieved from http://www
.prrac.org/pdf/CERDhealthEnvironmentReport.pdf

[160]International Covenant on Economic, Social and Cultural Rights, Dec. 16, 1966, 993 U.N.T.S. 3, (*entered into force* Jan. 3, 1976) [hereinafter ICESCR].

[161]Covenant on Economic, Social and Cultural Rights, Article 12(1), Dec. 16, 1966, 993 U.N.T.S. 3, (*entered into force* Jan. 3, 1976).

[162]Office of the United Nations High Commissioner for Human Rights, & The World Health Organization. The Right to Health. Fact Sheet no.31. Retrieved from http://www.ohchr.org/Documents/Publications/Factsheet31.pdf

[163]Little @297.

[164]International Covenant on Economic, Social and Cultural Rights, Dec. 16, 1966, 993 U.N.T.S. 3, (*entered into force* Jan. 3, 1976) [hereinafter ICESCR].

[165]International Covenant on Economic, Social and Cultural Rights, Dec. 16, 1966, 993 U.N.T.S. 3, (*entered into force* Jan. 3, 1976) [hereinafter ICESCR].

[166]International Covenant on Economic, Social and Cultural Rights, Dec. 16, 1966, 993 U.N.T.S. 3, (*entered into force* Jan. 3, 1976) [hereinafter ICESCR].

[167]International Covenant on Economic, Social and Cultural Rights, Dec. 16, 1966, 993 U.N.T.S. 3, (*entered into force* Jan. 3, 1976) [hereinafter ICESCR].

[168]Erdman, J. N. (1994). Human rights in health equity: Cervical cancer and HPV vaccines. *Southern University Law Review, 22,* 1, 371.

[169]Erdman, J. N. (1994). Human rights in health equity: Cervical cancer and HPV vaccines. *Southern University Law Review, 22,* 1, 371.

[170]United Nations Treaty Collection. Status of Treaties. International Covenant on Economic, Social and Cultural Rights. Retrieved from http://treaties.un.org/Pages/ViewDetails.aspx?src=TREATY&mtdsg_no=IV-3&chapter=4&lang=en

[171]United States Department of Labor. Family and Medical Leave. Retrieved May 10, 2010, from http://www.dol.gov/dol/topic/benefits-leave/fmla.htm

[172]United States Department of Labor. Family and Medical Leave. Retrieved May 10, 2010, from http://www.dol.gov/dol/topic/benefits-leave/fmla.htm

[173]Convention on the Elimination of All Forms of Discrimination Against Women Art. 12, Dec. 18, 1979, 1249 U.N.T.S. 13 (*entered into force* Sept. 3, 1981). Retrieved April 5, 2010, from http://www.un.org/womenwatch/daw/cedaw/text/econvention.htm#article12

[174]Convention on the Elimination of All Forms of Discrimination Against Women Art. 12, Dec. 18, 1979, 1249 U.N.T.S. 13 (*entered into force* Sept. 3, 1981). Retrieved April 5, 2010, from http://www.un.org/womenwatch/daw/cedaw/text/econvention.htm#article12

[175]Convention on the Elimination of All Forms of Discrimination Against Women Art. 12, Dec. 18, 1979, 1249 U.N.T.S. 13 (*entered into force* Sept. 3, 1981). Retrieved April 5, 2010, from http://www.un.org/womenwatch/daw/cedaw/text/econvention.htm#article12

[176]United Nations Treaty Collection. Status of Treaties. Convention on the Elimination of All Forms of Discrimination Against Women. Retrieved from http://treaties.un.org/Pages/ViewDetails.aspx?src=TREATY&mtdsg_no=IV-8&chapter=4&lang=en

[177]Kaiser Family Foundation. Putting Women's Health Care Disparities On The Map: Examining Racial and Ethnic Disparities at the State Level. Executive Summary. Retrieved May 9, 2010, from http://www.kff.org/minorityhealth/7886.cfm

[178]Convention on the Rights of the Child, Office of the United Nations High Commissioner for Human Rights. (Adopted and opened for signature, ratification and accession by General Assembly resolution 44/25 of 20 November 1989. entry into force 2 September 1990, in accordance with article 49; Not Ratified by US. Only Optional Protocol to the Convention on the Rights of the Child on the involvement of children in armed conflict was ratified.) Retrieved April 11, 2010, from http://www2.ohchr.org/english/law/pdf/crc.pdf

[179]Office of the United Nations High Commissioner for Human Rights. Convention on the Rights of the Child. Retrieved April 11, 2010, from http://www2.ohchr.org/english/law/pdf/crc.pdf

[180]Office of the United Nations High Commissioner for Human Rights. Convention on the Rights of the Child. Retrieved April 11, 2010, from http://www2.ohchr.org/english/law/pdf/crc.pdf

[181]Convention on the Rights of the Child, Office of the United Nations High Commissioner for Human Rights. Retrieved April 11, 2010, from http://www2.ohchr.org/english/law/pdf/crc.pdf

[182]Convention on the Rights of the Child, Office of the United Nations High Commissioner for Human Rights. Retrieved April 11, 2010, from http://www2.ohchr.org/english/law/pdf/crc.pdf

[183]U.S. Department of Health and Human Services. (2009). National Healthcare Disparities Report. Rockville, MD: Agency for Healthcare Research and Quality; 2009;AHRQ Publication No. 10-0004. Retrieved from http://www.ahrq.gov/qual/nhdr09/nhdr09.pdf

[184]U.S. Department of Health and Human Services. (2009). National Healthcare Disparities Report. Rockville, MD: Agency for Healthcare Research and Quality; 2009;AHRQ Publication No. 10-0004. Retrieved from http://www.ahrq.gov/qual/nhdr09/nhdr09.pdf

[185]U.S. Department of Health and Human Services. (2009). National Healthcare Disparities Report. Rockville, MD: Agency for Healthcare Research and Quality; 2009;AHRQ Publication No. 10-0004. Retrieved from http://www.ahrq.gov/qual/nhdr09/nhdr09.pdf

[186]U.S. Department of Health and Human Services. (2009). National Healthcare Disparities Report. Rockville, MD: Agency for Healthcare Research and Quality; 2009;AHRQ Publication No. 10-0004. Retrieved from http://www.ahrq.gov/qual/nhdr09/nhdr09.pdf

[187]Kinney, E. D. (2008). Recognition of the International Human Right to Health and Health Care in the United States. *Rutgers Law Review, 60*(335).

[188]United States Department of Labor. Retrieved April 3, 2010, from http://www.dol.gov/dol/topic/health-plans/erisa.htm

[189]United States Department of Labor. Retirement Plans, Benefits & Savings: Employee Retirement Income Security Act (ERISA). Retrieved May 14, 2010, from http://www.dol.gov/dol/topic/retirement/erisa.htm

[190]United States Department of Labor. Retirement Plans, Benefits & Savings: Employee Retirement Income Security Act (ERISA). Retrieved May 14, 2010, from http://www.dol.gov/dol/topic/retirement/erisa.htm

[191]United States Department of Labor. Retirement Plans, Benefits & Savings: Employee Retirement Income Security Act (ERISA). Retrieved May 14, 2010, from http://www.dol.gov/dol/topic/retirement/erisa.htm

[192]United States Department of Labor. Retirement Plans, Benefits & Savings: Employee Retirement Income Security Act (ERISA). Retrieved May 14, 2010, from http://www.dol.gov/dol/topic/retirement/erisa.htm

[193]United States Department of Labor. Retirement Plans, Benefits & Savings: Employee Retirement Income Security Act (ERISA). Retrieved May 14, 2010, from http://www.dol.gov/dol/topic/retirement/erisa.htm

[194]Teitelbaum, J., & Wilensky, S. (2007). *Essentials of health policy and law* (p. 135). Sudbury, MA. Jones & Bartlett Pub.

[195]Center for Medicaid and Medicare Services. EMTALA Overview. Retrieved April 3, 2010, from http://www2.cms.gov/EMTALA/

[196]Center for Medicaid and Medicare Services. EMTALA Overview. Retrieved April 3, 2010, from http://www2.cms.gov/EMTALA/

[197]Center for Medicaid and Medicare Services. EMTALA Overview. Retrieved April 3, 2010, from http://www2.cms.gov/EMTALA/

[198]Center for Medicaid and Medicare Services. EMTALA Overview. Retrieved April 3, 2010, from http://www2.cms.gov/EMTALA/

[199]Center for Medicaid and Medicare Services. EMTALA Overview. Retrieved April 3, 2010, from http://www2.cms.gov/EMTALA/

[200]U.S. Department of Health & Human Services. Retrieved April 4, 2010, from http://www.hhs.gov/ocr/privacy/

[201]42 USC 1395 cc (a)(1).

[202]Title VI of the 1964 Civil Rights Act, Pub. L. No. 88–352, 78 Stat. 252 (1964) (codified at 42 U.S.C. §2000d-200d-4 [2005]).

[203]Title VI of the 1964 Civil Rights Act, Pub. L. No. 88–352, 78 Stat. 252 (1964) (codified at 42 U.S.C. §2000d-200d-4 [2005]).

[204]Teitelbaum, J., & Wilensky, S. (2007). *Essentials of health policy and law* (p. 142). Sudbury, MA: Jones & Bartlett Pub.

[205]Teitelbaum, J., & Wilensky, S. (2007). *Essentials of health policy and law* (p. 142). Sudbury, MA: Jones & Bartlett Pub.

[206]Randall, V. R. (2006). Lifestyle changes: Keys to reducing health disparities among people of color: Article: Eliminating racial discrimination in health care: A call for state health care anti-discrimination law. *DePaul Journal of Health Care Law, 10*, 1, 9.

[207]Randall, V. R. (2006). Lifestyle changes: Keys to reducing health disparities among people of color: Article: Eliminating racial discrimination in health care: A call for state health care anti-discrimination law. *DePaul Journal of Health Care Law, 10*, 1, 9.

[208]Teitelbaum, J., & Wilensky, S. (2007). *Essentials of health policy and law* (p. 142). Sudbury, MA: Jones & Bartlett Pub.

[209]Robert, A., & Moy, D. R. (Eds.). (2006). *Legal manual for New York physicians.* (2nd ed., p. 187). Albany, NY: New York State Bar Association and Medical Society of New York.

[210]42 U.S.C. Section 12102(2).

[211]29 C.F.R. Section 1630.2(h)1.

[212]29 C.F.R. Section 1630.2(h)2.

[213]Robert, A., & Moy, D. R. (Eds.). (2006). *Legal manual for New York physicians.* (2nd ed., p. 187). Albany, NY: New York State Bar Association and Medical Society of New York.

[214]Robert, A., & Moy, D. R. (Eds.). (2006). *Legal manual for New York physicians.* (2nd ed., p. 187). Albany, NY: New York State Bar Association and Medical Society of New York.

[215]Robert, A., & Moy, D. R. (Eds.). (2006). *Legal manual for New York physicians.* (2nd ed., p. 187). Albany, NY: New York State Bar Association and Medical Society of New York.

[216]Teitelbaum, J, & Wilensky, S. (2007). *Essentials of health policy and law* (p. 143). Sudbury MA. Jones & Bartlett Pub.

[217]Bragdon v. Abbott, 524 U.S. 624 (1998).

[218]Bragdon, 524 U.S. at 628–29. In this case, there was not an absolute refusal to treat the patient because the dentist offered to fill the cavity at a hospital. Id. at 629. This

alternative, however, would have subjected the plaintiff to additional costs imposed by the hospital. Id. Moreover, there was no evidence that the defendant had privileges at any hospital. Id. at 651.

[219]Crossley, M. (2000). Symposium: The American With Disabilities Act: A ten-year retrospective: Becoming visible: The ADA's impact on health care for persons with disabilities. *Alabama Law Review, 52,* 51 citing 42 U.S.C. § 12182(a)(1994) states: "No individual shall be discriminated against on the basis of disability in the full and equal enjoyment of the goods, services, facilities, privileges, advantages, or accommodations of any place of public accommodation by any person who owns, leases (or leases to), or operates a place of public accommodation."

[220]Crossley, M. (2000). Symposium: The American With Disabilities Act: A ten-year retrospective: Becoming visible: The ADA's impact on health care for persons with disabilities. *Alabama Law Review, 52,* 51 citing 42 U.S.C. § 12181(7)(F).

[221]Crossley, M. (2000). Symposium: The American With Disabilities Act: A ten-year retrospective: Becoming visible: The ADA's impact on health care for persons with disabilities. *Alabama Law Review, 52,* 51 (2000) citing 42 U.S.C. § 12182(b)(3) (1994) provides the direct threat defense, which states that: Nothing in this subchapter shall require an entity to permit an individual to participate in or benefit from the goods, services, facilities, privileges, advantages, and accommodations of such entity where such individual poses a direct threat to the health or safety of others. The term "direct threat" means a significant risk to the health or safety of others that cannot be eliminated by a modification of policies, practices, or procedures or by the provision of auxiliary aids or services.

[222]Abbott v. Bragdon, 912 F. Supp. 580, 587–91, 595 (D. Me. 1995).

[223]Crossley, M. (2000). Symposium: The American With Disabilities Act: A ten-year retrospective: Becoming visible: The ADA's impact on health care for persons with disabilities. *Alabama Law Review, 52,* 51 citing Abbott, 912 F. Supp. at 584–85. In addition to the direct threat issue, another critical issue to the case was whether plaintiff's asymptomatic HIV infection qualified as disability under the ADA. Bragdon, 524 U.S. at 628. The Supreme Court affirmed the judgment of the First Circuit and the district court in holding that the HIV infection was an impairment that substantially limited the plaintiff (Abbott) major life activity of reproduction. Id. at 647.

[224]Crossley, M. (2000). Symposium: The American With Disabilities Act: A ten-year retrospective: Becoming visible: The ADA's impact on health care for persons with disabilities. *Alabama Law Review, 52,* 51 citing Abbott v. Bragdon at 649.

[225]Crossley, M. (2000). Symposium: The American With Disabilities Act: A ten-year retrospective: Becoming visible: The ADA's impact on health care for persons with disabilities. *Alabama Law Review, 52,* 51 citing United States v. Morvant, 898 F. Supp. 1157 (E.D. La. 1995); D.B. v. Bloom, 896 F. Supp. 166 (D.N.J. 1995).

[226]Teitelbaum, J., & Wilensky, S. (2007). *Essentials of health policy and law* (p. 143). Sudbury, MA:. Jones & Bartlett Pub.

[227]Vijeyarasa, R. (2009). Putting reproductive rights on the transitional justice agenda: The need to redress violations and incorporate reproductive health reforms in post-conflict development. *New England Journal of International and Comparative Law, 15,* 41 citing Fourth World Conference on Women, Sept. 4–15, 1995, Beijing Declaration and the Platform for Action, U.N. Doc. A/CONF.177/20 (Oct. 17, 1995). Retrieved from http://www.un.org/esa/gopher-data/conf/fwcw/off/a—20.en [hereinafter FWCW]

[228]Griswold v. Connecticut, 381 U.S. 479.

[229]Eisenstadt v. Baird, 405 U.S. 438.

[230]Roe v. Wade, 410 US 113 (1973).

[231]Planned Parenthood of Southeastern Pennsylvania v. Casy. 505 U.S. 833 (1992).

[232]Planned Parenthood of Southeastern Pennsylvania v. Casy. 505 U.S. 833 (1992).

[233]Stenberg v. Carhart, 530 U.S. 914 (2000).

[234]Jones, J. H. (2010). Women's reproductive rights concerning abortion, and governmental regulation thereof — Supreme Court cases. *American Law Reports Federal. 2d, 20,* 1.

[235]Jones, J. H. (2010). Women's reproductive rights concerning abortion, and governmental regulation thereof — Supreme Court cases. *American Law Reports Federal. 2d, 20,* 1.

[237]117 Stat. 1201(13) (Pub. L. No. 108-105) (2003).

[238]117 Stat. 1201(3)-(8) (Pub. L. No. 108-105) (2003).

[239]Carhart v. Gonzales, 413 F.3d 791.

[240]Carhart v. Gonzales, 413 F.3d 791.

[241]Carhart v. Gonzales, 413 F.3d 791.

[242]Gonzales v. Carhart, 127 S. Ct. 1610, 167 L. Ed. 2d 480, 20 A.L.R. Fed. 2d 673 (U.S. 2007).

[243]American College of Obstetricians and Gynecologists (2007, April 18). ACOG statement on the US Supreme Court decision upholding the Partial-Birth Abortion Ban Act of 2003. Press release. Retrieved May 14, 2010, from http://www.acog.org/from_home/publications/press_releases/nr04-18-07.cfm

[244]American College of Obstetricians and Gynecologists (2007, April 18). ACOG statement on the US Supreme Court decision upholding the Partial-Birth Abortion Ban Act of 2003. Press release. Retrieved May 14, 2010, from http://www.acog.org/from_home/publications/press_releases/nr04-18-07.cfm

[245]Institute of Medicine. (2002, March). Unequal treatment: What healthcare system administrators need to know about racial and ethnic disparities in Healthcare. Retrieved from http://www.iom.edu/~/media/Files/Report%20Files/2003/Unequal-Treatment-Confronting-Racial-and-Ethnic-Disparities-in-Health-Care/Disparities Admin8pg.ashx

CHAPTER 4

A Rights-Based Approach to Health Care Reform

Anja Rudiger and Benjamin Mason Meier

INTRODUCTION

Sixty-five years after the United States first gave serious consideration to universal health care, the political agenda has once again been dominated by health care reform. In considering the scope and content of a national health care system, international human rights law offers a normative framework for setting national health care policy. Human rights norms can guide policy decisions by delineating people's rights and associated duties of state and third party actors with regard to fulfilling the right to health care, thereby intervening in the debate on private and public responsibilities. This chapter seeks to describe the obligations imposed by the human right to health and how these have been applied to successive health care reform efforts in the United States. It argues that in the United States, these obligations require treating health care as a public good that is financed and administered publicly rather than left to the competing interests of the private market. The chapter concludes with a vision for shifting U.S. discourse and policy from the commodification of health care to the collective pursuit of a healthy society.

A RIGHTS-BASED APPROACH TO HEALTH CARE

Public health practitioners occasionally refer to health as a human right, but such rhetorical usage is not usually derived from the normative foundation presented in the international legal framework nor applied rigorously to health and health care policy decisions. As Jonathan Mann and Sophia Gruskin lamented more than a decade ago, the "lack of knowledge about human rights among health professionals . . . is the dominant problem" for the "nascent health and human rights movement."[1] Despite a recent rise in rights-based discourse, normatively driven efforts to improve public health and to ensure universal access to care have been held back by a lack of awareness of how legal norms inform public policy obligations arising from the right to health. Given the prevailing American view of health care as a commodity (to be purchased in the market) rather than as a public good and a human right (to be grounded in social justice), U.S. health reform has repeatedly faltered and health inequities have increasingly widened. Without rights-based obligations, U.S. advocates have lacked a legal and analytical basis to advance legislation for the common good and have forfeited policy to those with financial interest in maintaining the status quo.

To bridge the conceptual divide between health care and human rights, it is necessary that health advocates deepen their understanding of the application of rights to policy. Grounded in the inherent dignity and equality of all human beings, human rights are considered to be those claims that are inalienable, universal, and indivisible, with each claim of a rights-holder implicating correlative duties on a governmental duty-bearer. As codified in international law, human rights impose binding obligations on governments. Working through formal human rights obligations, rather than the nonobligatory language of morality or charity, rights discourses have long provided a legal and analytical framework for evaluating state health policies under the purview of the human right to health.[2] By applying the language of international law and incorporating the obligations of the right to health in national policy debates, public health advocates can invoke governmental duties to realize rights-based health care reform.

EVOLUTION OF HEALTH RIGHTS IN THE UNITED STATES

The evolution of health rights discourse in the United States has long avoided international human rights obligations while exposing a perceived—if fallacious and uniquely American—tension between personal freedom and health equity. With reflexive antipathy toward a human right to health care, the U.S. policy debate has largely excluded human rights obligations – to the detriment of universal health care reform. After 60 years in the evolution of health rights, are international legal obligations now ripe for application to U.S. health care reform?

Although the United States has faced political claims for universal health care for more than a century,[3] the international codification of a human right to health began in the aftermath of the Second World War. Addressing human rights at the end of the Depression and in the midst of the War, U.S. President Franklin Delano Roosevelt announced to the world that the post-War era would be founded on four "essential human freedoms": freedom of speech, freedom of religion, freedom from fear, and freedom from want.[4] It is the final of these "four freedoms," freedom from want, that heralded a state obligation to provide for the health of its people. With Roosevelt conceiving of these freedoms as the basis of a second American "Bill of Rights," this freedom from want would be couched in the language of liberty, with the understanding that "a necessitous man is not a free man" and the guarantee of a "right to adequate medical care and the opportunity to achieve and enjoy good health."[5]

Creating a formal international legal system of human rights, the United Nations proclaimed its Universal Declaration of Human Rights (UDHR) on December 10, 1948, establishing through it "a common standard of achievement for all peoples and all nations."[6] Defining a collective set of interrelated social welfare rights for all peoples, the nascent United Nations framed a right to health in the UDHR by which, "everyone has the right to a standard of living adequate for the health and well-being of himself and of his family, including food, clothing, housing and *medical care* [italics added] and necessary social services."[7] In preparing this right to health, derived by Eleanor Roosevelt from drafts of the American Law Institute, there was widespread international agreement that this human right to health included both universal access to modern health care and the conditions conducive to health, as reflected in the contemporaneous thinking of social medicine scholars on "underlying determinants of health."[8] With the U.S. government providing unprecedented medical care for its military servicemen and veterans and facing mounting pressure for implementing a comprehensive social security system, America was poised to join European nations in the post-War enactment of universal health care reform.

However, with the U.S. Congress shifting to Republican control in the 1946 midterm election, breaking up the "New Deal coalition" in U.S. liberal politics, the United States abandoned previous efforts to consider comprehensive health insurance and made its Cold War aversion to "socialized medicine" a hallmark of its policy in health. Aligning themselves with the political objections of the Republican Party, physician groups pressed fatal objections to the budding health and human rights movement, with the American Medical Association (AMA)—reminiscent of its opposition to the "public option" in the 2009 health care reform debate—objecting vigorously to what it characterized as governmental interference in private medical practice. In rejecting the human right to health as a basis for national health care reform,[9] repelling both Roosevelt's and Truman's domestic efforts to create a universal health insurance program,[10] the AMA would extend to international forums its well-funded advocacy of "personal freedom" against "socialized medicine."[11] Despite governmental recognition that "access to the means for the attainment and preservation of health is a basic human right,"[12] this well-funded political and professional opposition would combine to create a 20-year impasse in health reform, without any advancement in international law for health or any assumption of responsibility by the U.S. government.

Under these U.S. constraints in the midst of the Cold War, it would not be until 1966 that the United Nations codified the obligations of the UDHR in the International Covenant on Economic, Social and Cultural Rights (ICESCR), defining in it a "right of everyone to the enjoyment of the highest attainable standard of physical and mental health" that included governmental obligations to progressively realize "conditions which would assure medical service and medical attention to all in the event of sickness."[13] In this same human rights spirit of the 1960s—galvanizing U.S. movements for civil rights, labor, and the elderly against the inequities of market-based health insurance—the demand for universal health care would arise anew in U.S. policy discourse. Viewing health as a first-order obligation of government, President Lyndon Johnson argued that "[i]t is imperative that we give first attention to our opportunities—and *obligations* [italics added]—for advancing the Nation's health."[14] In accordance with this government responsibility, drawn from President John F. Kennedy's "New Frontier," the United States developed its Medicare and Medicaid systems under 1965 amendments to the Social Security Act. Promulgated over the strong objections of the Republican Party, AMA, and business interests,[15] Medicare would meet the needs of the elderly through guaranteed payment of care for anyone above the statutory age whereas Medicaid would provide for the indigent through matching contributions to state health programs for designated groups among the economically disadvantaged.

Although U.S. scholars and advocates would turn explicitly to a human right to health in the wake of the Medicare and Medicaid debates[16]—making ideological demands for a minimum level of universal medical care and putting forward systems analogous to those in Europe as a means of assuring more equitable medical services[17]—those references to rights would come to be interpreted, specifically by the medical profession, as the right to individual choice rather than as a governmental duty to realize health on an equitable basis.[18] As health care reform movements stagnated in the 1970s and 1980s—with the entrenched commercial interests of a consolidating health industry blunting any political efforts to consider public financing of universal care—health inequalities exploded under the market-based health care model.[19]

With the United States then widely perceived to be a system "in crisis," proposed health insurance reforms of the early 1990s sought to avoid the political contentiousness of advocates' efforts to advance a rights-based approach to health care. Given an understanding that the United States had fallen behind every other high-income country in providing for the health of its people (resulting in spiraling individual health care costs and diminishing public health outcomes), President Bill Clinton's proposals for health care reform explicitly avoided human rights language, focusing on market-based rationales for insurance reform.[20] Without a normative rationale for care, these 1993 efforts fell prey to the same misleading demonization of "socialized medicine" and financial interests of a profitable health care industry.

Although some advocates for rights-based reform in the 1990s referred to international legal norms, they lacked the benefit of a recognized analytical framework to set out the parameters of the then amorphous right to health. This changed in 2000 with the publication of General Comment 14 by the UN Committee on Economic, Social and Cultural Rights (CESCR). Seeking to develop a right to health commensurate with an evolving understanding of health care, the CESCR interpreted the ICESCR to find that the right to health is an "inclusive right extending not only to timely and appropriate health care but also to the underlying determinants of health." In providing for health care, General Comment 14 outlines that all health care services should be made available, accessible (physically and economically), acceptable, and of sufficient quality, including specifically,

> the provision of equal and timely access to basic preventive, curative, rehabilitative health services and health education; regular screening programmes; appropriate treatment of prevalent diseases, illnesses, injuries and disabilities, preferably at community level; the provision of essential drugs; and appropriate mental health treatment and care.[21]

Given these international efforts to clarify a human right to health care, U.S. scholars obtained a stronger platform to explore rights-based health care reform as part of a larger governmental mission of "leveling the social playing field with respect to health."[22] With the United States again pursuing health care reform under President Obama, advocates resumed the effort to create a stronger role for human rights in facilitating reform and in realizing health care, and ultimately health, for all.

HEALTH CARE REFORM DISCOURSE UNDER THE OBAMA ADMINISTRATION

Preceding the 2008 presidential campaign, several universal health care bills—including at least one of them granting an explicit right to health care[23]—had languished in Congress, along with a proposed constitutional amendment for the equal right to health care.[24] However, in the absence of federal legislation, momentum for reform was driven by states and local districts, which carried out practical experiments with incremental measures to improve access to health care. An entire field of advocacy organizations mobilized in parallel with states' actions to address the systemic failure to provide access to health care for all, which had led to an unconscionable exclusion from care on the one hand and unsustainable costs on the other. Several states (e.g., Massachusetts, Maine, and Vermont), many Democratic Party candidates in the 2008 elections, and most advocacy groups explicitly promoted "universal coverage" as a solution to the health care crisis.[25] However, they stopped short of recognizing the human right to health care or taking policy actions that would fulfill this right.

The political and social context of health care reform efforts under the Obama administration presented several new opportunities for advancing universal health care reform and the right to health care. The parameters of the debate briefly appeared to change when the right to health care was elevated to a prime-time topic in an October 2008 presidential debate, with then-Senator Obama confirming that health care should indeed be a right.[26] He was not the only leading politician to invoke a right to health care during this reform period, yet these assertions of such a right never advanced beyond rhetoric and did not indicate an understanding of human rights norms as codified in the international legal framework. Instead, as the debate progressed, policymakers agreed to pursue an "American solution," based on an outright rejection of universal health care models from other countries, while failing to recognize the commodification of health care as the homegrown root of the crisis. In a system where health services are sold for profit on the market and financed through private insurance and individual payments, access to and availability of health care inevitably remain restricted to those who can pay.

Despite the onset of an economic recession in late 2008, health care reform retained its prominent position on the policy agenda, as it was recast as integral to economic recovery. Access to health care was no longer a question of ensuring population health, let alone an issue of sharing costs and risks more equitably and thus fostering the redistributive processes on which functioning health systems rely. If reformers ever envisioned the universal and equitable protection of people's health as a key goal for society, economic arguments and cost considerations all but eviscerated this normative perspective and turned health reform into an exercise of better market management in collaboration with the health care industries that stood to benefit.

For human right to health advocates, this signaled the continuing hegemony of a familiar position in the century-old debate on universal health care in the United States. Health care was treated as a market commodity, economic rights morphed into consumer choice and corporate claims to "fair" (yet subsidized) competition, and personal responsibility for healthy behaviors trumped the government's obligation to secure equitable access to health care as a public good. Despite widespread popular agreement on the need for radical change of the U.S. health care system, reform efforts under the Obama administration were once again subjected to market imperatives combined with a uniquely American debate over the role of government and the allocation of public and private responsibilities.[27]

As in earlier federal efforts, the contemporary policy impasse is best illustrated by the contested nature of the function of government; in this case, exemplified in the proposal for a so-called public option – a public health insurance plan offered alongside private and for-profit plans. From a human rights perspective, an expansion of public responsibility for securing access can be considered a step toward greater accountability and health protection. However, in this case, reformers' proposals for a public "option" mirrored the operation of market-based, private coverage plans. In fact, proponents of a public plan, including President Obama, cast their support in the language of commodified health care, offering the government's participation in the marketplace as an injection of much-needed competition that would not threaten the market but enable it to thrive. The hegemony of the market discourse thus prompted advocates to frame their case for the "change" promised during Obama's presidential campaign as a fair and efficient market intervention rather than an effort to better protect the public's health. This adoption of a market-based approach—be it strategic or ideological—led to the exclusion of proposals for a universal single payer health care system, depicted once again as a foreign introduction of "socialized medicine."

Despite the single payer bills pending in Congress and state legislatures, and significant popular support for a national health care plan in the form of single payer, mainstream advocacy groups and the Democratic Party establishment dismissed single payer as facilitating "dislocation" and opted instead for protecting the interests of those enjoying relative stability and security under the existing system—primarily those with employer-based coverage and the health care industry itself.

This balancing act of protecting the status quo while advancing incremental reforms initially gave rise to the aspirational concept of shared responsibility, which could potentially be operationalized through collectively financed health care in the form of a social insurance system based on the solidarity needed to achieve universal access to care. However, subsequent plans to force individuals into the health insurance market in their role as consumers (not as equal members of society contributing to a shared public good) reduced shared responsibility to personal responsibility, effectively increasing the industry's customer base rather than improving access to actual care. The "rights" of insurance companies to engage in relatively unencumbered "free enterprise" received priority over the rights of people to have their fundamental needs met through collectively financed public services. A reform model that treats health care as a product sold via the insurance market for individual consumption, not only glosses over obvious "market failures"—such as the exclusion of those who cannot pay—but also pretends that each person values health services differently, based on his or her own personal preferences that can be expressed in a market exchange. This neglects our common need for the best available care and renders cross-subsidizing of the costs of such care difficult. It also indicates that the ingrained hostility to public services, especially those with a redistributive component, is not only a prerogative of American conservatives but extends across the policy spectrum and reveals the deep-seated ideological rift between the United States and its European counterparts.[28]

COMPONENTS OF A RIGHTS-BASED APPROACH
TO HEALTH CARE REFORM

Advocates for rights-based reforms seek to confront the subjugation of human needs to market forces by building a sustainable movement for an ideological shift away from a commodification of needs and toward a collective fulfillment of rights. Right to health advocates seek to establish health care as a terrain contested by rights-based claims for universality and equity, not by economic interests framed as matters of individual responsibility and choice.

During the health reform period under the Obama administration, advocates using a right to health framework ranged from single payer networks, such as Healthcare-NOW!, to the Human Right to Health Caucus of the US Human Rights Network and the Human Right to Health Care Coalition formed by Amnesty International, the Opportunity Agenda, the National Health Law Program (NHeLP), and the National Economic and Social Rights Initiative (NESRI).[29] While some activists were content to adopt the rhetorical power of human rights, others sought to operationalize international norms by adapting the analytical framework set out by the CESCR in General Comment 14 to the U.S. health care context. These latter activists argued that rights-based claims without substantiation in legal and policy analysis risked remaining caught in an empty cycle of ideological exchange. In contrast, marshalling the analytical force of the human rights framework could help change the terms of the debate through policy guidance informed by normative principles, rights-based indicators, and empirical evidence.

To maximize the relevance of human rights norms to the U.S. health care reform debate, rights-based advocates developed workable standards for health care reform based on the international normative indicators of accessibility, availability, acceptability, and quality of health care. Using these standards as an assessment tool (see Figure 4.1), advocates completed detailed human rights analyses of reform plans, showing that market-based proposals, including the bills adopted by the U.S. Senate and the House of Representatives,[30] failed to meet key human rights standards.[31] For example, insofar as *access* to care must be universal, equitable, affordable, and comprehensive, market-based proposals were unable to guarantee meaningful access in accordance with these international standards. None of the plans included everyone, nor did any propose to fund and distribute care equitably, or render it affordable by correlating contributions (or exemptions) with the ability to pay (or lack thereof). Moreover, in their focus on individual coverage "choices," rather than a collective goal of health protection, they cast comprehensive coverage as a "Cadillac" option, available only to the few and subject to a proposed excise tax.

Beyond revealing the shortcomings of reform plans that purport to increase access, human rights norms offer guidance on how a health care system should be financed to meet rights-based standards. To translate this into practice, NESRI has developed 10 human rights principles for financing health care (see Figure 4.2), tailored to the U.S. context and derived from the standards outlined in General Comment 14.

Starting with the fundamental yet much neglected principle that the purpose of a health system is to secure comprehensive protection of people's health—uncompromised by profit motives or other extraneous

FIGURE 4.1 Human Rights Assessment Tool for Health Care Reform

Summary Scorecard (Condensed Version)

Human Rights Principles		Proposal X	Proposal Y
Health care is a right			
Universal access to health, goods, facilities, and services	Universality		
	Affordability		
	Equity		
	Comprehensiveness		
Availability of health infrastructure and services everywhere			
Acceptability and dignity of care			
Quality of health care			
Accountability			

Assessment Standards (Condensed Version)

ACCESS
Access to care must be **universal** and must protect everyone's health on an **equitable** basis. Facilities, goods, and services must be **affordable, comprehensive,** and physically accessible for all where and when needed.

Universal
Health care must be equally accessible to every person living in the United States, guaranteed and continuous throughout people's lives.

Standards	Proposal X	Proposal Y
Everyone should have guaranteed access to health care. In an insurance system, this also implies that everyone receives comprehensive coverage.		
No one should be discriminated against on the basis of income, health status, gender, race, age, immigration status, or other factors.		
Access to care should be easy, continuous, and integrated for everyone.		

Affordable
Health care must always be affordable for everyone, with financial contributions based on the ability to pay, not on the use of services.

Standards	Proposal X	Proposal Y
Access to health services should be uncoupled from payment, with services funded through pooled contributions based on the ability to pay.		

(Continued)

FIGURE 4.1 Human Rights Assessment Tool for Health Care Reform *Continued*

Standard	Proposal X	Proposal Y
Prices charged by the private sector (e.g. insurers, providers, pharmacies) should be publicly regulated. There should be no financial barriers to care, including through deductibles or other out-of-pocket costs.		
Public subsidies should be designed to enable equitable access and incentivize comprehensive and quality services.		
In an insurance system, risk pools should be as broad as possible to share costs and risks equitably and increase affordability for all.		

Equitable
Health care facilities, goods, and services must be distributed equitably, with resources allocated and accessed according to needs.

Standards	Proposal X	Proposal Y
Disparities in access to care, and different tiers of access or coverage, should be eliminated.		
Access to care should be on the basis of clinical need, not privilege, payment, employment, immigration status, or any other factor.		
Health care should be recognized as a public good, which everyone can readily access based on their needs.		
The public financing and administration of the health care system should be expanded as the strongest vehicle for guaranteeing equal access.		

Comprehensive
Everyone must get all screenings, treatments, therapies, drugs, and services needed to protect their health.

Standards	Proposal X	Proposal Y
In an insurance system, coverage benefits for every person must be comprehensive and encompass all preventive, remedial, rehabilitative and palliative care, including mental health, dental and vision care, prescription drugs, and reproductive health.		
Health care services should not be restricted for certain groups, and no one should be penalized for his or her health status or behavior.		

(Continued)

FIGURE 4.1 Human Rights Assessment Tool for Health Care Reform *Continued*

AVAILABILITY

Adequate health care infrastructure (e.g., hospitals, community health facilities, trained health care professionals), goods (e.g., drugs, equipment), and services (e.g., primary care, mental health care) must be available in all geographical areas and to all communities.

Standards	Proposal X	Proposal Y
Health care infrastructure and resources should be distributed equitably to ensure that health care is available where it is needed.		
Health care professionals should be brought into underserved areas and fields.		
Hospitals and community health centers should be supported in underserved areas.		
Everyone should be able to have a regular primary care provider and to select providers of their choice.		

ACCEPTABILITY AND DIGNITY

Health care institutions and providers must respect dignity, provide culturally appropriate care, and be responsive to needs based on gender, age, culture, language, and different ways of life and abilities. They must respect medical ethics and protect patient confidentiality and privacy rights.

Standards	Proposal X	Proposal Y
Health services should be responsive to patients' needs and culturally appropriate.		
Language services should be routinely provided.		
Patient privacy rights and patient control over personal data should be strengthened.		

QUALITY

All health care must be medically appropriate and of good quality, guided by quality standards and control mechanisms, and provided in a timely, continuous, safe, and patient-centered manner.

Standards	Proposal X	Proposal Y
Uniform quality standards and independent quality control should be enforced for all insurers and providers.		
Disparities in quality of care received by different population groups should be eliminated.		
In an insurance system, payments to providers should not depend on a patient's insurance source, but instead be linked to appropriate, coordinated, and patient-oriented care and to health outcomes.		

(Continued)

FIGURE 4.1 Human Rights Assessment Tool for Health Care Reform *Continued*

ACCOUNTABILITY		
Private companies and public agencies must be held accountable for protecting the right to health care through enforceable standards, regulations, and independent compliance monitoring.		
Standards	**Proposal X**	**Proposal Y**
Insurers, providers, manufacturers, and public agencies should operate transparently, with democratic oversight and regulation.		
People should have adequate information to navigate the health system easily, and they should be able to participate in health system decision making.		
Private companies and public agencies should be held accountable for meeting the populations' health needs.		

interests—rights-based guidance then sets out the parameters for financing universal and equitable access. Universality requires that health care is financed in a way that includes every resident and avoids separating people into different tiers. The principle of equity requires that health care be treated as a public good and shared equitably by all, not as a market commodity sold only to those who can pay.[32] As government is responsible for ensuring equal access to public goods for all, rights-based access to care is best achieved through public financing and administration. Although the international norms allow the possibility of a public, private, or mixed system (GC 14 at par. 36), there is overwhelming empirical evidence, both in the United States and abroad,[33] that governments have been unable to fulfill their obligation to protect against private actors, such as insurance companies, undermining the right to health care (GC 14 at par. 33). Instead, private or privately administered financing has consistently led to inequities and disincentives to providing appropriate coverage and care, because such market-based mechanisms must prioritize business imperatives over health concerns. As a result, evidence confirms that highly commodified systems are positively correlated with ill health.[34] The right to health requires the removal of all barriers interfering with access to health services (GC 14 at par. 21); therefore, access should be free at the point of use and financed in an equitable and collective way through progressive taxation or social insurance contributions. This also entails that insurance coverage may be a sufficient but not a necessary way to facilitate access to care. Coverage can fulfill this intermediary role only if it is based on the principle of income and

FIGURE 4.2 Human Rights Principles for Financing Health Care

A. Definition of Principles

1. **Focused on health:** Health care financing must be completely aligned with the central purpose of a health system: protecting people's health.
2. **Universal and unified:** Health care financing must secure automatic access to care for everyone and avoid separating people into different tiers.
3. **Public:** Health care is a public good that should be publicly financed and administered.
4. **Free:** At the point of access, health care services must be provided without charges or fees.
5. **Equitable:** Health care financing must be equitable and nondiscriminatory.
6. **Centered on care:** Care should be financed as directly as possible, without intermediaries. Insurance coverage, if used as a vehicle for financing care, works only if based on the principle of risk and income solidarity.
7. **Responsive to needs:** Resources must be allocated equitably, guided by health needs.
8. **Rewarding quality:** Financing mechanisms must reward the provision of quality, appropriate care, and the improvement of health outcomes.
9. **Cost-effective:** Resources must be used effectively and sustainably to protect the health of all.
10. **Accountable:** Financing mechanisms and procedures must be accountable to the people.

B. Scorecard for Health Care Financing Proposals

Human Rights Financing Principles	Proposal X	Proposal Y
Focused on health, with comprehensive services		
Universal and unified		
Public		
Free at the point of access		
Equitable		
Centered on care		
Responsive to needs		
Rewarding quality		
Cost-effective		
Accountable		

risk solidarity, with those who happen to enjoy better health or higher incomes contributing at a level that helps support the entire system.

Rights-based financing guidelines also address the indicators of availability, acceptability, and quality by requiring financing mechanisms to allocate resources based on needs, to reward the provision of quality and appropriate care that improves health outcomes, and to use resources cost-effectively to benefit the whole of society while prioritizing investments for disadvantaged groups.[35] Finally, of particular significance to the U.S. health care financing debate are the procedural standards common to all human rights, requiring nondiscrimination, transparency, participation, and accountability. In a market-based system that commodifies needs, few procedural protections are available, whereas in a rights-based system, all financing mechanisms and procedures must be developed with and overseen by the people for whose benefit they exist.

These health care financing standards, derived from the international framework, are embedded in an overarching human rights narrative that is centered on the principles of universality, equity, and accountability. In a society that relegates the fulfillment of human needs to residual programs for the poor, universality is an important but often overlooked standard. The denial of economic and social rights affects everyone (albeit not equally), as does the call for solidarity to provide public goods collectively. The principle of equity is essential to challenging the health system's reliance on inherently unequal market distribution, driven by individual purchasing power rather than collective need.[36] Although this has not gone unnoticed by policymakers, evidenced by public funding for insurance programs such as Medicare and Medicaid as well as public health initiatives, these interventions effectively prop up a regressively financed system that continuously produces new inequities. As a result, health disparities in the United States remain far greater than in comparable high-income states, at the same time that any government involvement that could potentially rectify this is demonized. A rights-based emphasis on accountability can address the practical concerns that may contribute to these antigovernment sentiments. In a market-based system, accountability amounts to no more than buyer's choice, and government is seen as simultaneously remote and overbearing. In a rights-based system, however, institutions have a duty to enable people to participate in decision-making and exercise monitoring and oversight functions, which are crucial prerequisites for ensuring the system's legitimacy.

Outside the rights-based advocacy community, the principle of accountability remains largely limited to calls for basic transparency and information, and advocates' arguments for universality and equity tend to be muddled both along and across predictable fault lines. For example, moderate reformers seeking to supplement their market-based defense of a public insurance option with a normative argument have appealed to solidarity grounded in "the social contract that binds us to each other,"[37] whereas single payer advocates, whose proposals require social solidarity, have attempted to show that their plan would benefit self-interested individuals.[38]

Using a human rights analysis, however, advocates can link rights with responsibilities, individual and community needs with collective contributions, and government involvement with people's participation in a way that builds support for the right to health care and fundamental U.S. health system reform.

CONCLUSION

Grounded in an analytical framework of human rights standards, advocates for rights-based health reform are able to address both the policy and practical implications of commodified health care and counter the ideological hegemony of individualism that resides within the "free market" paradigm. By envisioning health care as a public good, financed and administered collectively to realize the social goal of a healthy society, rights-based activists in the United States can create a powerful narrative to elevate the public sphere as an enabler of needs fulfillment, and a protector against inequitable market forces, thereby transcending the prevailing perception of human rights as protections only against the state. This may ultimately pave the way not only for the fulfillment of the right to health care but also for the recognition of the underlying social determinants of health and thus the realization of a synoptic right to health. If we are to progressively realize this right, we need to redouble our efforts to include health care reform advocates in a broader movement for social and economic rights in the United States.

NOTES

[1]Mann, J., & Gruskin, S. (1997). The 2nd International Conference on Health and Human Rights: Bridge to the future. *Health & Human Rights, 1*(1).

[2]Daniels, N. (1985). *Just health care.* Boston: Cambridge University Press.

[3]Birn, A. E., Brown, T. M., Fee, E., & Lear, W. J. (2003). Struggles for national health reform in the United States. *American Journal of Public Health, 93*(1), 86–91.

[4]Congressional Record. (1941). 87: 44, 46–47. In S. I. Rosenman (Ed.), *The public papers and addresses of Franklin D. Roosevelt: 1940.* 1941. 672.

[5]President Franklin Roosevelt's Message on the State of the Union, Jan. 11, 1944. *Congressional Record.* 1944; 90: 55, 57.

[6]*Universal Declaration of Human Rights.* G.A. Res. 217A(III), U.N. GAOR, 3d Sess., at 71, U.N. Doc. A/810; 1948: Article 7.

[7]Universal Declaration of Human Rights. (1948). Article 25(1).

[8]Humphrey, J. P. (1984). *Human rights and the United Nations: A great adventure.* Dobbs Ferry, NY: Transnational Publishers.

[9]Hearings of the Committee on Foreign Affairs, Subcommittee on National and International Movements, House of Representatives, 13, 17 June, 3 July 1947.

[10]Sunstein, C. R. (2004). *The second Bill of Rights: FDR's unfinished revolution and why we need it more than ever.* New York: Basic Books.

[11]Peon, M. (1979). *Harry S. Truman versus the Medical Lobby: The genesis of medicare.* Columbia: University of Missouri Press.

[12]President's Commission on the Health Needs of the Nation. (1953). Washington, DC: U.S. Government Printing Office; p. 3.

[13]International Covenant on Economic, Social and Cultural Rights (1966). Article 12.

[14]U.S. Department of Health, Education, and Welfare. (1966). *Proceedings of the White House Conference on Health, November 3 and 4, 1965* (p. 3). Washington, DC: U.S. Government Printing Office.

[15]Birn, A. E., Brown, T. M., Fee, E., & Lear, W. J. (2003). Struggles for national health reform in the United States. *American Journal of Public Health, 93*(1), 86–91.

[16]Szasz, T. S. (1969). The right to health. In D. S. Burris (Ed.), *The right to treatment.* New York: Springer.

[17]For example Sidel, V. W., & Sidel, R. (1977). *A healthy state: An international perspective on the crisis in United States medical care.* New York: Pantheon Books.

[18]Fried, C. (1976). Equality and rights in medical care. *Hastings Report, 6,* 29–34.

[19]Bovbjerg, R. R., Griffin, C. C., & Carroll, C. E. (1993). U.S. health care coverage and costs: Historical development and choices for the 1990s. *Journal of Law, Medicine & Ethics, 21*(2), 141–162.

[20]Chapman, A. R. (1994). *Health care reform: A human rights approach.* Washington: Georgetown University Press.

[21]U.N. Committee on Economic, Social and Cultural Rights. (2000). The right to the highest attainable standard of health, CESCR General Comment 14. 22d Sess., Agenda Item 3, U.N. Doc. E/C.12/2000/4. 2000.

[22]Yamin, A. (2005). The right to health under international law and its relevance to the United States. *American Journal of Public Health, 95*(7), 1156–1161. See also Irwin, A., Rubenstein, L., Cooper, A., & Farmer, P. (2008). Fixing the U.S. healthcare system: What role for human rights. In C. Soohoo, C. Albisa, & M. F. Davis (Eds.), *Bringing human rights home.* Westport, CT: Greenwood Publishing Group.

[23]HR 3000, The Josephine Butler United States Health Service Act, introduced by Rep. Barbara Lee in the 110th Congress and in previous congressional periods.

[24]House Joint Resolution 30 (H.J. Res. 30), a resolution for a constitutional amendment introduced by Rep. Jesse Jackson Jr. in 2004.

[25]Rudiger, A. (2010). From private profits to public goods? A human rights assessment of health care reform. In M. Major (Ed.), *Where do we go from here? American democracy and the renewal of the radical imagination* (pp. 49–69). Lexington Books/Rowman and Littlefield.

[26]Commission on Presidential Debates. (2008). *Debate Transcript, October 7 2008: The Second McCain-Obama Presidential Debate.* Retrieved October 2008, from http://www.debates.org/pages/trans2008c.html

[27]This is also illustrated in several conflicting polling results on the role of government: In a *New York Times*/CBS poll from June 2009, 72% of the public supported a government-run health plan alongside private plans, but in the same poll 56% said the government is already "doing too many things better left to businesses and individuals," June 12–16, 2009 New York Times/CBS poll (polling results on health. Retrieved from

http://graphics8.nytimes.com/packages/images/nytint/docs/latest-new-york-times-cbs-news-poll-on-health/original.pdf; general polling results retrieved from http://graphics8.nytimes.com/packages/images/nytint/docs/latest-new-york-times-cbs-news-poll/original.pdf)

[28]This rift is also illustrated in polling results (e.g., an international poll conducted every 10 years found that support for the government's responsibility to provide health care has consistently been higher in Europe (between 50% and 90%, with lows in Germany and highs in Britain) than in the United States (between 36% in 1985 and 56% in 2006), although the significant increase of support in the United States should also be noted. Leibniz Institute for the Social Sciences, International Social Survey Programme (http://www.gesis.org/en/services/data/survey-data/issp/modules-study-overview/role-of-government/)

[29]Amnesty International USA. Retrieved from http://www.amnestyusa.org/demand-dignity/health-care-is-a-human-right/page.do?id=1021217 This page lists the organizations that have affirmed that health care is a human right and endorsed the principles of universality, equity, and accountability.

[30]In late 2009, the U.S. Senate passed the Patient Protection and Affordable Care Act (H.R. 3590) and the House of Representatives passed the Affordable Health Care for America Act (H.R. 3962). No final bill had passed both chambers at the time of writing.

[31]National Economic and Social Rights Initiative. (2008). *Pursuing a new vision for health care: A human rights assessment of the presidential candidates' proposals.* Retrieved from http://www.nesri.org/Human_Rights_Assessment.pdf; National Economic and Social Rights Initiative. (2008). *A human rights assessment of the presidential nominees' health plans.* Retrieved from http://www.nesri.org/Human_Rights_Assessment2.pdf; National Economic and Social Rights Initiative. (2008). *A human rights assessment of single payer plans.* Retrieved from http://www.nesri.org/Single_Payer_Human_Rights_Analysis.pdf; National Economic and Social Rights Initiative. (2009). *Do federal health care reform bills meet human rights standards?* Retrieved from http://www.nesri.org/BillAssessment-1.pdf; National Economic and Social Rights Initiative. (2009).

[32]For an in-depth argument for health care as a public good, see also Fisk, M. A. (2000). Case for taking health care out of the market. In A. Anton, M. Fisk, & N. Holmstrom (Eds.), *In defense of public goods.* Westview Press.

[33]For international evidence see, for example, Oxfam International, *Blind Optimism: Challenging the myths about private health care in poor countries,* Oxfam Briefing Paper, February 2009. http://www.oxfam.org/policy/bp125-blind-optimism

[34]See, for example, Mackintosh, M., & Koivusalo, M. (2005). Health systems and commercialization: In search of good sense. In M. Mackintosh & Koivusalo, M. (2005). *Commercialization of health care: Global and local dynamics and policy responses.* Palgrave Mcmillan.

[35]National Economic and Social Rights Initiative. (2009). *Human rights principles for financing health care.* Retrieved from http://www.nesri.org/Human_Rights_Principles_for_Financing_Health_Care.pdf

[36]For an in-depth analysis of the maldistribution of health care in a market economy, see Hart, J. T. (1971). The inverse care law. *Lancet, 1*(7696), 405–412.

[37]Hacker, J. S. (2009). Sharing risks in a new era of responsibility. In Health and income security Brief No 13. (National Academy of Social Insurance: April 2009).

[38]McCanne, D. (2009). Kaiser Health Tracking Poll, Quote of the Day—The official blog of Physicians for a National Health Program (PNHP). Retrieved from http://www.pnhp.org/blog/2009/06/08/kaiser-health-tracking-poll/

CHAPTER 5

Rights-Based Approaches and Millennium Development Goals

Elvira Beracochea, Monika Sawhney, and Ujwal Chhetry

INTRODUCTION

Realizing human rights, particularly the right to health, requires States to develop policies, allocate resources, and create necessary infrastructure. In the case of health, this requires the delivery of promotive and preventive programs and quality and safe health services to all. At the global scale, this responsibility is usually shared between developing and developed countries (with developed countries typically serving as donors and trade partners).

With or without assistance from developed countries, some developing countries have created strategies more or less effective in ensuring the right to health of their citizens. Cuba[1] for example, has developed an army of more than 33,000 doctors that covers the entire population through a network of about 500 clinics with coverage of 30,000–60,000 citizens each. Bangladesh,[2] on the other hand, relies on a network of village health volunteers, government-run health centers, and nongovernmental organizations (NGOs) that provide services. However, like millions of people in developing countries, the lowest quintile in the socioeconomic scale in Bangladesh die at a much higher rate in spite of the existing affordable preventive and curative interventions.

Until the year 2000, there had not been a list of accepted measureable goals to gauge development progress toward ensuring access to health care for all. That year, the United Nations (UN) General Assembly, along with

FIGURE 5.1 The Eight Millennium Development Goals

Goal 1: Eradicate extreme poverty and hunger
Goal 2: Achieve universal primary education
Goal 3: Promote gender equality and empower women
Goal 4: Reduce child mortality
Goal 5: Improve maternal health
Goal 6: Combat HIV/AIDS, malaria, and other diseases
Goal 7: Ensure environmental sustainability
Goal 8: Develop a global partnership for development

147 heads of state (189 nations in total), approved the Millennium Declaration (MD). The MD is not a binding treaty. However, it does announce the public commitment of the signing nations to a global development agenda. In addition to defining essential values such as freedom, equality, solidarity, tolerance, respect for nature, shared responsibility for international relations, peace, and disarmament, the MD further defined which goals to strive for first. Those goals are listed in Figure 5.1.

Several international organizations, including the UN family, World Health Organization (WHO), United Nations Development Programme (UNDP), United Nations Population Fund (UNFPA), United Nations International Children's Emergency Fund (UNICEF), and other agencies, started to refocus their programs on contributing to reach the Millennium Development Goals (MDGs). In 2002, the United Nations commissioned the Millennium Project[3] to determine rapid and affordable ways to reach the MDGs. The Millennium Project researchers identified 18 targets and 48 indicators to be reached by 2015 (those were later expanded to 21 and 60, respectively). The project promoted "Quick Wins" (see Figure 5.2) as simple, effective, and affordable interventions, which made it easy for countries, donors, and UN agencies to agree on best development practices that could yield rapid results.

One of the most important results of the MDGs is that every year, progress reports on each indicator in each country are available online for all to see and use.[4] The latest data suggest that health systems in most countries need to improve if they are to realize the right to health (Backman et al., 2008). It is the disease burden that prevents progress in most MDGs (Stuckler, Basu, & McKee, 2010).

In response to the MDGs, the United States embarked in disease control programs to address AIDS and malaria, and other European and Asian donors also started various programs. However, without a global plan (as Kent

FIGURE 5.2 "Quick Wins"

QUICK WINS

- Eliminate school and uniform fees to ensure that all children, especially girls, are not out of school because of their families' poverty. Lost revenues should be replaced with more equitable and efficient sources of finance, including donor assistance.
- Provide impoverished farmers in sub-Saharan Africa with affordable replenishments of soil nitrogen and other soil nutrients.
- Provide free school meals for all children using locally produced foods with take-home rations.
- Design community nutrition programs that support breastfeeding and provide access to locally produced complementary foods and, where needed, micronutrient (especially zinc and vitamin A) supplementation for pregnant and lactating women and children under five.
- Provide regular annual deworming to all schoolchildren in affected areas to improve health and educational outcomes.
- Train large numbers of village workers in health, farming, and infrastructure (in 1-year programs) to provide basic expertise and services to rural communities.
- Distribute free, long-lasting, insecticide-treated bed nets to all children in malaria endemic zones to cut decisively the burden of malaria.
- Eliminate user fees for basic health services in all developing countries, financed by increased domestic and donor resources for health.
- Expand access to sexual and reproductive health information and services, including family planning and contraceptive information and services, and close existing funding gaps for supplies and logistics.
- Expand the use of proven effective drug combinations for AIDS, TB, and malaria. For AIDS, this includes successfully completing the 3 by 5 initiative to bring antiretrovirals to 3 million people by 2005.
- Set up funding to finance community-based slum upgrading and earmark idle public land for low-cost housing.
- Provide access to electricity, water, sanitation, and the Internet for all hospitals, schools, and other social service institutions using off-grid diesel generators, solar panels, or other appropriate technologies.
- Reform and enforce legislation guaranteeing women and girls property and inheritance rights.
- Launch national campaigns to reduce violence against women.
- Establish, in each country, an office of science advisor to the president or prime minister to consolidate the role of science in national policymaking.
- Empower women to play a central role in formulating and monitoring MDG-based poverty reduction strategies and other critical policy reform processes, particularly at the level of local governments.
- Provide community-level support to plant trees to provide soil nutrients, fuelwood, shade, fodder, watershed protection, windbreak, and timber.

Note. From "Quick Wins," UN Millennium Project Web site. Available from http://www .unmillenniumproject.org/documents/4-MP-QuickWins-E.pdf discusses in chapter 6), results have been uneven, particularly when it comes to MDGs 4 and 5—child and maternal, respectively. To this date, consensus on a global health plan has not emerged. In 2010, the Obama administration developed the Global Health Initiative,[5] a more comprehensive approach that will focus on 20 countries. If successful, it will likely set the standard for development assistance in health. However, in spite of having a focus on women and girls, the initiative does not seem to have a rights base.

The MD was developed at a time when government-funded social services decreased and the role of the private sector expanded. State-sponsored services, which were highly subsidized, were instead distributed through an unregulated private sector. This transition brought choice (although of varying quality) to those that could afford and access it, mostly in urban areas, in contravention of human rights principles and law. Consequently, vulnerable groups fell through the cracks of weakened health systems that did not recognize equal rights for all (Fox & Meier, 2009; Hickey & Mitlin, 2009). The impact of these structural adjustment policies is still evident in many countries.

"The current global economic crisis is evidence that the neoliberal economic policies of the past 3 decades have not worked to help developing countries get ahead in development and protect the rights of all their citizens" (Balakrishnan, Elson, & Patel, 2010, p. 27). Moreover, the impact of the current financial crisis on the most vulnerable populations also demonstrates that social and economic development programs and the realization of the right to health need a legal framework to guide decisions and efforts.

MILLENNIUM DEVELOPMENT GOALS AND HUMAN RIGHTS DOCUMENTS

Manfred Nowak describes the human rights approach as one that is based "on the explicit recognition of a legally binding normative framework with rights, entitlements, duties, responsibilities, and accountability" (Scheinin & Suksi, 2005, p. 4). In this section, we will briefly discuss how MDGs complement established human rights documents.

As discussed in chapters 1 and 2, Article 12 of the International Covenant on Economic, Social and Cultural Rights (ICESCR) and General Comment 14 of the UN Committee on Economic, Social and Cultural Rights (CESCR) provide a legal framework for the realization of the universal right to health. In addition, the Declaration on the Right to Development,[6] proclaimed by the United Nations in 1986, and the MD constitute the legal bases for the right to participate in the development process and for governments and donors to provide development assistance to reach global development goals. Sengupta (2004) states that the "right to development is a right to both the process and the outcome of the process" (p. 51), which needs to be realized with equity and accountability.

The MD and the Declaration on the Right to Development can also provide a framework to address the social determinants of health[7] that go beyond the provision of health care. They can obligate governments and the international community to scale up public health systems, while reducing inequities in health through poverty-reducing economic growth (Fox & Meier, 2009, p. 17). As Fox and Meier note, "the human right to development offers a legal framework by which to restructure the system to meet global justice imperatives for health" (p. 117). This is the legal framework that should guide public health work and all development assistance projects and partnerships between developed and developing nations to ensure public health programs and services address what really makes people sick.

In addition to this legal framework, public health professionals involved in the implementation of a global rights-based approach (RBA) need to adhere to the Paris Declaration (PD) on Effectiveness and Accountability of 2005[8] and the Accra Agenda for Action.[9] Although not a legally binding document, the PD has been endorsed by more than 120 countries and more than 90 donor and development assistance organizations. The PD provides five practical principles for concerted global development actions: ownership, harmonization, alignment, managing for results, and mutual accountability. Various related indicators measure the extent to which decisions and actions respect and empower developing countries; these ensure that donors do not drive the development process. The principles of the PD agree with the spirit of partnership and cooperation espoused by the Declaration on the Right to Development and the eighth MDG regarding global partnerships.

The MDGs are rights based in that they meet the following criteria:

- Action oriented—all policies and programs should contribute directly to realization of one or several human rights
- Guidance—human rights standards and principles should guide all actions to be taken
- Empowerment—by raising the capacity of duty bearers
- Accountability (of each of the actors)—ensuring the rights of people who are supposed to be benefiting, also take into account the cost per beneficiary per program that is being implemented
- Efficiency and effectiveness—demonstrate effectiveness of the work done and achievement of the MDGs through efficient use of our global resources

TABLE 5.1 Millennium Development Goals and Human Rights: Complementary Frameworks and International Legal Basis

Millennium Development Goals	Key Related Human Rights Standards
Goal 1: Eradicate extreme poverty and hunger	UDHR Article 25(1), ICESCR Article 11
Goal 2: Achieve universal primary education	UDHR Article 25(1), ICESCR Articles 13 and 14, CRC Article 28(1)(a), CEDAW Article 10, CERD Article S (e)(v)
Goal 3: Promote gender equality and empower women	UDHR Article 2, CEDAW, ICESR Article 3, CRC Article 2
Goal 4: Reduce child mortality	UDHR Article 25, CRC Articles 6, 24 (2)(a), ICESCR Article 12 (2)(a)
Goal 5: Improve maternal health	UDHR Article 25, CEDAW Articles 10(h), 11(f), 12, 14(b), ICESCR Article 12, CRC Article 24(2)(d), CERD Article 5(e)(iv)
Goal 6: Combat HIV/AIDS, malaria, and other diseases	UDHR Article 25, ICESCR Article 12, CRC Article 24, CEDAW Article 12, CERD Article S (e)(iv)
Goal 7: Ensure environmental sustainability	United Nations Framework Convention on Climate Change, 1992
	Kyoto Protocol to the United Nations Framework Convention on Climate Change, 1997
Goal 8: Develop a global partnership for development	UN Charter Articles 1(3), 55 and 56, UDHR Articles 22 and 28, ICESCR Articles 2(1), 11(1), 15(4), 22 and 23, CRC Articles 4, 24(4) and 28(3)

Note. CEDAW, Convention on the Elimination of All Forms of Discrimination Against Women; CERD, Convention on the Elimination of All Forms of Racial Discrimination; CRC, Convention on the Rights of the Child; ICESCR, International Covenant on Economic, Social and Cultural Rights; UDHR, Universal Declaration of Human Rights; UN, United Nations.

Table 5.1 summarizes the complementary frameworks of the MDGs and key human rights documents.

BARRIERS TO IMPLEMENTING RIGHTS-BASED APPROACHES

From a public health perspective, there are two main barriers to the implementation of an RBA on a global scale: the project-based type of assistance and the public health needs-based approach. First, most donors provide their assistance through projects that are implemented by contractors or their own staff. Although many projects play a capacity-building and change agent role in the implementation of public health improvements, these improvements are not implemented by the national professionals who are actually in charge of the country's health services and programs, but by project staff. Consequently, capacity building is something that the project staff does with some degree of assistance by the national staff. Projects usually have short-term objectives focused on delivering outputs (such as numbers of people trained or children immunized) and are not focused on the long-term goal: a continuous development process of achieving progressive impact. Handover is usually done at the end of the project, but there is little evidence of lasting sustainable capacity transfer a few years after a project ends.

In addition, coordination and harmonization of development and public health methods vary from donor to donor, from one agency or implementing contractor to another. Each donor has its own development approach and there is often confusion as to what is the best and most efficient approach to improve specific health programs. Development efforts need to undergo rigorous evaluations and harmonization of plans and activities in consultation with all stakeholders, particularly women.

Second, public health professionals are used to identifying and prioritizing needs. As discussed in chapter 1, the needs-based approach considers the needs of the majority. RBAs consider the needs of all citizens. In an RBA, it is the people whose rights are not being fulfilled that need to be prioritized. Unfortunately, many public health professionals do not always see that ensuring everyone's right to health (particularly the rights of the most vulnerable) is their role. A change of mindset and processes will be needed. Specific examples of what this reorientation can be like can be found in the chapters by Nichola Cadge and Ariel Frisancho, which discuss the experiences of Save the Children and Cooperative for Assistance and Relief Everywhere (CARE), respectively.

USING RIGHTS-BASED APPROACHES TO MEET THE MILLENNIUM DEVELOPMENT GOALS

The use of an RBA to meet the MDGs, especially the goals related to improvement of reproductive, maternal, and child health requires the concerted action of various actors: right holders, duty bearers, rights-based advocates, and rights-based service providers.

Right Holders

Supported by the human rights framework, the rights of the vulnerable and the poorest of the poor are the focus of the MDG agenda. With the ultimate goal of fulfilling the right to development and the right to health for all, the targets of 2015 set the floor of what needs to be progressively fulfilled, not the ceiling. In developed countries, laws, consumers' rights, and a strong civil society usually advance the democratic process voicing the needs of those who are underserved and vulnerable, women in particular (Hunt & Bueno de Mesquita, 2007). However, in developing countries there is usually a dearth of development processes or structures where the voice of the vulnerable can be heard. The development process needs to include the creation of mechanisms for right holders to have a voice and actively participate in the development process.

Duty Bearers

Duty bearers include governments, donors, and public health professionals. Governments are the main duty bearers when it comes to human rights, including the right to health. Donors share the responsibility for global development (Articles 55–56 of UN Charter). Most of the donors have agreed to the principles of the PD. Therefore, they have accepted the need to empower developing countries to take ownership of their development process and the responsibility of being mutually accountable for the results.

As an example, the Global Fund to Fight AIDS, Tuberculosis and Malaria allows countries to take ownership and responsibility for the grants received. Developed countries contribute to the Global Fund, which ties performance-based conditions to the release of funds and deploys funds for health system development and improvement as well as service delivery for the three target diseases. In addition, the Global Fund requires representation of all stakeholders (including women's groups, civil society, and representatives of those affected by the disease in each country), which adds a welcomed degree of transparency and participation. The Global Fund is an example of how developed countries can contribute to the development process without having to implement projects. Similar performance-based mechanisms (Loevinsohn, 2008) have demonstrated their effectiveness. The creation of other creative financing mechanisms such as "cash on delivery"[10] would allow countries to implement the quick wins and other effective development interventions in the MDG agenda. Scaling up the use of these innovative mechanisms also requires an RBA and a mindset change in the way most donors work, from attribution to contribution, and sharing the responsibility for results instead of taking credit for all that their funds purchased (Gostin, 2001).

The public health professional working for a government or donor agency then becomes a duty bearer who needs to be up to date with these new tools to implement an RBA. An effective duty bearer role is essential for the success of the RBA. Governments need to empower public servants to do all they can to fulfill the rights of all citizens, creating partnerships at various levels, coordinating all stakeholders, and sharing information and progress indicators. Donors that adopt an RBA need to create the incentives for their staff to innovate and implement new funding mechanisms. It is incumbent on public health and development professionals to advocate and develop new tools for donors to use RBAs.

The importance of accountability of all these duty bearers can be better appreciated from a global perspective of their impact. Consider this scenario: Approximately 500,000 women die every year of pregnancy-related conditions, mostly in South Asia and sub-Saharan Africa. What would happen if a global network of 1,000 partnerships—including governments, donors, NGOs, private providers, and civil society organizations (CSOs)—were created and worked together so that each had the duty and accountability for preventing 500 maternal deaths?

Rights-Based Advocates

The public health professional working for an NGO, CSO, or advocacy agency is in charge of gathering the information and evidence that will give voice to those that are not being served. There are numerous organizations advocating for human rights and development. Although many have started to converge around various issues related to their individual missions, they are not organized into networks and they lack a concerted strategy. In the next few years, we expect to see the creation of international networks of international and country level organizations (see, for example, the People's Health Movement at http://www.phmovement.org) that would sit at the table with duty bearers and advocate for fulfillment of the right to health and the right to development.

Rights-Based Service Providers

Public health professionals who provide services or manage programs using RBA must find new ways to serve those whose rights need to be protected and design innovative programs to reach them. Unfortunately, a global shortage of human resources prevents rapid response; production and deployment of health workers is not strategically managed from a global perspective and the "brain drain" follows the market demand and supply (Beaglehole, 2004).

The WHO, UNICEF, UNDP, and other UN agencies have all embraced RBAs, and the MDGs and are contributing to advocacy and global capacity building efforts. Greater leadership and coordination of approaches is required to avoid potential and real duplication of efforts. For example, United States Agency for International Development (USAID), Joint United Nations Programme on HIV/AIDS (UNAIDS), WHO, and UNICEF are all involved in orphan care and pediatric AIDS.

The World Bank and the International Monetary Fund have been criticized for lack of responsibility in their lending practices, including the conditionalities (conditions attached to loans, debt relief, and other financial arrangements) and for not contemplating the social impact of these measures. Further oversight and transparency of these global financial institutions would allow the development of rights-based financial approaches that strengthen health systems and reduce poverty.

Private voluntary organizations, faith-based organizations (FBOs), and NGOs in general are changing the way development assistance is provided. Funding through various charity and partnership mechanisms contributes to development in much larger proportion (83%) than Official Development Assistance (ODA; 17%; Adelman, 2009). Most of these organizations have their own codes of ethics, but most make no explicit reference to the protection and fulfillment of human rights. Leadership and alignment are necessary to bring the power of this enormous sector to bear in favor of global development goals and the universal right to health. This is an area where public health professionals have a unique opportunity to inform sound strategy decisions.

Educational and research institutions not only train the next generation of development and public health professionals but also function as knowledge generators and stewards of our collective experience. The responsibility of universities (particularly schools of public health) in helping realize the rights to health and development has not been well understood or explored in a way that would allow us to leverage their knowledge and expertise toward implementing the MDGs.

In sum, there is a need to change the paradigm; to "relocate the locus of control and authority" (Gordon & Sylvester, 2004, p. 48). The assumption that development aid always brings improvement can and should be challenged; and the definition of "improvement" is subjective (Gordon & Sylvester). Usually in the development process, the values of the Western developed countries are imposed. How can we avoid ineffective aid? The answer is through RBA approaches. Ambassador Jan Cedergren (Sweden), chair of the Development Assistance Committee (DAC), reiterated the recurring message from the discussions, that "gender equality, environment sustainability and human rights are fundamental cornerstones for achieving good development results" (PD, 2005, p. 7).

CASE STUDY

Calcutta Kids[11]—Nongovernmental Organization Playing the Role of Right Advocate

The Government of India has been implementing the Universal Declaration of Human Rights (UDHR) since its conception phase and has signed all five human rights instruments: ICESCR, International Covenant on Civil and Political Rights (ICCPR), Convention on the Elimination of All Forms of Racial Discrimination (CERD), Convention on the Elimination of All Forms of Discrimination Against Women (CEDAW), and Convention on the Rights of the Child (CRC). Moreover, the Indian constitution also echoes most of the elements of UDHR, especially "fundamental rights" (Part III), which encompasses the "right to equality; right to particular freedoms; right against exploitation; freedom of religion; cultural and educational rights and right to constitutional remedies" (Centre for Development and Human Rights, 2004, p. 126).

The proportion of people below the national poverty line in India in 1990 was 37.2%; by 2004–2005 it had gone down to 27.5%. If it continues to decrease at this pace, India will be able to achieve MDG 1, "eradicate extreme poverty and hunger" (Central Statistical Organisation, 2009). The absolute number of poor in the country has declined from 320 million in 1993–1994 to 301 million in 2004–2005. The rights of these remaining 301 million poor must be fulfilled. Despite improvements in maternal and infant mortality, a quarter of all maternal deaths still take place in India and 1 out of 4 infant deaths also take place in India.

What can be done? The answer is a combination of strategies grounded in RBA that includes all stakeholders, each accountable for a share of the work. Calcutta Kids is an example of an organization following such an approach. This NGO works with women and children in the underserved slums in and around Kolkata, India. The focus includes increasing access to health and nutrition services, providing health information, and encouraging positive health changing

(Continued)

(*Continued*)

behaviors. Their primary objective is to initiate community-based programs that advance the promotion and delivery of good health care, medical advocacy, and health education.

Calcutta Kids is committed to the principles of sustainable development and to the creation of responsible government structures ultimately capable of meeting the basic human needs of its citizens. Starting with about 40 children, the goal of Calcutta Kids is to enable a small proportion of needy children to receive the health care they need and to enjoy the rights they deserve. Imagine a network of organizations like Calcutta Kids united to account for the rights of every child in Kolkata. Like many NGOs, Calcutta Kids respects, protects, and fulfills the rights of children, but it cannot help all the children in need in Kolkata. A network of organizations working in partnership could if they were willing to demonstrate their progress and results and be accountable for the effectiveness, efficiency, and quality of the services to the children they serve. The strength of an RBA is in the number of individuals and organizations that joins in its implementation and accounts for its results.

CONCLUSION

This chapter has examined the elements of an RBA to reach the MDG and improve the effectiveness of development aid. In sum, we recommend that public health professionals consider the following recommendations to include RBA elements in their everyday work.

- What is your role? We all play a role in reaching the MDGs. Are you a duty bearer, right holder, advocate, a provider, or a combination of these? Reflect on your career and the leadership role you play. How do you respect, protect, and fulfill the rights to health and development?
- Consider the implementation of an RBA to achieve MDGs. Supranational structures and networks have started to be formed that can have global impact on the poorest of the poor if based on an RBA legal framework. Get familiar with the language of the MD, PD, Global Fund, and the Global Health Initiative and look for ways to advocate for the MDGs wherever you work.

- Maternal health, child health, and reproductive health rights are lagging behind. Make it a priority to use public health tools to identify those whose rights are not protected.
- Promote ownership of the development process and social transformation by playing a coach's role, not the "expert's" role. Create opportunities that allow people to find their own solutions, empower themselves, exercise their voice, and influence the development processes.
- Strengthen democratic governance by participating and supporting your State in identifying and fulfilling its responsibilities to its citizens.
- Become familiar with the UDHR and other international legal documents and refer to them when planning and allocating resources. These documents provide sustainability through universal ethics. In this way, our public health work will translate the principles of international declarations and conventions into entitlements and concrete action and results.
- Consider the elements of implementing an RBA to reach the MDG as you read the next chapter, Global Plans of Action for Health. What can you apply now to contribute to reach the MDGs?

REFERENCES

Adelman, C. (2009). Global philanthropy and remittances: Reinventing foreign aid. *Brown Journal of World Affairs, 15*(2), 23–33.

Backman, G., Hunt, P., Khosla, R., Jaramillo-Strouss, C., Fikre, B. M., Rumble, C., et al. (2008). Health systems and the right to health: An assessment of 194 countries. *Lancet, 372*(9655), 2047–2085.

Balakrishnan, R., Elson, D., & Patel, R. (2010). Rethinking macro economic strategies from a human rights perspective. *Development, 53*, 27–36.

Beaglehole, R. (2004, September). Challenging the public health workforce. *Scandinavian Journal of Public Health, 3*, 241–242.

Centre for Development and Human Rights. (2004). *The right to development: A primer.* New Delhi: Sage Pub.

Fox, A. M., & Meier, B. M. (2009). Health as freedom: Addressing social determinants of global health inequities through the human rights to development. *Bioethics, 23*, 112–122.

Gordon, R. E., & Sylvester, J. H. (2004). Deconstructing development. *Wisconsin International Law Journal.* Retrieved February 17, 2010, from http://works.bepress.com/ruth_gordon/1

Gostin, L. (2001). A vision of health and human rights for the 21st century: A continuing discussion with Stephen P. Marks. *Journal of Law, Medicine & Ethics, 29*(2), 139–140.

Hickey, S., & Mitlin, D. (2009). *Rights-based approaches to development: Exploring the potential and pitfalls.* Sterling, VA: Kumarian Press.

Hunt, P., & Bueno de Mesquita, J. (2007). *Reducing maternal mortality. The contribution of the right to the highest attainable standard of health.* Essex, UK: Human Rights Centre University of Essex.

Loevinsohn, B. (2008). *Performance-based contracting for health services in developing countries: A toolkit.* Washington, DC: The World Bank.

Scheinin, M., & Suksi, M. (2005). *Human rights in development Yearbook 2002: Empowerment, participation, accountability, and non-discrimination: Operationalising a human rights-based approach to development.* Dordrecht, The Netherlands: Martinus Nijhoff Publishers.

Sengupta, A. (2004). The human right to development. *Oxford Development Studies, 32*(2), 179–203.

Stuckler, D., Basu, S., & Mckee, M. (2010). Drivers of inequality in Millennium Development Goal progress: A statistical analysis. *PLoS Medicine, 7*(3): e 1000241.

Villanova University Legal Working Paper Series villanovalwps-1004, Villanova University School of Law.

OTHER RESOURCES

Andreassen, B.-A., & Marks, S. P. (Eds.). (2006). *Development as a human right: Legal, political, and economic dimensions* (2nd ed.). Cambridge, MA: Harvard University Press.

Beaglehole, R., Bonita, R., Horton, R., Adams, O., & McKee, M. (2004). Public health in the new era: Improving health through collective action. *Lancet, 363*(9426), 2084–2086.

Center for Strategic International Studies. (2010). *Report of The CSIS Commission on Smart Global Health Policy.* Washington, DC: CSIS.

Clapham, A., & Robinson, M. (2009). *Realizing the right to health.* Zürich: Rüffer & Rub.

Mann, J. M. (1999). *Health and human rights: A reader.* New York: Routledge.

Sen, A. K. (2000). *Development as freedom.* New York: Anchor Books.

UN Committee on Economic, Social, and Cultural Rights. (2000). The right to the highest attainable standard of health, CESCR General Comment 14. 22d Sess., Agenda Item 3, U.N. Doc. E/C.12/2000/4.

NOTES

[1]World Health Organization. Retrieved from http://www.who.int/bulletin/volumes/86/5/08-030508/en/index.html

[2]South-East Asia Regional Office (WHO,India). Retrieved from http://www.searo.who.int/LinkFiles/Bangladesh_CountryHealthSystemProfile-Bangladesh-Jan2005.pdf

[3]UN Millennium Project. Retrieved from http://www.unmillenniumproject.org/

[4]Millennium Development Goals Indicators. Retrieved from http://millenniumindicators.un.org/unsd/mdg/default.aspx

[5]Global Health Initiative. Retrieved from http://www.pepfar.gov/ghi/index.htm

[6]Office of the High Commissioner for Human Rights. Retrieved from http://www2.ohchr.org/english/law/pdf/rtd.pdf

[7]World Health Organization. (2008). Closing the Gap in a Generation: Health Equity Through Action on the Social Determinants of Health. Retrieved from http://whqlibdoc.who.int/publications/2008/9789241563703_eng.pdf

[8]Organisation for Economic Co-operation and Development. Retrieved from http://www.oecd.org/dataoecd/11/41/34428351.pdf

[9]Accra Agenda for Action. Retrieved from http://siteresources.worldbank.org/ACCRAEXT/Resources/4700790-1217425866038/AAA-4-SEPTEMBER-FINAL-16h00.pdf

[10]Birdsal, N., & Savedoff, W. D. (2010). *Cash on delivery: A new approach to aid*. Washington: Center for Global Development.

[11]Calcutta Kids. Retrieved from http://www.calcuttakids.org/

CHAPTER 6

Global Plans of Action for Health

George Kent

INTRODUCTION

Health is not only a series of separate national issues; it is also a global issue. The globalization process has accelerated the intensity and diversity of ways in which actions in one part of the globe can affect health conditions in other parts. Even if there were no such linkages, health everywhere should be a matter of global concern in moral terms. The fact that life is nasty, brutish, and short in many places should trouble all of us.

International human rights law calls on us to view health and related issues as global in scope. The *United Nations Charter* says, in Article 55:

> With a view to the creation of conditions of stability and well-being which are necessary for peaceful and friendly relations among nations based on respect for the principle of equal rights and self-determination of peoples, the United Nations shall promote:
>
> a. higher standards of living, full employment, and conditions of economic and social progress and development;
> b. solutions of international economic, social, health, and related problems; and international cultural and educational cooperation; and
> c. universal respect for, and observance of, human rights and fundamental freedoms for all without distinction as to race, sex, language, or religion.

Article 56 then says:

> All Members pledge themselves to take joint and separate action in co-operation with the Organization for the achievement of the purposes set forth in Article 55.

On this basis, the core document of the modern global human rights system, the *Universal Declaration of Human Rights*, says in Article 28:

> Everyone is entitled to a social and international order in which the rights and freedoms set forth in this Declaration can be fully realized.

Thus, the Charter and the Declaration clearly acknowledge the responsibility of the global community, taken as a whole, for the realization of human rights. They recognize that the primary obligations of states with regard to human rights are internal, but that they have external obligations as well.

The global community encompasses all agencies that act globally, including international governmental and nongovernmental organizations, transnational business enterprises, and nation-states in their external relations. The global community is a large, inclusive concept, comparable to the state. States manifest themselves by having their constituent members and their people form governments that manage a specific population and territory. Similarly, it is up to the collectivity of all people, acting through their states, to devise effective forms of global governance. This gives the global community the voice and the visibility it needs.

It is now primarily through the United Nations and its associated agencies that the countries of the world carry out the functions of global governance. Action is frequently taken in the name of the global community, on matters of security and trade, for example. If the global community can take responsibility for issues relating to trade, there is no reason why it cannot take comparable responsibility for issues such as health and nutrition. The European Union provides a suggestive model of ways in which institutional arrangements can be made to address specific issues for a group of separate nations.

The global community is not an independent entity with its own will and its own voice. It should be understood as the agent of the collectivity of all people, acting through their states and other agencies, and subordinate to that collectivity. At present, the global community is not explicitly and directly a subject of international law. Its obligations should be spelled out more clearly in the law (Kent, 2008).

If everyone is entitled to an international order that will ensure the full realization of all human rights, there is an obligation to work on envisioning and establishing such an order.

The global perspective is clearly acknowledged in General Comment 14, an authoritative interpretation of the meaning of the right to health (United Nations Economic and Social Council, 2000). International obligations of states are spelled out in Paragraphs 38–42 and the roles of international organizations are covered in Paragraphs 63–65. Paragraph 38 begins:

> States parties should recognize the essential role of international cooperation and comply with their commitment to take joint and separate action to achieve the full realization of the right to health. In this regard, States parties are referred to the Alma-Ata Declaration which proclaims that the existing gross inequality in the health status of the people, particularly between developed and developing countries, as well as within countries, is politically, socially and economically unacceptable and is, therefore, of common concern to all countries.

Thus, the global community taken as a whole must be viewed as sharing in the obligation to ensure the realization of the right to health and other human rights. The rights and the correlative obligations do not end at national borders. Each state has external obligations relating to the health of people elsewhere. For example, states must ensure that their exports do not endanger the health of people in the countries that import their products. In addition, states acting together through international agencies such as the World Health Organization (WHO) and the World Trade Organization also have obligations to ensure the realization of the right to health and other human rights.

Although it is clear that there are such global obligations, work needs to be done to clarify their specific content. The argument here is that the best way to clarify those obligations is through a multilevel planning process. Health goals need to be set (such as the goals stated in the Millennium Development Project, discussed in chapter 5), and strategies need to be worked out for achieving those goals.

Concrete obligations for ensuring realization of the right to health for all can be identified through the formulation of jointly prepared plans for realizing that goal.

Once the global community knows, through planning, what steps are required to reach the goal, then there is an obligation to take those steps. If there are several different ways to reach the goal, choices may be made among them, but there is an obligation to choose some path that can realistically be expected to reach the goal. There are choices that can be made with regard to means, but there is no choice with regard to the obligation to move decisively toward the goal of realizing the right to health for all.

There is a need for global, national, and local plans of action that could be expected to ensure realization of the right to health for all. Not only moral considerations but also a fair interpretation of human rights law and principles require that planning (Kent, 2008).

THE LACK OF GLOBAL HEALTH PLANS

It is easy to find progress reports on the Millennium Development Project (Millennium Development Goals, 2006; United Nations Department of Economic and Social Affairs, 2006; World Bank, 2006; United Nations Development Programme [UNDP], 2009; World Economic Forum, 2006). Many people have the impression that there is a global Millennium Development Project underway. A rather vague overall plan for such a project was prepared in 2005, but it was not adopted (UN Millennium Project, 2005a). The reality is that at the global level, there is only a small advocacy office in the UNDP in New York that calls for more effective work at the national level. The lack of programmatic global action is illustrated by a report focused specifically on nutrition issues under Millennium Development Goal 1. The report offered several generalized recommendations but had little to say about how they would be implemented (UN Millennium Project, 2005b).

There is a document called the *Global Strategy for Infant and Young Child Feeding* (WHO, 2003) and another called the *Global Strategy on Diet, Physical Activity and Health* (WHO, 2004). Whether they are global and whether they are strategies is debatable, because they really focus on national programs. For example, the Global Strategy on Infant and Young Child Feeding said, "The primary obligation of governments is to formulate, implement, monitor and evaluate a comprehensive *national policy* [italics added] on infant and young child feeding" (WHO, 2003, ¶ 36). It did not say what their obligations are to children outside their national jurisdictions. International organizations were called on to do various things (WHO, 2003, ¶¶ 47–48), but these were not set out as specific duties to be carried out in a programmatic way. The document did not say what was to be done about nations that do not prepare a suitable national policy on infant and young child feeding. (Policies related specifically to women and children's health are covered in more detail in chapters 10 and 11.)

The need for truly global plans is especially clear when dealing with refugees, because by definition, they are no longer under the jurisdiction of their home countries. The United Nations' refugee agency functions under the United Nations High Commissioner for Refugees (UNHCR). It has published UNHCR's *Strategic Plan for Nutrition and Food Security 2008–2012* (UNHCR 2008). Strategic Objective 1 is "To protect the right of UNHCR's PoCs [Persons of Concern] to sufficient food which relies upon access to adequate nutrition and food security." The "key strategies" are as follows:

(1.1) Policies, guidelines and programmes to improve nutrition (including micronutrients), infant and young child feeding and food security.
(1.2) Ensure provision of a general ration where required, which is sufficient in terms of quantity, quality, regularity and equity.
(1.3) Support to food security through strategies to enhance self reliance.
(1.4) Provide essential non food items where required. (UNHCR, 2008, §IV ¶7)

This is not a summary of a detailed narrative elsewhere in the document. It is the entire strategy for protecting refugees' right to food.

Whether or not plans are global in scope, we should ask whether documents such as these from WHO, the United Nations International Children's Emergency Fund (UNICEF), and UNHCR really offer strategies. The view taken here is that a serious strategy is a detailed plan of stepwise action under which designated actors use specific resources to arrive at a concrete target within a specified time. On this basis, something called the Global Strategy for Infant and Young Child Feeding should describe a plan of action at the global level. There should be clearly stated goals, a management body, well-specified indicators of progress toward the goals, explanations of how the actions are expected to relate to outcomes, and a description of the global commitment of resources to be used by the managers as they pursue the goals.

A good plan would include provisions for having the management body monitor the progress and make adjustments if the trajectory is not on target. If there is no provision for midcourse corrections, the plan is not serious. No captain would launch a ship without having some means for steering it.

It might be useful to compare these documents with the Global Strategy and Plan of Action on Public Health, Innovation and Intellectual Property (World Health Assembly, 2008). This document is more detailed, identifying different "stakeholders," specifying the actions they are expected to take, and the time frame in which they are to be carried out. There are also explicit provisions for monitoring their performance. The document does not offer precise goals or a fully detailed strategic plan, but it does move in that direction.

A serious strategy would give us confidence that the goal would in fact be reached within the specified time frame. Achievement of the goal is what one expects from a plan for building a bridge or sending a mission to the moon, and it is also what one should expect from serious plans about health.

The Global Strategy for Infant and Young Child Feeding offers sensible advice on how infants and young children should be fed. If the document had been called "Recommendations for Infant and Young Child Feeding," there would be no reason to quarrel with it. The issue raised here, illustrated by the Millennium Development Project and the Global Strategy for Infant and Young Child Feeding, is that there seems to be a steady pattern of misrepresentation. There is much talk about what appear to be grand global efforts to promote good health, although in fact, there are no serious global programs, programs that could realistically be expected to achieve clearly stated goals.

There have been many cases of lofty rhetoric but meager plans at the global level. For example, the campaign for "A World Fit for Children," launched by the UN Special Session on Children in May 2002, offered a plan of action whose main function was to affirm that the major work was to be done through National Plans of Action (United Nations General Assembly, 2002). There was no real acceptance of responsibility or commitment of resources by the global community as a whole.

For a time, it appeared that the Ending Child Hunger and Undernutrition Initiative (ECHUI) led by the World Food Programme and UNICEF (ECHUI Website, 2007) might launch a truly global effort to address the massive problem of children's malnutrition in a serious way. However, almost all the action was to take place at the national level. The operational approach was "to strengthen national capacities for integrating and scaling up the delivery within national policy frameworks and programmes of a focus set of 'anti-hunger interventions' " (ECHUI Framework, 2007, p. 13). There was no explanation of what was to be done about children in countries whose governments were unwilling or unable to do what needs to be done. There was some discussion of social safety nets within countries, but no discussion of the idea of a global safety net for children. There was no specific global goal for the reduction of child hunger and malnutrition. ECHUI's successor, the Renewed Efforts Against Child Hunger and Undernutrition (REACH) program, with its modest resources and aspirations, is limited in much the same ways (REACH, 2010).

Poor health persists in the world partly because many national governments lack the capacity or the will to do what needs to be done to solve the problems. Solutions cannot then be based on the assumption that every country has the capacity and the will. Perhaps many governments and their programs could be strengthened, but that would take time and well-designed programs for the purpose.

So long as poor health is treated solely as a series of national problems, global programs are doomed to failure. Serious plans of action need a strong global component that complements the national efforts.

THE QUESTIONABLE SUCCESS OF GLOBAL HEALTH PROGRAMS

The illusion of global action is propelled in part by the fact that when things are going bad globally, it is no one's fault, but when things take a turn for the better, international agencies are quick to claim credit for it. For example, in September 2007, there was much trumpeting when UNICEF announced that for the first time, the number of children who die before their fifth birthdays each year fell to less than 10 million in 2006 (McNeil, 2007). Some said that the improvements were meager and questionable (Murray, Laakso, Shibuya, Hill, & Lopez, 2007). However, UNICEF was quick to say, "global efforts to promote child immunization, breast-feeding and anti-malaria measures had helped cut the death rate of children under age 5 by nearly a quarter since 1990 and more than 60 percent since 1960" (Dunham, 2007).

These programs certainly have helped, but by how much? The United States Agency for International Development (USAID) used to boast that child mortality rates were declining in most of the nations in which its child survival program was working. That might have been because there has been a steady worldwide decline in child mortality rates almost everywhere, a decline that has been occurring independently of any specific interventions. Where there are no extraordinary events such as widespread armed conflict or massive epidemics such as HIV/AIDS, child mortality rates go down. Showing that there have been improvements is not the same as showing that a particular program or action has produced those improvements. Some of these "outcomes" would have taken place just as well in the absence of the programs or actions.

Most of the progress reports relating to the Millennium Development Project describe trends on indicators of interest, but they do not show that these results were related in any direct way to the activities of the project. We need to know not only whether there has been some improvement in key indicators, but also whether the improvements were the result of the activities. How are actions linked to outcomes?

These are questions that should be asked where there is in fact a plan of action that is being carried out. At the global level, however, usually it is not a story of failing plans of action, but of absent plans of action. There is a huge difference. There is no way to assess the progress of plans that have not been made.

FUNDS NEED PLANS AND PLANS NEED FUNDS

International assistance levels are low compared with the levels of need, and in relation to the promises that have been made. The weakness of the global commitments is illustrated by the promise made in 1970 at the United Nations General Assembly that donor governments would raise their Official Development Assistance to 0.7% of their Gross National Income by the mid-1970s (United Nations General Assembly, 1970, ¶ 43). That commitment has been reaffirmed many times, but the reality is that their assistance reached an all-time high of only 0.33% in 2005, less than half the target level, 3 decades after the target date (Organisation for Economic Co-operation and Development [OECD], 2006; United Nations Economic and Social Council, 2006, ¶ 2).

The *Economist* magazine described the Millennium Development Goals as "Ends Without Means" (Economist, 2004, p. 72), undoubtedly referring to the inadequate supply of money for the work. However, the project also lacks adequate plans for using the money. The same can be said with regard to Official Development Assistance. The commitment to reaching a specific percentage of Gross National Income has never been tied to specific action plans. Much of the money that is provided is spent on things that should not really be counted as development work, such as restoring war-damaged facilities in Iraq.

There is a need for money, but there is also a need for real commitments to concrete plans, specific courses of action that are seriously expected to achieve the goals that are set out. The summit conferences on health do sometimes set out plans of action, but over time, we often find that they had little substance. There are many broken promises in terms of funding and in terms of planning. It just might be that if there were more serious planning at the global level, more nations would be willing to put money into the effort. If serious accountability is included as part of the package, as envisioned in the Paris Declaration and the Accra Agenda for Action, we could envision serious and effective global strategies (OECD, 2009).

HEALTH IS A SHARED OBLIGATION

The director of the United Nations Millennium Campaign (the advocacy arm of the project), speaking about the prospects for meeting the Millennium Development Goals by 2015, argued, "any country where the leaders are serious about realizing the goals in the next 10 years can in fact make it happen" (Sandrasagra, 2006). That is a doubtful proposition. In any case, the Millennium Development Project should explain what is to be done to ensure the achievement of the Millennium goals where national governments are either unwilling or unable to do what needs to be done. The global community cannot discharge its obligations simply by pointing to the obligations of national governments. If human rights such as the human right to health are treated as if rights and duties end at national borders, the entire human rights project is undermined.

Everyone agrees that national governments carry the *primary* obligations for the realization of their own people's human rights. However, the global community now acts as if these were *exclusively* the obligations of national governments, and not obligations that are shared by all in some measure.

At times, the fact that authority is decentralized is used as a rationale for evading responsibility. In the United States, for example, authority regarding health and education rests primarily with the states of the United States. As a result, children in Mississippi, for example, remain worse off than most other American children. Globally, children in Niger remain near the bottom of the global list because the powerful treat problems like health and nutrition mainly as problems of the separate nations.

Decentralization can be a way of retaining inequality. People tend to localize issues when they do not want to accept responsibility for what really ought to be viewed as problems of the larger group. At some point, it becomes inescapably obvious that some issues simply cannot be addressed on a local basis, as in the case of climate change, for example. By now, it should be obvious that matters such as health and hunger cannot be addressed only on a local basis.

In terms of governance, the primary responsibility for dealing with such issues lies with national governments. It is the states, represented by their governments, that sign and ratify the international human rights agreements, and thus it is the states that are the primary duty bearers from the perspective of human rights law. The right to food guidelines published by the FAO acknowledge, "States have the primary responsibility for their own economic and social development, including the progressive realization of the right to adequate food in the context of national security" (Food and Agriculture Organization [FAO], 2005, p. 33). The guidelines then go on to say that national development efforts should be supported by an enabling international environment. The relevant international agencies "are urged to take actions in supporting national development efforts for the progressive realization of the right to adequate food in the context of national food security" (FAO, 2005, p. 33). However, although human rights law and the right to food guidelines acknowledge the obligations to cooperate and assist internationally, there is no claim that the cooperation and assistance must achieve any particular level. The global community has not taken on clear and concrete obligations comparable to those it calls on the separate nations to take on.

International agencies such as the WHO and the FAO sometimes recognize the need to formulate long-range action plans. However, their action plans are mostly inward looking, for their own organizations, not for the world. An external evaluation of the FAO reinforces this approach. It shows much more interest in strengthening FAO's standing in the world than in finding ways to address the world's food issues more effectively (FAO, 2007). If these organizations do not take the lead by facilitating the global planning that is needed, who will?

CONCLUSION

There is a need for serious global planning to deal with major health issues. However, it is commonly assumed that the proposed action program is to be embedded within the existing institutional structures. That structure also needs to be critically reviewed and changed as necessary. Laurie Garrett argues:

> today more money is being directed toward the world's poor and sick than ever before. But unless these efforts start tackling public health in general instead of narrow, disease-specific problems—and unless the brain drain from the developing world can be stopped—poor countries could be pushed even further into trouble, in yet another tale of well-intended foreign meddling gone awry. (Garrett, 2007)

Vicente Navarro has sketched out his views of the ideal national health system (Navarro, 2007). He is concerned not simply with the delivery of medical care, but also with the political, economic, social, and cultural determinants of health, the lifestyle determinants, and the socializing and empowering determinants. Although he focuses on national systems, his approach could help us to think about the ideal global health system. Clarifying that design would help us to appreciate the extent to which our present global system falls short. There is a need for comprehensive institutional arrangements—local, national, regional, and global—to ensure the realization of the right to health and related rights for all.

Global health is ultimately a challenge of global governance. We are not going to get significant improvements in global health unless we see it as a genuinely global issue and plan accordingly.

REFERENCES

Dunham, W. (2007). Medical journal hits U.N. agencies on health data. *Reuters*. Retrieved August 31, 2010, from http://uk.reuters.com/article/homepageCrisis/idUKN20208875._CH_.242020070920

ECHUI Framework. (2007). Global framework for action to end child hunger and undernutrition. *"Zero" Draft*. Retrieved August 31, 2010, from http://www.box.net/shared/zky1gvof65

ECHUI Website. (2007). Retrieved August 31, 2010, from http://endingchildhunger.blogspot.com/

Economist. (2004, September 11). Economics focus: Ends without means. *Economist*, 72.

Food and Agriculture Organization of the United Nations. (2005). Voluntary guidelines to support the progressive realization of the right to adequate food in the context of National Food Security. Retrieved August 31, 2010, from http://www.fao.org/docrep/meeting/009/y9825e/y9825e00.htm

Food and Agriculture Organization of the United Nations. (2007). *FAO: The challenge of renewal: Report of the independent external evaluation of the Food and Agriculture Organization of the United Nations (FAO)*. Retrieved August 31, 2010, from http://www.fao.org/unfao/bodies/IEE-Working-Draft-Report/K0489E.pdf

Garrett, L. (2007, January/February). The challenge of global health. *Foreign Affairs*. Retrieved August 31, 2010, from http://www.foreignaffairs.org/20070101faessay86103/laurie-garrett/the-challenge-of-global-health.html

Kent, G. (Ed.). (2008). *Global obligations for the right to food*. Lanham, MD: Rowman & Littlefield.

McNeil, D. G., Jr. (2007, September 13). Child mortality at record low; further drop seen. *New York Times*. Retrieved August 31, 2010, from http://www.nytimes.com/2007/09/13/world/13child.html?ex=1347336000&en=1f0d2cd7f97947ce&ei=5088&partner=rssnyt&emc=rss

Millennium Development Goals. (2006). The millennium development goals: Progress in Asia and the Pacific 2006. *United Nations Economic and Social Commission for Asia and the Pacific, United Nations Development Program, and Asian Development Bank* (Annual Report). Retrieved August 31, 2010, from www.mdgasiapacific.org

Murray, C. J., Laakso, T., Shibuya, K., Hill, K., & Lopez, A. D. (2007). Can we achieve Millennium Development Goal 4? New analysis of country trends and forecasts of under-5 mortality to 2015. *Lancet, 370*(9592), 1040–1054.

Navarro, V. (2007). What is a national health policy? *International Journal of Health Services: Planning, Administration, Evaluation, 37*(1), 1–14.

Organisation for Economic Co-operation and Development. (2006, April 4). Aid flows top USD 100 billion in 2005. *OECD*. Retrieved August 31, 2010, from http://www.oecd.org/document/40/0,2340,en_2649_201185_36418344_1_1_1_1,00.html

Organisation for Economic Co-operation and Development. (2009). The Paris Declaration and Accra Agenda for Action. *OECD*. Retrieved August 31, 2010, from http://www.oecd.org/document/18/0,3343,en_2649_3236398_35401554_1_1_1_1,00.html

Renewed Efforts Against Child Hunger and Undernutrition. (2010). REACH: Ending child hunger and undernutrition. Retrieved August 31, 2010, from http://www.reach-partnership.org/home

Sandrasagra, M. (2006, June 12). Development: Nine years, eight goals, no time to waste. *Inter Press Service News Agency*. Retrieved August 31, 2010, from http://www.ipsnews.net/print.asp?idnews=33583

UN Millennium Project. (2005a). Investing in development: A practical plan to achieve the millennium development goals. *United Nations Development Programme*. Retrieved August 31, 2010, from http://www.unmillenniumproject.org/reports/index.htm

UN Millennium Project. (2005b). Halving hunger: It can be done. *Earthscan/Millennium Project and United Nations Development Programme*. Retrieved August 31, 2010, from http://www.unmillenniumproject.org/reports/tf_hunger.htm

United Nations Development Programme. (2009). End poverty 2015: Millennium development goals. *UNDP*. Retrieved August 31, 2010, from http://www.un.org/millenniumgoals/index.shtml

United Nations Department of Economic and Social Affairs. (2006). The millennium development goals report 2006 (Annual report). *DESA*. Retrieved August 31, 2010, from http://mdgs.un.org/unsd/mdg/Resources/Static/Products/Progress2006/MDGReport2006.pdf

United Nations Economic and Social Council. (2000). Substantive issues arising in the implementation of the International Covenant on Economic, Social and Cultural Rights: General Comment No. 14 (2000): The right to the highest attainable standard of health (article 12 of the International Covenant on Economic, Social and Cultural Rights) *ECOSOC E/C.12/2000/4*. Retrieved August 31, 2010, from http://www.unhchr.ch/tbs/doc.nsf/385c2add1632f4a8c12565a9004dc311/40d009901358b0e2c1256915005090be?OpenDocument

United Nations High Commissioner for Refugees. (2008). UNHCR's strategic plan for nutrition and food security 2008–2012. *UNHCR*. Retrieved August 31, 2010, from http://www.unhcr.org/cgi-bin/texis/vtx/search?page=search&docid=4885998c2&query=strategic%20plan%20for%20nutrition

United Nations Economic and Social Council. (2006). Review of trends and perspectives in funding for development cooperation: Note by the Secretary General. *ECOSOC E/2006/60*. Retrieved August 31, 2010, from http://www.un.org/esa/coordination/ecosoc/E-2006-60%20SG%27s%20note%20on%20Funding.pdf

United Nations General Assembly. (1970). International development strategy for the second United Nations Development Decade. *UN General Assembly Resolution 2626 (XXV)*. Retrieved August 31, 2010, from http://daccess-ods.un.org/access.nsf/Get?Open&DS=A/RES/2626(XXV)&Lang=E&Area=RESOLUTION

United Nations General Assembly. (2002). Resolution S-27/2. A world fit for children. *United Nations A/Res/S-27/2*. Retrieved August 31, 2010, from http://www.unicef.org/specialsession/docs_new/documents/A-RES-S27-2E.pdf

World Bank. (2006). Global monitoring report 2006: Strengthening mutual accountability—Aid, trade, and governance (Annual report). *World Bank*. Retrieved August 31, 2010, from http://web.worldbank.org/WBSITE/EXTERNAL/EXTDEC/EXTGLOBALMONITOR/EXTGLOBALMONITOR2006/0,,menuPK:2186472~pagePK:64218926~piPK:64218953~theSitePK:2186432,00.html

World Economic Forum. (2006). Global governance initiative: Annual report 2006. *WEF*. Retrieved August 31, 2010, from http://www.weforum.org/pdf/Initiatives/GGI_Report06.pdf

World Health Assembly. (2008). Global strategy and plan of action on public health, innovation and intellectual property. *WHA*. Retrieved August 31, 2010, from http://www.who.int/gb/ebwha/pdf_files/A61/A61_R21-en.pdf

World Health Organization. (2003). Global strategy for infant and young child feeding. *WHO*. Retrieved August 31, 2010, from http://www.who.int/child_adolescent_health/documents/9241562218/en/

World Health Organization. (2004). Global strategy on diet, physical activity and health. *WHO*. Retrieved August 31, 2010, from http://www.who.int/dietphysicalactivity/goals/en/index.html

PART II

Rights-Based Approaches and Professional Development

CHAPTER 7

Ethical Issues and Rights-Based Approaches: Balancing Dual Loyalties

Leslie London, Leonard Rubenstein, and Laurel Baldwin-Ragaven

INTRODUCTION

Dual loyalty (DL) exists when there is a clinical role conflict between professional duties to a patient and obligations (express or implied) to a third party. Most typically, DL arises when a health professional, employed in a closed institutional setting (such as the military or prison context) is asked to deploy his or her skills for purposes of advancing the interests of the authorities, rather than as part of a clinical assessment or therapeutic intervention for a patient.

The phenomenon of DL and the threat it poses to clinical medical practice is both well recognized and is increasingly receiving policy attention in terms of ethical and human rights guidelines. However, the equivalent conflict of interest in the public health sphere is more complex. This is principally because of the population approach in public health. Unlike clinical medicine, involving patient–provider interactions covered by a set of semienforceable ethical codes applicable to the professional, the targets groups in public health practice are often vulnerable populations for which ethical codes are largely underdeveloped or difficult to apply. Further, many public health professionals are not members of any clinical discipline governed by specific ethical codes.

In this chapter, we explore this problem by highlighting examples of DL applicable to a broader public health context, illustrating the similarities and differences with the problem of the clinical DL. We propose expanding guidelines developed for the latter context, specifically oriented to the protection of human rights, to a public health environment. In doing so, we argue that even if this imposes additional accountability on public health professionals, this is entirely appropriate to a public health tradition with deep historical roots in social processes that recognize the social determinants of health and a commitment to health as a right.

ETHICS AND HUMAN RIGHTS IN HEALTH PROFESSIONAL PRACTICE

Ethical obligations are deeply rooted in the practice and traditions of the health professions. Although egregious violations of such adherence have and continue to occur (Bloche, 1986; Bloche & Marks, 2005; British Medical Association [BMA], 1986; Cilasun, 1991; Iacopino, Heisler, Pishevar, & Kirschner, 1996; McLean & Jenkins, 2003; Miles, 2004; Rayner, 1987; Reis et al., 2004; Singh, 2003; Stover & Nightingale, 1985), there is, today, little dispute over the primacy of respect for patient dignity and autonomy as part of the ethical obligations of all health professionals. Unlike the days when Uruguayan doctors could justify their participation in torture by claiming that "I was confined to my function. I ignored some aspects and there were some aspects I didn't want to know . . . It wasn't my purpose. I am a doctor" (cited in Bloche, 1987, p. 16). Almost all ethical codes globally have reached consensus that health professionals should not countenance torture, should never use their clinical skills to inflict harm on those deemed to be threats to the state, and should act independently in their clinical care of their patients.

In so far as respect for human rights is integral to the social compact of health professionals, a host of developments in medical ethics have likewise highlighted the importance of human rights to health professional practice. These include professional and scientific ethical guidelines (Amnesty International, 2009; United Nations Educational, Scientific and Cultural Organization [UNESCO], 2005; WMA, 1956, 1975, 1985, as updated), how-to manuals for health professionals incorporating human rights approaches (BMA & the Commonwealth Medical Trust, 2007; Open Society Institute and Equitas, 2007; Physicians for Human Rights, 2005; 2008), and human rights standards for investigations of torture (UN Office of the High Commissioner for Human Rights, 2004). To comply with ethical practice, therefore, health professionals delivering clinical care need to be cognizant of human rights in their professional practice and avoid actions that may result in the abuse of their patients' human rights.

Although human rights approaches to health and medical ethics are closely synergistic, there are important differences to note. The field of bioethics provides frameworks and guidance for ethical reasoning in health care, aimed at maximizing the likelihood of morally acceptable choices when resolving difficult moral dilemmas. Decisions about end-of-life care, about when it is justified to break patient confidentiality, and about access to scarce resources for treatment, all typically demand of the clinician careful ethical reasoning. The most common approach is the application and balancing of one or more of four principles (beneficence, nonmaleficence, autonomy, and justice) to reach a morally justifiable decision, the so-called principle-based approach (Beauchamp & Childress, 1994), although other approaches, such as virtue-based, utilitarian, communitarian, and case-based approaches may also apply.

Common to each of these approaches is the idea that there is no pre-existing "correct" answer to the question of what is "right" or "wrong"; rather, ethical reasoning enables the clinician to reach a morally correct response in the face of challenging and disparate choices. Indeed, in ethical reasoning, there is no a priori guidance regarding which principle should dominate when more than one principle are at stake. Historical traditions in North America, however, tend in practice to privilege individual autonomy over other principles (Baum, Gollust, Goold, & Jacobson, 2007; Emanuel, Wendler, & Grady, 2000); but, even there, none of the principles has inherent primacy nor is their interpretation universally clear (Takala, 2001). As a result, there is scope for enormous variability in moral decision making. Although moral disagreements per se are not a bad thing and should not make us sceptical about bioethical reasoning, such disagreements become problematic when human rights are at stake.

Human rights, by contrast, provide a more prescriptive framework for resolving morally problematic conflicts. With their foundation in the concept of universal entitlements to a common humanity as well as international law, human rights move away from a process that attempts to reconcile values and emotions with logic to one based on normative standards. Where a course of action can be shown to be a violation of patient rights, or will be likely to lead to violations, such actions are explicitly proscribed (and within the legal framework liable to legal sanction). Built over decades of recognition of and engagement with protecting vulnerable peoples' dignity and freedoms, human rights "can be seen as primarily ethical demands" (Sen, 2004, p. 319) that encapsulate universal agreement on how to manage relationships of power—a sort of a moral shorthand for an expression of universal ethics for health professionals as well as states (Adorno, 2002).

Of course, this characterization has the potential to oversimplify the complexity of both the human rights and medical ethics frameworks.

Much of bioethics has coalesced around generating ethical guidelines that represent consensus about the position that clinicians should take when facing difficult ethical choices, the deontology of health professions. Such guidelines provide benchmarks for ethical behavior against which health professional actions can and often are adjudicated, thereby approaching a more normative use of bioethics.

For example, the proscription of medical participation in torture has been confirmed as part of a global ethical consensus (World Medical Association, 1975). At the same time, a human rights approach often must take into account conflicts among competing rights and interests, so that human rights are not absolute standards and their application will require careful case-based analysis and the application of moral reasoning. However, broadly speaking, holding clinicians accountable to human rights standards provides a more normative framework to determine acceptable professional behavior. In contrast, bioethics takes into account a wide range of ethical concepts and constructs with more open-ended outcomes; indeed, it has been argued that human rights are only one of many competing ethical factors and cannot nor should not be treated as any more important than other ethical considerations (Benatar, 2006).

THE PROBLEM OF DUAL LOYALTY

One particular situation where the ethical obligations of clinicians toward vulnerable patients has been rather unclear is that of the problem of DL, where a health professional facing competing obligations may allow third-party pressures to lead him or her to become complicit, either actively or passively, in the violations of human rights of his or her patients (Rubenstein, London, Baldwin-Ragaven, & the Dual Loyalty Working Group, 2002).

For example, the evidence that U.S. health professionals shared confidential clinical information about prisoner–detainees and advised on interrogation techniques in Iraq and Guantanamo Bay (Bloche & Marks, 2005; Clark, 2006; Lifton, 2004; Miles, 2004; Singh, 2003) demonstrates more recent examples in a long litany of health professional's involvement in torture and abusive treatment of detainees. However, DL conflicts are also present in contexts where the violations of human rights may be less egregious, for example, in the conduct of disability assessments where state or third-party insurer interests may take preference over patient health needs, or where health practitioners may implement health policies that violate patient rights in the mistaken belief that such policies are necessary for the social good, as was the case with excesses in the implementation of reproductive health policies in India to curb population growth (cited in Rubenstein et al., 2002).

In all these examples, what is characteristic is the use of clinical skills to advance third-party interests, where these third-party interests are implied to represent some social objective. Resolution of these role conflicts is rarely considered in medical ethics; indeed, it is often masked by the Hippocratic notion that "the health of my patient shall be my first consideration" when in reality, third parties frequently have considerable stake in the outcomes of health professional activities. Further, the DL conflict is often exacerbated by structural factors (e.g., the health professional's employment contract, professional isolation, role conflict, and the presence of institutional discrimination against vulnerable groups) as well as bias and stigma in society more broadly.

To address this problem, an international working group developed a set of guidelines (see http://physiciansforhumanrights.org/library/report-dualloyalty-2006.html) that drew both on existing ethical codes internationally as well as on international human rights standards to assist health professionals in managing the DL conflicts they face (Rubenstein et al., 2002). Central to this approach is the notion that health personnel should not be instruments by which states and other third parties commit human rights violations or be facilitators of such violations. Procedurally, therefore, the clinician does not attempt to balance ethical principles but strives to follow human rights standards, and ideally does so with institutional mechanisms in place to protect clinical judgment and independence.

Guidelines developed by the workgroup include general guidelines and guidelines specific to "high-risk" environments, such as prisons, the military, forensics, occupational, and refugee settings. In formulating the guidelines, the workgroup located the prevention of DL conflicts in the context of institutional factors that allow health professionals to subvert their loyalty to patients and become complicit in violations of human rights. These factors (listed in Figure 7.1) imply that a structural response to address the problem of DL is needed, so that individual health professionals are not held solely responsible for standards of behavior that are not feasible nor practical, under onerous circumstances or where health professionals' lives are under threat (Lucas & Pross, 1995).

For example, where military doctors receive no support from professional organizations to insist on clinical independence and are not protected from victimization by law, it is neither realistic nor practical to expect them to stand up to harassment and intimidation when asked to participate in torture (London, Rubenstein, Baldwin-Ragaven, & Van Es, 2006). A range of institutional interventions are therefore needed to create an enabling environment for individual health professionals to make choices that protect patient rights.

FIGURE 7.1 **Institutional Factors Facilitating Violations of Human Rights Under Dual Loyalty**

- Employment or other relationships of the health professional to an employer or third party that compromise his or her clinical independence through pressure or sense of obligation.
- Demands on health professionals that compromise their ethical and human rights obligations to their patients.
- Lack of support from the profession for health workers facing pressures to compromise ethical and human rights standards and absence of peer support.
- Lack of accountability for health professional involvement in violations of human rights.
- Absence of mechanisms to protect health workers from victimization or to seek redress in the event of victimization.
- Lack of awareness among health professionals of the problem of dual loyalty and human rights.
- Omission from the training programs of health professionals, including undergraduate, postgraduate, and continuing education, on the problem of dual loyalty and human rights.
- Secrecy governing professional practice and health research where dual loyalty conflicts are masked.
- Absence of advisory, problem solving, and ombudsman services for health professionals at risk.
- Absence of monitoring systems to document violations and the pressures faced by health professionals.

Source: Rubenstein et al., 2002

PUBLIC HEALTH AND DUAL LOYALTY

What the DL workgroup also recognized is that application of strategies to prevent violations of human rights is much more easily accomplished when applied to individualized clinical care than to public health interventions. As noted here, certain difficulties arise when extending the DL framework to the public health field.

Firstly, where a health professional has a defined patient, or even a group of patients, the moral choices about how best to avoid abuse of their patients' rights is much more clearly informed by ethical and human rights guidelines. However, many public health professionals provide services to vulnerable communities or populations, rather than individuals, for which ethical codes are largely underdeveloped or difficult to apply. Moreover, the nature of public health professionals' services often has a long-term time frame: the benefits (or harms) may not be immediately traceable to the actions of the public health official and both the services and their beneficiaries are more difficult to define.

For example, fluoridation of drinking water may prevent dental caries at a population level, but, unlike a screening intervention, there is no direct evidence that the individuals who benefited from the public health intervention were those who consumed the fluoridated water. The benefits accruing to the group occur at the population level, and reflect the "population approach" first popularized by Geoffrey Rose (1985), which emphasizes shifting the population distribution of a risk factor as key to prevention of disease in individuals. Given that water fluoridation is an invasion of privacy and limits choice (about the contents of our drinking water in public systems), evaluation of the trade-off of the rights of some in the community against the rights of the collective requires different approaches.

When public health officials are engaged in policy decisions at a population level, the language of public health is usually concerned with issues of equity, efficiency, and effectiveness, in varying proportions depending on the character of the health system. However, decisions made based on technical considerations have widespread ramifications for the rights of patients and communities. The practice of public health clearly impacts on, or has the potential to impact substantially on the human rights of large numbers of people but takes place through the lens of public policy making rather than through a traditional professional–patient/client relationship. Indeed, it takes place outside of any recognized professional compact that typifies the usual health professional's position.

Secondly, whereas clinical practice can only be permitted if the professional is licensed with an appropriate professional board or council, many public health professionals may not be health professionals by training or, even if they have a professional degree in a health discipline, may be practicing entirely nonclinically in a context where their professional degree is essentially a conduit to their public health role. Most jurisdictions do not afford the same degree of professional recognition or regulation, and therefore accountability, to the discipline of public health as they do for clinical disciplines where direct patient care is involved. In the most extreme example, many ministers of health may be doctors or nurses, but act by providing political leadership in health matters. Should they be held to account to professional standards for the human rights consequences of the policies they adopt? What of epidemiologists, toxicologists, geologists, psychologists, or social scientists working in public health whose research or opinions inform policy decisions and programs?

Such contradictions are the subject of the remainder of this chapter, which explores through several case studies how DL conflicts play out in a population health context and how best public health practitioners can manage DL in their practice.

CASE STUDY
Health Professionals in Security Force Interrogations

Medical participation in torture of detainees by security forces has been well documented (Baldwin-Ragaven, De Gruchy, & London, 1999; Bloche, 1986; BMA, 1992; Cilasun, 1991; Iacopino et al., 1996; McLean & Jenkins, 2003; Rayner, 1987; Stover & Nightingale, 1985) and its DL conflicts have been well characterized (Rubenstein et al., 2002). Clinicians provide support to interrogation by advising on interrogation methods, sharing clinical information, resuscitating severely ill and injured prisoners, and, in some cases, helping to cover up evidence of the prisoner's torture. Further, simply by the seemingly innocent act of treating a detainee, the health professional may indirectly assist the interrogation process through rendering the detainee fit to undergo further interrogation and abuse. In all these examples, the health professional is present in some way—at, before, or after the interrogation—and uses his or her clinical acumen to serve a purpose other than patient care for the detainee, a purpose deemed legitimate by powerful third-party forces who may well threaten the health professional, either directly or indirectly.

However, there is also a nonclinical DL at play in the interrogation context, which is akin to a public health context. The most recent example of this problem is illustrated in the involvement of U.S. health professionals in supporting the interrogation of detainees in the "war on terror." It is now well established that physicians and psychologists assisted interrogation and torture of detainees in U.S. custody through such means as examining detainees to determine their vulnerabilities, reviewing and approving individual interrogation plans involving isolation and sleep deprivation, monitoring interrogations and providing feedback to interrogators, and in some cases, sharing medical records with interrogators (Miles, 2009). What is less well known is how CIA medical personnel at its Office of Medical Services (OMS) reviewed each proposed "enhanced" interrogation method and made determinations whether its use would amount to the infliction of severe mental pain and suffering. According to documents released in 2009 from the CIA and the U.S. Department of Justice, OMS reviewed and specifically approved the use of stress positions, dousing with cold water, isolation, sleep

(Continued)

(Continued)

deprivation, "walling," water boarding, and other techniques. In these reviews, health personnel were not acting in a clinical capacity in relation to a detainee but were responding to a request to establish policy on a group basis—for application in a prisoner population. Their opinions were then employed by the Justice Department's Office of Legal Counsel (OLC) to claim that the methods did not meet the legal definition of torture (i.e., infliction of severe physical or mental pain or suffering). In doing so, they deflected responsibility from and, indeed, gave cover to lawyers who provided legal authorization for the use of torture.

Thus, for example, the OLC reported that OMS expressed the view that "the shackling does not result in any significant physical pain for the subject" despite the fact that "in some cases, the detainee's hands may be raised above the level of his head" for up to 2 hours (U.S. Department of Justice, OLC, 2005, p. 11). Similarly, the lawyers wrote that OMS told them that "We do not believe that placing a detainee in a dark, cramped space for the limited period of time involved here could reasonably be considered a procedure calculated to disrupt profoundly the senses so as to cause prolonged mental harm" (U.S. Department of Justice, OLC, 2005, p. 33). Perhaps most extraordinarily of all, the lawyers noted that "however frightening the experience, OMS personnel have informed us that the waterboard technique is not physically painful" (U.S. Department of Justice, OLC, 2005, p. 42) and that "OMS's professional judgment that use of the waterboard on a healthy individual subject to these limitations would be 'medically acceptable'"(U.S. Department of Justice, OLC, 2005, p. 14). OMS also provided guidelines for the clinical management of people subjected to these and other techniques.

Although the authors of these medical opinions have not been revealed, it is likely that they had no contact with detainees and thus were quite removed from behaviors that typically exemplify medical participation in torture or from relationships that would be subject to professional ethics in the clinical domain. Instead, they exercised a policy role, engaging in a form of pseudo medical analysis that provided cover for lawyers and justification for medical personnel on the scene to provide medical support for the infliction of torture. As such, their role was no less monstrous than had they been at the side of the torturers advising interrogators when and how to proceed with simulated drowning, suspensions, or confinement in a box. Indeed, their behavior may have been even more monstrous than that of the individual clinician whose contact was probably limited to a handful of detainees and who was informed that more knowledgeable authorities had determined he or she was not a party to the infliction of severe pain or suffering (Rubenstein & Xenakis, 2010).

CASE STUDY
HIV Policy in the Context of AIDS Denialism

In 2000, a community-based nongovernmental organization (NGO) opened a rape counseling and care service at a local hospital in Mpumalanga Province of South Africa, a region with particularly high HIV rates. The NGO collaborated with the health managers and clinicians at the hospital to facilitate access to postexposure prophylaxis for HIV infection for the rape survivors in terms of a national policy on victim empowerment. The project represented a successful collaboration between the health services and civil society at a time when the country's president was expressing doubts about the toxicity of antiretroviral medications (ARVs) and courting "AIDS dissidents'" views. Rather than supporting the provision of care to patients in need, the provincial minister of health (known as the member of the executive council [MEC] for health in the province), who was a member of the ruling African National Congress' Health Committee, responded by criticizing the NGO program and insisting on stopping the provision of ARVs to rape survivors. Although the exact reasons for the rise of AIDS denialism under President Thabo Mbeki's rule remains a matter of conjecture, it is well recognized that the evolution of this discourse reflected a power struggle between political leaders and civil society voices over how to define the terms of the response to the HIV epidemic in South Africa (London, 2002a; Schneider & Fassin, 2002).

It was in this context that the MEC for health in the province pressed repeatedly for disciplinary action against the NGO and against senior staff who had supported the initiative, finally dismissing the doctor in charge of the hospital, Dr. Thys Von Mollendorff, for "gross insubordination" because he gave access to the NGO to provide ARVs to rape survivors. Coupled with this victimisation, there was extensive protest action by a health workers trade union allied to the African National Congress against all health personnel in the facility who were seen to be in support of the ARV program, extending to frank harassment at times (Von Mollendorff, 2009).

Writing subsequently about his experience, Dr. Von Mollendorff (2009) describes his conflict as follows:

> We were torn between dual loyalties: should we obey the political head of the Department of Health or put our patients first? For me

(Continued)

(*Continued*)

> as a physician, patients always come first and, as a public officer,
> I was required to act according to the Public Service Regulations
> (4.1.3): "An employee shall put the public's interest first in the
> execution of his or her duties." (p.82)

Although subsequently reinstated by a Labour Court ruling, and vindicated by the collapse of the regime of AIDS denialism at the highest political levels in South Africa with the removal of Thabo Mbeki from the South African presidency, Von Mollendorff never returned to the public service or to work in Mpumalanga Province. However, his case represents a clear example of how a clinician manager, when facing a situation of DL, needed to be aware of the human rights implications of his actions, and also how the decision to act in the context of a DL conflict may have considerable personal cost.

In addition, the provincial minister of health, whose vigor in denying access to ARVs for rape survivors was entirely driven by an ideological agenda dictated from her political leadership, was a qualified nurse by training. Should a health administrator, a public health official, or even a political leader in health be subject to specific ethical and human rights obligations by virtue of being a health professional, or should he or she be considered to be acting in a public capacity independent of his or her professional status? The provincial minister of health was never reported to the South African Nursing Council for her actions, nor was any political action taken against her for having obstructed care for rape survivors. Indeed, there is no forum for hearing such claims about these kinds of human rights violations outside the political realm.

The accountability of public officials and leaders who are also health professionals is perhaps best summarized by a reader of a daily newspaper in Cape Town writing at the height of AIDS denialism in South Africa about the conduct of the then minister of health:

> A minister of health is supposed to advise a president . . . on
> the validity of medical research. What are Tshabalala-Msimang's
> medical qualifications? . . . Did she swear the Hippocratic Oath
> and sign the Geneva Convention as all of us newly graduated doc-
> tors did? . . . It seems that loyalty to the party overrides the deaths
> of thousands of our people and our raped babies. (Bain, 2003)

CASE STUDY
Abstinence-Only Sex Education

Although financial support for programs promoting sexual abstinence has been in place in the United States for more than 2 decades, the period since the mid-1990s under President George W. Bush saw a major expansion of federal funding for abstinence programs with a shift to funding programs that teach abstinence only and restrict the availability of other information on the prevention of teenage pregnancy and sexually transmitted infections, including HIV (Santelli et al., 2006). The policy limited federal funding for health education to only those public schools that adopted a curriculum, which met stringent criteria including the promotion of abstinence outside of marriage as its exclusive purpose and the exclusion of any advocacy or information on alternative contraceptive use other than to highlight their failure rates. As a result, studies conducted by the CDC of school-based health education programs found that by 2000, 96% of high schools in the United States taught abstinence as the best way to avoid pregnancy, HIV, and STDs (cited in Santelli et al., 2006) and the figure in 2006 was only marginally lower at 88% (Kann, Telljohann, & Wooley, 2007).

There is convincing support for the argument that the policy was not based on evidence, nor has its implementation been monitored in the same way for effectiveness that other comprehensive sexual education programmes have been (Ott & Santelli, 2007). Indeed, many studies have shown that abstinence only programmes have been ineffective in reducing sexual and reproductive health risks (Kohler, Manhart, & Lafferty, 2008; Santelli et al., 2006; Trenholm et al., 2008). Rather, the policy has been driven by ideological assumptions based on moral and religious beliefs, which have been given preferential influence on presidential decision making, in conflict with current scientific evidence (Santelli, 2008). Studies have shown that the restrictions imposed on providing information about alternatives to abstinence has prevented adolescents' access to measures known to be effective (Darroch, Landry, & Singh, 2000; Starkman & Rajani 2002) as well as violating rights of adolescents to complete and accurate information on sexual and reproductive health, which is recognized as instrument to realizing the human right to the highest attainable standard of health (Ott & Santelli; Santelli et al., 2006). In its implementation, the policy has also led to discrimination and stigma against teen pregnancies and sexual orientations other than heterosexuality and has promoted homophobia and gender stereotypes (Ott & Santelli; Santelli et al., 2006).

(Continued)

(Continued)

Here, the DL dilemma is one in which public health officials are forced, because of withholding of financial subsidies, to pursue the implementation of preventive programs that are neither effective nor consistent with human rights of a target population. Similar arguments could be made regarding the DL pressures facing public health professionals working in international health programs funded by U.S. federal grants. The third-party pressure is institutional and operates far from the level of an individual patient. Indeed, as a preventive program, there are no patients, only a vulnerable population of adolescents. By enabling programs that limit access to accurate information, adolescents are being deprived of known interventions that could prevent STIs and pregnancy, and thereby are at risk of serious violations of their human rights, leaving the public health official involved deeply conflicted.

RESPONDING TO DUAL LOYALTIES IN PUBLIC HEALTH

The similarities and contrasts among the different cases reflect, firstly, the diversity of practice in the public health context, as well as the difficulties in formulating a uniform response to the problem, where professional obligations intersects so obviously with ethical policy making (Danis, Clancy, & Churchill, 2002) and where population approaches to health change the nature of professional accountability (Cassel & McParland, 2002; Emanuel, 2002).

Reich and Roberts (2002) describe three approaches to public health ethics namely, utilitarianism, human rights approaches, and communitarianism, but do not offer guidance as to which approach might be preferable or how such approaches should be applied. Nancy Kass (2001) developed an approach to consider ethical implications in public health programs and policy development. This approach reflects in large measure those human rights constructs that have served to underpin analogous tools arising from the health and human rights domain (Gostin & Mann, 1999; International Federation of Red Cross and Red Crescent Societies & Francois-Xavier Bagnoud Centre for Health and Human Rights, 1999; London, 2002b). These tools[1] examine the consonance of public health policy with human rights by focusing on rendering the policy goals explicit and exploring questions of effectiveness, burdens (both known and potential, and both health and rights burdens), fairness in implementation, the existence, and effectiveness of alternatives as well as their relative intrusiveness. Although preoccupied primarily with analyzing the trade-offs inherent in public health policies that limit individual rights when pursuing the public good, they also extend to identifying which policies best advance health as a socioeconomic right and how health policies should do so. Rather than leaving it to the public health practitioner's intuition, they provide a set of benchmarks against which a public policy choice can be tested when facing a DL conflict so as to ensure a utilitarian argument for the public good does not unreasonably result in violations of individuals or vulnerable populations' rights.[2]

Other developments have proposed the framework of reasonableness for accountability (Daniels, 2000) to provide guidance for difficult ethical resource allocation decisions in public health, emphasizing reasonableness of process to circumvent difficulties in reaching consensus on substantive outcomes. More recently, Baum et al. (2007) proposed a framework aimed at preempting ethical conflicts in public health practice through reflection on six considerations aimed at avoiding the creation of ethical tensions.

Therefore, although a range of tools and frameworks exist for ethical and human rights analysis in public health practice, they provide little direct guidance linking the public health practitioners' professional obligations to how best to resolve the DL problem in the public health context. Rather, they provide the tools needed for public health professionals to weigh considerations that are frequently case and context specific when facing a DL conflict. It is precisely these tools that will enable the public health practitioner to negotiate a practice choice that maximizes human rights outcomes, much as clinical practitioners are expected to put the interests of their patients first.

In situations of a clinical DL conflict (such as pressure to assist in interrogation of a "terrorist"), health professionals are often asked to interpret the interests of the state or a third party as being more morally compelling than that of a single vulnerable individual and typically do not possess either the information or the skills to make such an interpretation. How is a health professional to judge a claim that a detainee is a "terrorist" or someone who has planned to cause mass destruction, and who should therefore be subjected to unusual and inhumane forms of interrogation, to prevent such atrocities, for example? The DL project proposed that health professionals should not be drawn into making such judgments. Moreover, where limitations of individual rights are proposed to benefit the public good, frequently framed persuasively by utilitarian arguments, any "decision to depart from fidelity to the patient should be within a recognized framework of exceptions" (Rubenstein et al., 2002, p. 65). Translated into the public health context, this means (a) the application of well-established tools for measuring the justification for such limitations (Gostin & Mann, 1999; International Federation of Red Cross and Red Crescent Societies & Francois-Xavier Bagnoud Centre for Health and Human Rights, 1999; Kass, 2001 ; London, 2002b) and (b) doing so in the context of a recognized framework for evaluating policies that are, drawing on Daniels' (2000) arguments, transparent and trustworthy.

CONCLUSION

The general guidelines proposed by the DL project (see Table 7.1) might then be adapted to a public health context by drawing analogies between guidelines geared for individual patient care and the principles that should apply in the public health context.

For example, whereas measures that raise awareness or that require enhanced training, exercise of independent judgment, self-reflection, maintenance of confidentiality, and building a community of practice would apply equally to both domains, certain guidelines are specific to the nature of public health practice. Therefore, for example, the skills critically needed would not necessarily be those that help to alert a clinician to a potential abuse of a patient in a treatment situation, but rather tools that enable the public health practitioner to understand a rights-based approach to balancing public good and individual rights and to act appropriately. Similarly, whereas a clinical DL may have to grapple with ensuring that third-party pressures do not result in substandard care to individuals or even groups, a typical public health DL is one where, because of the invisibility of claims of poor and marginalized communities, there is an incentive to respond to the needs of political more powerful groups.

Modern public health practice recognizes that health is both an end (a right) in and of itself but is also instrumental to human development (Beaglehole, Bonita, Horton, Adams, & McKee, 2004), so there will be circumstances where, notwithstanding rights being inalienable, limits may justifiably be placed on individual rights in order to advance the public good where the public good is itself the realization of public health as a right. But such limitations must be consonant with human rights principles and must recognize the indivisibility of civil and political rights with socioeconomic entitlements, even in the context of priority setting among many public health needs (Hunt, 2007). Public health professionals, therefore, need to be

TABLE 7.1 Dual Loyalties: Guidelines for Public Health Professional Practice

Clinical Dual Loyalty	Public Health Dual Loyalty
Study and training in human rights to enable familiarity with implications of human rights for clinical practice.	Study and training in human rights to enable familiarity with implications of human rights for public health practice.
Develop skills to identify situations where dual loyalty conflicts threaten human rights and where independent professional judgment may be compromised.	Develop skills to identify situations where dual loyalty conflicts threaten human rights and if and how limitations on rights may be justified within a human rights framework.
Place the protection of the patient's human rights and well-being first; resist demands to subordinate patient human rights to third-party interests.	Place the protection of the human rights (individual and collective) first; resist demands to subordinate human rights to third-party interests.
Ensure that the provision of care be at least equal to the current standard of care for vulnerable patients, if not increased access to care.	Ensure that the needs of the most marginal groups and communities are not displaced by the needs of more powerful stakeholders in health policies and programs; to do so, interrogate the different interests driving the adoption of the particular program or policy and who is not in the agenda-setting process.
Exercise independent clinical judgment in therapeutic or evaluative services.	Exercise independent judgment in one's public health discipline.
Be aware of how professional skills may be misused to violate the human rights of individuals and take appropriate steps to avoid this misuse; self-reflection.	Be aware of how professional skills may be misused to violate the human rights of individuals and communities, and take appropriate steps to avoid this misuse; self-reflection.
Recognize that passive participation in violations of a patient's human rights is a breach of loyalty to the patient.	Recognize that passive participation in violations of the human rights of individuals or one or more collectives is a breach of professionalism (regardless of current presence/absence of deontological codes of conduct).
Only depart from loyalty to the patient within a framework of exceptions established by a standard-setting authority competent to define the human rights obligations of a health professional; any such departure should be disclosed to the patient.	Conduct public health practice where rights of groups are considered against others within a framework of exceptions established by a standard-setting authority competent to define the human rights obligations of a public health professional; in decision-making processes transparent to the public.

(Continued)

TABLE 7.1 Dual Loyalties: Guidelines for Public Health Professional Practice *Continued*

Clinical Dual Loyalty	Public Health Dual Loyalty
Maintain confidentiality of medical information except where the patient consents to disclosure or where an exception recognized by competent authorities in medical ethics permits disclosure.	Maintain confidentiality of identifiable medical information except where the patient consents to disclosure or where an exception recognized by competent authorities in medical ethics permits disclosure.
Resist state demands to participate in a violation of the human rights of patients.	Resist state demands to participate in a violation of the human rights of patients or collectives (e.g., particular communities, ethnic minorities).
Act with an understanding of health professionals' collective obligation to uphold human rights and well-being of the patient.	Act with an understanding of public health professionals' collective obligation to uphold human rights and well-being of patients and collectives.
Take advantage of opportunities for support from local, national, and international professional bodies to meet their ethical and human rights duties to the patient.	Take advantage of opportunities for support from local, national, and international professional bodies to meet ethical and human rights obligations to communities.
Report violations of human rights that interfere to appropriate authorities, both civil and medical.	Report violations of human rights that interfere to appropriate authorities, both civil and medical.
Act individually and collectively to bring an end to policies and practices that prevent the health professional from providing core health services to some or all patients in need.	Act individually and collectively to bring an end to policies and practices that prevent the health professional from providing core health services to some or all patients in need.
Support colleagues individually and collectively—through professional bodies—when the state acts to impede or threaten their ability to fulfill their duty of loyalty to patients.	Support colleagues individually and collectively—through professional bodies—when the state acts to impede or threaten their ability to fulfill their obligations toward the human rights of patients and collectives.

Source: Adapted from Rubenstein et al., 2002

able to make such assessments or to access support to do so. For example, many recent responses to the problem of extreme drug-resistant TB (Boggio et al, 2008; Sakoane, 2007; Singh, Upshur, & Padayatchi, 2007) have been singularly lacking in insight into the appropriateness of coercive measures for achieving the public health objective of control of drug-resistant TB

(London, 2009) resulting, in practice, in wholly inappropriate pursuit of patient confinement as a strategy of immediate rather than "last resort" (Amon, Girard, & Keshavjee, 2009). When confronted with requirements to develop or implement public health policies that infringe human rights, the public health official is ethically required to resist them just as a clinician faced with a demand to participate in torture must; and the community of peers should offer support in maintaining a human rights stance (Rubenstein et al., 2002). Of course, resistance may take less overt form, varying from turning to professional peers and organizations for support through to considering whistle-blowing to draw attention to the policy.

Lastly, we have raised the question about particular accountability of public officials and leaders who happen also to be health professionals, both to the public through civil society oversight and to the profession of public health. Should they be held to a higher level of accountability than the general public, or a professional from a nonmedical discipline? Notably, the International Covenant on Economic, Social and Cultural Rights (1966) frames citizen responsibility in terms of "duties to other individuals and to the community to which he belongs . . . to strive for the promotion and observance of the rights recognized in the present Covenant." Ordinary citizens, whether they are health professionals or not, are expected to act in accordance with a rights-based social contract. Moreover, to the extent the officials are agents of the state, they must respect, protect, and fulfill human rights. We would argue that the particular and additional responsibility for health professionals in relation to human rights, whether in a clinical or public health role, is to ensure that the professional does not become an instrument for the violation of rights. Inasmuch as that imposes additional accountability on health professionals, then health professionals do carry an added burden. However, such a commitment is essential if we are to live up the ideals of a public health tradition with deep historical roots in social processes that recognize the social determinants of health, and the role that health plays, both as an end in itself and as an instrumental to human development.

REFERENCES

Adorno, R. (2002). Biomedicine and international human rights law: In search of a global consensus. *Bulletin of the World Health Organization, 80*, 959–963.

Amnesty International. (2009). *Ethical codes and declarations relevant to the health professions* (5th Rev. ed.). London: Amnesty International. AI index: ACT 75/001/2009. Retrieved December 28, 2009, from http://www.amnesty.org/en/library/info/ACT75/001/2009/en

Amon, J. J., Girard, F., & Keshavjee, S. (2009). Limitations on human rights in the context of drug-resistant tuberculosis: A reply to Boggio et al. Health and Human Rights. *Perspectives.* Retrieved August 31, 2010, from http://hhrjournal.org/blog/wp-content/uploads/2009/10/amon.pdf

Bain, J. E. (14 March, 2003). Where's the evidence? Letter to the editor. *Cape Times.*

Baldwin-Ragaven, L., De Gruchy, J., & London, L. (1999). *An ambulance of the wrong colour: Health professionals, human rights, and ethics in South Africa.* Cape Town: University of Cape Town Press (Pty) Ltd.

Baum, N. M., Gollust, S. E., Goold, S. D., & Jacobson, P. D. (2007). Looking ahead: Addressing ethical challenges in public health practice. *The Journal of Law Medicine & Ethics,* 35(4), 657–67, 513.

Beaglehole, R., Bonita, R., Horton, R., Adams, O., & McKee, M. (2004). Public health in the new era: Improving health through collective action. *Lancet,* 363(9426), 2084–2086.

Beauchamp, T. L., & Childress, J. F. (1994). *Principles of biomedical ethics.* New York: Oxford.

Benatar, D. (2006). Bioethics and health and human rights: A critical view. *The Journal of Medicine & Ethics,* 32(1),17–20.

Bloche, M. G. (1986). Uruguay's Military Physicians: Cogs in a System of State Terror. *Journal of the American Medical Association,* 255, 2788–2793.

Bloche, M. G. (1987). *Uruguay's military physicians: Cogs in a system of state terror.* Washington: American Association of the Advancement of Science.

Bloche, M. G., & Marks, J. (2005). Doctors and interrogators at Guantanamo Bay. *New England Journal of Medicine,* 353, 1.

Boggio, A., Zignol, M., Jaramillo, E., Nunn, P., Pinet, G., & Raviglione M. (2008). Limitations on human rights: Are they justifiable to reduce the burden of TB in the era of MDR- and XDR-TB? *Health and Human Rights,* 10, 121–126.

British Medical Association. (1986). Working party on the involvement of doctors in torture. Involvement of doctors in torture: Conclusions and recommendations. *Lancet,* 15, 1(8481), 628–629.

British Medical Association. (1992). Medicine betrayed: Participation of doctors in human rights abuses. London: Zed Books.

British Medical Association, & the Commonwealth Medical Trust. (2007). *The right to health: A toolkit for health professionals.* Author.

Cassel, C. K., & McParland, E. (2002). Accountability: Regulating health care as a public good. In M. Danis, C. Clancy, & L. Churchill (Eds.), *Ethical dimensions of health policy* (pp. 249–262). New York: Oxford University Press.

Cilasun, U. (1991). Torture and the participation of doctors. *Journal of Medical Ethics,* 17 (Suppl.), S21–S22.

Clark, P. A. (2006). Medical ethics at Guantanamo Bay and Abu Ghraib: The problem of dual loyalty. *The Journal of Law Medicine & Ethics,* 34(3), 570–80, 481.

Daniels, N. (2000). Accountability for reasonableness. *British Medical Journal,* 321(7272),1300–1301.

Danis, M., Clancy, C., & Churchill, L. (Eds). (2002). Ethical Dimensions of Health Policy. New York: Oxford University Press.

Darroch, J. E., Landry, D. J., & Singh, S. (2000). Changing emphases in sexuality education in U.S. public secondary schools, 1988–1999. *Family Planning Perspective, 32*(5), 204–211, 265.

Emanuel, E. J., Wendler, D., & Grady, C. (2000). What makes clinical research ethical? *The Journal of the American Medical Association, 283,*2701–2711.

Emanuel, E. J. (2002). Patient v. population: Resolving the ethical dilemmas posed by treating patients as members of populations. In M. Danis, C. Clancy, & L. Churchill (Eds.) *Ethical dimensions of health policy* (pp. 227–245). New York: Oxford University Press.

Gostin, L., & Mann, J. M. (1999). Toward the development of a human rights impact assessment for the formulation and evaluation of public health policies. In J. M. Mann, et al., (Eds), *Health and human rights: A reader* (pp. 54–71). New York, NY: Routledge.

Hunt, P. (2007). UN Report of the Special Rapporteur on the right of everyone to the enjoyment of the highest attainable standard of physical and mental health. United Nations General Assembly, 62nd session, Agenda item 72b, UN doc. A/62/214, 8th August 2007. Accessed at http://www.essex.ac.uk/human_rights_centre/research/rth/docs/GA2007.pdf on August 31st 2010.

Iacopino, V., Heisler, M., Pishevar, S., & Kirschner, R. H. (1996). Physician complicity in misrepresentation and omission of evidence of torture in postdetention medical examinations in Turkey. *The Journal of the American Medical Association, 276*(5), 396–402.

International Covenant on Economic, Social and Cultural Rights. (1966). New York: United Nations.

International Federation of Red Cross and Red Crescent Societies & the Francois-Xavier Bagnoud Centre for Health and Human Rights. (1999). The Public Health-Human Rights Dialogue. In J. M. Mann et al. (Eds.), *Health and human rights: A reader* (pp. 46–53). New York, NY: Routledge.

Kann, L., Telljohann, S. K., & Wooley, S. F. (2007). Health education: Results from the School Health Policies and Programs Study 2006. *The Journal School Health, 77,* 408–434.

Kass, N. E. (2001). An ethics framework for public health. *American Journal of Public Health, 91,* 1776–1782.

Kohler, P. K., Manhart, L. E., & Lafferty, W. E. (2008). Abstinence-only and comprehensive sex education and the initiation of sexual activity and teen pregnancy. *The Journal of Adolescent Health, 42*(4), 344–351. Epub 2008 Jan 31.

Lifton, R. J. (2004). Doctors and torture. *The New England Journal of Medicine, 351*(5), 415–416.

London, L. (2002a). Dual loyalties, health professionals and HIV policy in South Africa. (Editorial Opinion). *South African Medical Journal, 92,* 882–883.

London, L. (2002b). Human rights and public health: Dichotomies or synergies in developing countries? Examining the case of HIV in South Africa. *Journal of Law, Medicine and Ethics, 30,* 677–691.

London, L. (2009). Confinement for extreme drug-resistant TB (XDR-TB): Balancing protection of health systems, individual rights and the public's health. *International Journal of Tubercle and Lung Disease, 13*(10), 1200–1209.

London, L., Rubenstein, L., Baldwin-Ragaven, L., & Van Es, A. (2006). Dual loyalty among military health professionals: Human rights and ethics in times of armed conflict. *Cambridge Quarterly of Health Care Ethics, 15*(4), 381–391.

Lucas, T., & Pross, C. (1995). Caught between conscience and complicity: Human rights violations and the health professions. *Medicine and Global Survival, 2*(2), 106–114.

McLean, G. R., & Jenkins, T. (2003). The Steve Biko affair: A case study in medical ethics. *Developing World Bioethics, 3*(1), 77–95.

Miles, S. H. (2004). Abu Ghraib: Its legacy for military medicine. *Lancet, 364,* 725–729.

Miles, S. H. (2009). Oath betrayed: America's torture doctors (2nd ed.). Berkeley: UC Press.

Open Society Institute and Equitas. (2007). Health and Human Rights. A resource guide for the Open Society Institute and Soros Foundations Network. Retrieved December 19, 2009, from http://equalpartners.info/

Ott, M. A., & Santelli, J. S. (2007). Abstinence and abstinence-only education. *Current Opinion in Obstetrics and Gynecology, 19*(5), 446–452.

Physicians for Human Rights. (2005). Examining asylum seekers. A health professional's guide to medical and psychological evaluations of torture. Cambridge, MA: Author.

Physicians for Human Rights. (2008).The right to health and health workforce planning. A Guide for Government Officials, NGOs, Health Workers, and Development Partners. Cambridge, MA: Author.

Rayner, M. (1987). *Turning a blind eye: Medical accountability for torture in South Africa.* Washington, DC: American Association for the Advancement of Science.

Reis, C., Ahmed, A. T., Amowitz, L. L., Kushner, A. L., Elahi, M., & Iacopino, V. (2004). Physician participation in human rights abuses in southern Iraq. *The Journal of the American Medical Association, 291*(12), 1480–1486.

Roberts, M. J., & Reich, M. R. (2002). Ethical analysis in public health. *Lancet, 359*(9311),1055–1059.

Rose, G. (1985). Sick individuals and sick populations. *International Journal of Epidemiology 14,* 32–38.

Rubenstein, L., & Xenakis, S. (2010). Roles of CIA physicians in enhanced interrogation and torture of detainees. *Journal of the American Medical Association, 304*(5), 569–570.

Rubenstein, L. S., London, L., Baldwin-Ragaven, L., & the Dual Loyalty Working Group. (2002). Dual Loyalty and Human Rights in health professional practice. Proposed guidelines and institutional mechanisms. A project of the International Dual Loyalty Working Group. Physicians for Human Rights and University of Cape Town. Boston. Retrieved August 31, 2010, from http://physiciansforhumanrights.org/library/report-dualloyalty-2006.html

Sakoane, R. (2007). XDR-TB in South Africa: Back to TB sanatoria perhaps? *PLoS Medicine* 4(4), e160.

Santelli, J. S., Ott, M. A., Lyon, M., Rogers, J., Summers, D., & Schleifer, R. (2006). Abstinence and abstinence-only education: A review of U.S. policies and programs. *The Journal of Adolescent Health*, 38(1), 72–81.

Santelli, J. S. (2008). Medical accuracy in sexuality education: Ideology and the scientific process. *American Journal of Public Health*, 98(10), 1786–1792.

Schneider, H., & Fassin, D. (2002). Denial and defiance: A socio-political analysis of AIDS in South Africa. *AIDS*, 16(Suppl. 4), S45–S51.

Sen, A. (2004). Elements of a theory of human rights. *Philosophy and Public Affairs* 32/4

Singh, J. A. (2003). American physicians and dual loyalty obligations in the "war on terror." *British Medical Center Medical Ethics*, 4, E4.

Singh, J. A., Upshur, R., & Padayatchi, N. (2007). XDR-TB in South Africa: No time for denial or complacency. *PLoS Medicine*, 4(1), e50.

Starkman, N., & Rajani, N. (2002). The case for comprehensive sex education. *AIDS Patient Care STDS*, 16(7),313–8.

Stover, E., & Nightingale, E. O. (Eds.). (1985). *The breaking of bodies and minds.* New York: W.H. Freeman and Co.

Takala, T. (2001). What is wrong with global bioethics? On the limitations of the four principles approach. *Cambridge Quarterly of Healthcare Ethics*, 10, 72–77.

Trenholm, C., Devaney, B., Fortson, K., Clark, M., Bridgespan, L. Q., & Wheeler, J. (2008). Impacts of abstinence education on teen sexual activity, risk of pregnancy, and risk of sexually transmitted diseases. *Journal of Policy Analysis and Management*, 27(2), 255–276.

UN Office of the High Commissioner for Human Rights. (2004). *Manual on the effective investigation and documentation of torture and other cruel, inhuman or degrading treatment or punishment ("Istanbul Protocol")*. HR/P/PT/8/Rev.1, Retrieved December 19, 2009, from http://www.unhcr.org/refworld/docid/4638aca62.html

United Nations Educational, Scientific and Cultural Organization. (2005). Universal Declaration on Bioethics and Human Rights. Adopted by UNESCO's General Conference on 19 October 2005. Retrieved December 19, 2009, from http://portal.unesco.org/en/ev.php-URL_ID=31058&URL_DO=DO_TOPIC&URL_SECTION=201.html

U.S. Department of Justice, Office of Legal Counsel. Memorandum for John A. Rizzo, Senior Deputy General Counsel, CIA. May 10, 2005.

Von Mollendorff, T. (2009). Daring to care: A doctors' persecution in Mpumalanga. In K. Cullinan & A. Thom (Eds.), *The virus, vitamins, and vegetables: The South African HIV/AIDS mystery* (p. 82). Auckland Park: Jacana Media.

World Medical Association. (1956). *Regulations in times of armed conflict.* Adopted by the 10th World Medical Assembly, Havana, Cuba, October 1956, and Edited by the 11th World Medical Assembly, Istanbul, Turkey, October 1957, and Amended by the 35th World Medical Assembly, Venice, Italy, October 1983 and The WMA General Assembly, Tokyo 2004, and Editorially revised at the 173rd Council Session, Divonne-les-Bains, France, May 2006. Retrieved August 31, 2010, from http://www.wma.net/en/30publications/10policies/a20/index.html

World Medical Association. (1975). Declaration of Tokyo. Guidelines for Physicians Concerning Torture and other Cruel, Inhuman or Degrading Treatment or Punishment in Relation to Detention and Imprisonment. *Adopted by the 29th World Medical Assembly, Tokyo, Japan, October 1975, and editorially revised at the 170th Council Session, Divonne-les-Bains, France, May 2005 and the 173rd Council Session, Divonne-les-Bains, France, May 2006.* Retrieved August 31, 2010, from http://www.wma.net/en/20activities/10ethics/20tokyo/index.html

World Medical Association. (1985). *Statement on non-discrimination in professional membership and activities of physicians.* Adopted by the 37th World Medical Assembly, Brussels, Belgium, October 1985 and editorially revised with a name change at the 170th Council Session, Divonne-les-Bains, France, May 2005. Retrieved August 31, 2010, from http://www.wma.net/en/30publications/10policies/f10/index.html

ENDNOTES

[1]These tools draw substantively on the Siracusa Principles, which provide criteria by which to assess the compatibility of a rights limitation with a human rights framework. The principles were formulated at a meeting of experts in international law in Sirucusa and adopted by the UN Commission on Human Rights in 1984. UN Commission on Human Rights. (2009, December 30). The Siracusa Principles on the Limitation and Derogation Provisions in the International Covenant on Civil and Political Rights, 28 September 1984, E/CN.4/1985/4. Retrieved from http://www.unhcr.org/refworld/docid/4672bc122.html

[2]For examples of the application of such tools, see Gostin, L., Mann, J. M. (1994). Toward the development of a human rights impact assessment for the formulation and evaluation of public health policies. *Health and Human Rights, 1*(1),58–80; Heymann, S. J., Sell, R. L. (1999). Mandatory public health programs: To what standards should they be held? *Health and Human Rights, 4*(1),193–203; Mathews, S. (2006). Criminalizing deliberate HIV transmission—Is this good public health? *South African Medical Journal, 96*(4), 312–314; London, L. (2002). Human rights and public health: Dichotomies or synergies in developing countries? Examining the case of HIV in South Africa. *The Journal of Law Medicine & Ethics, 30*(4), 677–691.

CHAPTER 8

A Rights-Based Approach to Research: Assessing the Right to Water in Haiti

Margaret L. Satterthwaite and Amanda M. Klasing

INTRODUCTION

A human rights-based approach (RBA) to public health creates the space for partnerships between public health practitioners and human rights advocates by providing a shared framework and discourse from which to approach interventions and advocacy to improve public health. Employing the rights framework both in project design and implementation and in developing community health assessments and studies aimed at demonstrating the status of enjoyment of rights goes beyond ensuring that interaction at the community level respects human rights; it provides a framework for analyzing the role of multiple actors in the realization or violation of the human rights in question. This careful assessment of how relevant actors have an impact on human rights allows for accurate understandings of structural inadequacies in local systems and widens the frame from intervention to include advocacy and coordination of efforts among local and national government actors, international donors, and nongovernmental organizations (NGOs).

Thus, the strength of the RBA is twofold. First, it provides a methodology for practitioners to ensure that their own actions place the "rights holder," the individual, at the center of those interventions designed to improve access to rights. Placing the rights holder at the core of development ensures that the individual's voice is heard in the corridors of power that influence his or her human rights, including local and national government bodies, international agencies, and private organizations. Second, a rights framework provides a lens—that of international law—for understanding the status of the rights in question and for identifying which actors, the so-called duty bearers, are legally responsible in a given situation for advancing those rights.

This chapter presents an example of how to leverage these two strengths both to ensure that studies and interventions are themselves rights respecting and to design rights-based programs aimed at improving access to water in a sustainable way by bolstering the capacity of duty bearers to fulfill their obligations toward rights holders. The authors draw from the human rights report *Wòch Nan Soley: The Denial of the Right to Water in Haiti* and the underlying study on which the report was based to demonstrate how cross-disciplinary rights-based methodologies can be used in a community-based study to develop human rights advocacy aimed at changing the structures that lead to violations of the rights to water and health. The authors (who were the primary investigator [PI; Klasing] and faculty supervisor [Satterthwaite] for the study) also explore how traditional human rights and public health research methodologies can be united to collect and analyze community data in a way that it respects the human rights of participants of the study while also gathering data about the status of the rights in question.

THE RIGHT-TO-WATER STUDY IN PORT-DE-PAIX, HAITI

Under international human rights law, the fulfillment of the right to water requires that water be *available*, meaning that it should be sufficient for personal and household use; it must be of a *quality* that makes it safe and free from contaminants harmful to human health; and it must be physically and economically *accessible* to all without discrimination. Haiti has some of the worst water in the world, and its people struggle to realize their right to water. The United Nations Development Programme (UNDP) has ranked Haiti at 154th out of 177 countries for water, sanitation, and nutritional status (UNDP, 2006) and the Water Poverty Index, an index developed to express the links between household welfare and water availability, ranked Haiti at 147th place out of 147 countries (Lawrence, Meigh, & Sullivan, 2002, p. 11). In July 1998, the Inter-American Development Bank (IADB) approved $54 million in loans to the Haitian government for water and sanitation projects designed to improve potable water and sanitation services and to establish a regulatory framework for the development of wastewater services (IADB, 1998). The original loan contract documents identified two communities as recipients of first-year projects to improve potable water: Les Cayes and Port-de-Paix.

In a report assessing the predicted impact of the project in Port-de-Paix, the IADB projected overwhelmingly positive results in improving socioeconomic and health conditions in the community, including an anticipated reduction of gastrointestinal disease, a significant benefit to poverty reduction, up to a 90% decline in the cost of water to the poor, an increase in the availability of potable water, and a reduction of time required to collect water. In short, the IADB identified the most "evident" impact of the project to be "an overall improvement in the quality of life" caused by the "reasonable access to affordable supplies of good quality drinking water" (IADB, 1997, p. 19).

Unfortunately, after approval of the loan, the IADB withheld its disbursement, and those of other social sector loans for health, roads, and education because of the pressure from the U.S. government, which acted based on its views of the political situation in Haiti. Disturbed by the obvious public health impacts of the blocking of these loans, Zanmi Lasante, a sister organization based in Haiti of Partners In Health, began advocating for the disbursal of the loans, viewing this work as an important complement to its daily provision of health care to the poor in Haiti. Soon, Zanmi Lasante joined forces with Partners In Health as well as the Robert F. Kennedy Center for Justice & Human Rights and the New York University Center for Human Rights and Global Justice to demand accountability for the human rights impact that the withholding of the loans had on the people of Haiti. To continue their advocacy, the organizations recognized that data concerning the status of the right to water would provide ammunition in their advocacy but found that relevant data did not exist. A study was designed to collect data on the human rights impact—specifically on the right to water and directly related rights, such as the right to health, life, and education—of the lack of ready access to potable water in Port-de-Paix, because without money from the loans, the water project in Port-de-Paix could not begin. The study incorporated a rights-based framework into its design and implementation, meaning that it was intended to fully respect the rights of those in the community where the study was conducted.

No model existed for the study in Port-de-Paix, because the data sought was rights-based data—data that would go beyond traditional potable water indicators by providing both information about the status of the rights in question and the corresponding obligations of the state and other actors. To guarantee, the study could adequately demonstrate the responsibility of states involved in the decision to block the IADB loans and the resulting impact on human rights in the community, analysis of the data had to be firmly grounded in the legal obligations and duties set out in human rights law. Further, through robust legal analysis, the data could illustrate the nexus between violations of the human right to water and other human rights, particularly the right to health. The study also followed an RBA in its implementation, through which the partner organizations actively sought to encourage participation of community members to aid in capacity building and to increase awareness about the right to water.

Study Design and Methodology

The study was primarily designed by lawyers to support a legal analysis of the violation of the right to water and other related rights because of acts or omissions of relevant duty bearers. Public health professionals, medical doctors, and medical anthropologists provided assistance with randomization techniques, and survey design and modeling; however, the legal team, with a law student with social scientific training as the PI, relied on legal norms to develop the research instruments. Close collaboration between the legal team and a Haitian bioethicist encouraged the development of innovative ways to ensure the study itself was rights respecting.

The study combined qualitative and quantitative methodologies for data collection. Each research instrument for the study was designed to elucidate the extent to which the people of Port-de-Paix could access their right to water, and the ways that the duty bearers were or were not shouldering their obligations related to the right to water and associated rights. The main quantitative data was gathered through a survey of households chosen by probability randomization techniques. The survey data was augmented by quantitative and qualitative data drawn from in-depth medical interviews with a second set of randomly chosen households to further investigate the incidence of waterborne illness. Focus groups were conducted with key informants familiar with the water systems in Port-de-Paix. In addition, participant observation and informal interviews provided important context for the qualitative data. Lastly, to gather information about one of the most important aspects of the right to water—water quality—samples of water from different sources in the city were tested for chemical and bacterial contamination and pH levels. Additional contextual data was collected through traditional human rights methodologies, including a Freedom of Information Act lawsuit that dislodged documents concerning the blocking of the IDB loans, interviews with government officials, and desktop research concerning the legal, regulatory, and physical infrastructure in place in Haiti relevant to the right to water.[1]

Legal Accuracy and the Identification of Duty Bearers

One of the key advantages of the RBA is that it allows researchers and advocates to design recommendations responsive to their findings that are based on a solid legal foundation. Public health professionals, like their human rights counterparts, should be comfortable conversing in and situating the right to health and related rights, such as the right to water, within the appropriate legal framework so that they can effectively partner with—and/or call on—the appropriate actors to make the changes needed to achieve rights fulfillment. Human rights law is derived from multiple sources, including domestic law, international and regional human rights treaties, and customary international law. Under this legal framework, the state is the primary guarantor of human rights, which is why the state is considered the main duty bearer in any rights-based study or intervention. This means that the state has the duty to ensure the protection and realization of human rights for persons within its territory or under its jurisdiction. The nature of this duty can be understood in three parts: the responsibility to respect, the responsibility to protect, and the responsibility to fulfill. States have the obligation to respect human rights—that is, to refrain from directly interfering in the enjoyment of human rights; to protect—that is, to prevent third parties (including other states, private companies, and NGOs) from interfering in the enjoyment of human rights; and to fulfill—that is, to take steps to ensure the realization of human rights for all, including through direct provision of services where individuals or communities cannot access their rights in other ways.

The legal strength of the RBA emanates from the accurate identification of appropriate duty bearers who can be called on to take concrete steps to improve rights. What this means in practical terms for public health research is that studies should be designed to focus on the fundamental human rights guaranteed to individuals and to identify which actors—under international law and given the factual circumstances at play in a given situation—have corresponding obligations to ensure access to those rights. Although local and national governments will always remain the primary duty bearers, in the context of highly indebted poor countries, the relevant duty bearers will often also include elements of the international community that are engaged in on-the-ground work or in the funding of relevant services.

Studies using the RBA should identify all powerful actors, including international agencies and NGOs, which may have taken on roles similar to those traditionally played by the government, for instance the delivery of basic health care, water, or food. Analyzing the activities of those powerful actors under human rights law will often bring to light important capacity gaps on the part of the relevant duty bearers responsible for protecting human rights, such as the common inability of local or national government agencies to regulate or coordinate the work of NGOs, donors, or the private sector. Such capacity gaps deprive the state, as primary duty bearer, of the abilities it needs to protect and fulfill rights, which can lead to aid dependency and lack of democratic control over the infrastructure needed to fulfill basic rights. Studies that take these complex interactions into consideration will help ensure that interventions to improve access to rights not only provide direct services to communities but also contribute to the capacity of the primary duty bearer—the state—to fulfill those rights in the end.

A rights-based study may need to take on a mixed methodology approach to accurately collect the data necessary to analyze relationships among rights holders and various duty bearers. For example, in the Port-de-Paix study, researchers used the household study and medical interviews to determine the status of the right to water and its impact on health. Focus groups, informant interviews, a lawsuit, and desktop research on laws and regulations were used to identify the relevant duty bearers, capacity gaps, and powerful actors impacting the right to water. A complete understanding of these relationships helped researchers formulate legally accurate recommendations that spoke to the lived reality of rights holders and to identify advocacy targets.

RIGHTS-RESPECTING STUDY DESIGN

In addition to using the human rights framework as a lens to design studies aimed at elucidating the status of rights fulfillment and the obligations of duty bearers, the RBA should be used to ensure that public health studies, assessments, and interventions are themselves rights respecting. This can be done through the adoption of several RBA principles: empowerment, indivisibility and interdependence, nondiscrimination and attention to vulnerable groups, accountability, and participation. In the next section, the authors briefly discuss how the Port-de-Paix study was designed both to be rights respecting and to gather relevant data to demonstrate the status of the right to water.

Empowerment

The principle of empowerment requires that studies and interventions operate from the recognition that individuals are entitled to enjoy their fundamental human rights. This means that public health researchers and service providers should treat beneficiaries of programming as rights holders rather than recipients of charity. In the Port-de-Paix study, empowerment was addressed in two ways. First, legal research and key informant interviews were designed to assess whether community members were able to access water *as a right*—that is, whether the right to water was protected by law, regulation, and government practice. The results of this assessment were included in the study report. Second, the PI and enumerators worked to empower community members as they implemented the study, educating participants about their rights as participants and about the purpose of the study, as well as providing education to the larger community advocacy goals of the project and the human right to water.

Indivisibility and Interdependence

The principle of indivisibility and interdependence recognizes that all human rights—from civil and political to economic, social, and cultural— are interrelated and that the fulfillment of one right is dependent on the fulfillment of other rights. Further, the denial or violation of one right will have an impact on the enjoyment of other rights. In the case of the right to water, this principle is particularly clear, as water is not only an independent right, but also a necessary component to the realization of many other rights, including the rights to health, to an adequate standard of living, to life, to food, and even to education. In the Port-de-Paix study, researchers sought not only to demonstrate the status of the right to water, but also to reveal the status of interrelated rights, especially the right to health. Data on the interrelated rights was gathered through the household survey and in-depth medical interviews. Researchers worked to ensure that the study respected the interrelated nature of rights by avoiding the artificial separation of results about water from those concerning health.

Nondiscrimination and Attention to Vulnerable Groups

The principle of nondiscrimination is one of the cornerstones of the human rights framework, requiring that public health studies and interventions uncover and address vulnerabilities and incapacities caused by different forms of discrimination. The Port-de-Paix study design sought to both ensure that vulnerable groups had access to participation in the study and that the data collected would address the diverse experiences of community members in accessing the right to water. To make certain that all in the community had a fair opportunity to participate in the household study, investigators employed a complex randomization process that used global positioning system (GPS) waypoints to guarantee that all households within the community had a roughly equal chance to share their experience through the survey. In addition, focus group discussions were divided up both by age and gender, allowing investigators to explore the variable ways in which men, women, boys, and girls have or lack access to the right to water. Some questions in the household survey and in-depth medical interviews also sought to elucidate whether there were discriminatory impacts of the denial of the right to water in Port-de-Paix. Study results demonstrated, for example, that women and girls shoulder a disproportionate share of the responsibility for collection of water.

Accountability

The principle of accountability obliges public health researchers and practitioners to identify the relationships of accountability that should exist between duty bearers and rights holders and to design interventions aimed at strengthening those relationships. As explored earlier, this means analyzing the legal standards that apply to various duty bearers and collecting data to identify where accountability breaks down. In the Port-de-Paix study, the household survey, focus groups, and informant interviews sought information about which actors were responsible for blocking or furthering access to potable water. The legal analysis then placed these relationships into the framework of international human rights law, allowing the final report to make recommendations concerning which duty bearers should take on different roles in respecting, protecting, and fulfilling the right to water.

Another element of accountability was the relationship of accountability the researchers sought to construct between study participants and investigators. This relationship was fostered in part through transparency—the study team made known its objectives through community meetings and publicly available information about the study—and in part through individual interactions with participants. With respect to the latter, informed consent procedures were key. For example, the study team altered the standard informed consent protocol by providing an explanation of the purpose of the study that addressed the participants as rights holders. At the suggestion of community members, the team also adapted the traditional consent form to create a kind of "contract" that both the participant and the investigator signed, with a copy to be kept by each party; the accountability of the researchers were stressed through the provision of this form to the participants alongside the investigators' contact information.

Participation

Active, free, and meaningful participation of individuals is central to the human rights framework and essential to the RBA. In relation to public health interventions, the principle requires that communities be involved in the entire life cycle of a project—from needs assessment to implementation and evaluation. The Port-de-Paix study included questions in the household survey designed to elicit information about opportunities for community members to participate in decisions concerning the water system—opportunities that are required to ensure compliance with the right to water. The study was also designed with significant participation from community members, whose views were sought through informal discussions, pilot focus groups, and community meetings. Participation was emphasized in the preparation of the report's recommendations as well: recommendations were, in part, based on community members' own suggestions, solicited through targeted focus groups commenting on preliminary findings of the study.

STUDY RESULTS AND OUTCOMES

The study yielded unsurprisingly dismal results concerning the quality, quantity, and accessibility of water in Port-de-Paix. In the years waiting for the IADB loans to be disbursed and the water system project to be implemented, the public water system in Port-de-Paix had collapsed. To meet their water needs, households in Port-de-Paix rely heavily on water provided by private vendors who pump water from the same water table as the heavily polluted Trois Rivières river into tanker trucks that distribute water throughout the community. Purchasing water from these private vendors is prohibitively expensive for many families, with almost 87% of the families surveyed indicating that there are times when the household cannot afford water. When families cannot afford to purchase water, they collect it directly from usually polluted rivers and streams. When households can afford water, it is often contaminated, as private vendors do not treat water as a matter of practice. Water testing conducted during the study confirmed this with 14 out of 19 samples tested from various sites testing positive for coliform bacteria. The state of the water system in Port-de-Paix has measurable impacts on the population and their associated human rights, including the right to health. In-depth medical interviews uncovered a recent case of typhoid in 15% of households interviewed.

The results of the study demonstrate that the water in Port-de-Paix is inadequate to meet the basic daily needs of the population, but because the study employed a rights-based methodology, investigators could determine that the situation in Port-de-Paix also represented a case of unfulfilled human rights. Demanding that duty bearers fulfill their rights obligations requires a heightened legitimacy in fact-finding gained via the implementation of a rigorous methodology. The results gathered in the study completed years of legal and factual research on the failure of the international community—and especially the IADB and the U.S. government—to fulfill its human rights obligations regarding the people of Haiti. The four partner organizations responsible for the study launched a report in summer 2008 that included the key findings of their research, including the results of the study, and called for accountability for the acts that led to the denial of the right to water. The report became an important advocacy tool in advancing the economic, social, and cultural rights of Haitians.

The release of the report opened up dialogue with the IADB, which had previously shut down constructive communication with these organizations in the years since it had taken action to block the loans. The IADB, faced with the facts that its actions had real consequences for the human rights of the people of Haiti, began cooperating with the advocacy organizations to move the water projects in question forward. The report also piqued the interest of members of the U.S. Congress, leading to the possibility of further investigations into the United States' role in blocking the loans. In addition, agencies of the United States, including United States Agency for International Development (USAID) and the Department of State, have engaged with the authors of the report concerning the United States' obligations in Haiti and the Department of State's views on the RBA to development.

The report has also served as an important coalition-building tool. The organizations have shared the report more widely with the human rights advocacy community as an example of rigorous documentation of violations of economic, social, and cultural rights. At the 5th World Water Forum in Istanbul, Turkey, the organizations shared the report with representatives of leading private and international organizations focused on water, including several agencies of the United Nations. Individual authors have presented the report to numerous grassroots and university human rights organizations to synergize support for the fulfillment of economic, social, and cultural rights generally, and the right to water in Haiti specifically.

The results of a rights-based study alone will not ensure the fulfillment of human rights; however, as the right to water study demonstrates, employing an RBA can create opportunities for important advocacy to address the human rights issues covered by a study. A rights-based study does not end with an analysis of the results, but can serve as a catalyst for advocacy to change the human rights situation reflected in the study results.

CONCLUSION

An RBA to community health assessments and public health research, including studies concerning access to potable water, offers several important advantages by providing a framework for analyzing the role of multiple actors in the realization and violation of the right and for assessing structural inadequacies in relevant local systems. Further, an RBA grounded in a strong legal analysis provides the data and discourse necessary to widen the frame from ensuring that program implementation is rights respecting to ensuring that intervention efforts contribute to the capacity of local, national, and international duty bearers to fulfill their human rights obligations. In this way, the RBA helps transform short-term responses into durable solutions. Most importantly, by ensuring that public health studies and assessments are rights respecting, practitioners take steps to promote the entitlements of rights holders in question and not act in a manner that would frustrate rights holders' access to their fundamental human rights.

REFERENCES

Inter-American Development Bank. (1997, July). *Potable water and sanitation sector reform and investment program environmental assessment annex II* (IDB Document No. HA-0014/ENV-SUM A-II). Retrieved August 4, 2010, from http://idbdocs.iadb.org/wsdocs/getdocument.aspx?docnum=454841

Inter-American Development Bank. (1998, August 12). *Potable water and sanitation sector reform and investment program* (IDB Document No. 1010/SF-HA). Retrieved September 7, 2010, from http://www.unhchr.ch/tbs/doc.nsf/0/3d02758c707031d58025677f003b73b9

Lawrence, P., Meigh, J., & Sullivan, C. (2002). The water poverty index: An international comparison. *Keele Economic Research Papers, 2002/19*. Keele, UK: Keele University.

United Nations Development Programme. (2006). *Human development report 2006: Beyond scarcity: Power, poverty and the global water crisis*. New York: Author.

OTHER RESOURCES

New York University School of Law Center for Human Rights & Global Justice, Partners in Health, Robert F. Kennedy Center for Justice & Human Rights, & Zanmi Lasante. (2008). Wòch Nan Soley: The denial of the right to water in Haiti. Retrieved September 7, 2010, from http://www.chrgj.org/projects/docs/wochnansoley.pdf

United Nations Committee on Economic, Social and Cultural Rights. (2002). *General comment no. 15: The right to water* (U.N. Doc. E/C.12/2002/11). Retrieved September 7, 2010, from http://www.unhchr.ch/tbs/doc.nsf/0/3d02 758c707031d58025677f003b73b9

Varma, M. K., Satterthwaite, M. L., Klasing, A. M., Shoranick, T., Jean, J., Barry, D., et al. (2009). Wòch nan Soley: The denial of the right to water in Haiti. *10 HEALTH & HUM. RTS. 67.* Retrieved September 7, 2010, from http://www .hhrjournal.org/index.php/hhr/article/view/82/152

NOTES

[1]For study results, see Center for Human Rights and Global Justice. (2008). Robert F. Kennedy Memorial Center for Human Rights, Partners In Health, and Zanmi Lasante *Wòch Nan Soley: The denial of the right to water in Haiti.* Retrieved from http://www.chrgj.org/projects/docs/wochnansoley.pdf; and http://parthealth.3cdn.net/0badc680352663967e_v6m6b1ayx.pdf

CHAPTER 9

Using the Right to Food to Teach Human Rights

George Kent

INTRODUCTION

Teaching about the human right to health or food or anything else could be done by working through the basic international human rights treaties and trying to unravel their meaning. This is difficult because there is consensus on some elements and not on others, so their meaning is unclear. Moreover (as discussed in chapter 6), those agreements state broad principles and leave it to individual governments to make the rights more concrete in their national laws. Not only the law but also much of the literature on rights is remote and abstract. This chapter will explore the core meaning of *rights*, using the right to food as an illustration. What is the meaning of the right to something . . . whatever that something might be?

KEY ELEMENTS OF RIGHTS SYSTEMS

People sometimes use the word *rights* as shorthand for *human rights*. That is unfortunate because there are many different kinds of rights: property rights, contract rights, consumer rights, and so forth. A hospital may have a patients' bill of rights, and prisoners may have their own rights. Rights may be established by a local institution, a local government, or a national government. Organizations of many different kinds set out rights for their members. Local rights apply only in particular jurisdictions, and do not necessarily involve international agencies or national governments, so they are not *human* rights.

Rights-based social systems can be conceptualized as a generic abstract form. The core elements of such systems are not plainly articulated in the literature on rights. In my view, in any well-developed rights system, there are three major roles to be fulfilled: the rights holders, the duty bearers, and the agents of accountability. The task of the agents of accountability is to make sure that those who have the duties carry out their obligations to those who have the rights. Thus, to describe or design a rights system, we need to know the following:

A. The nature of the rights holders and their rights;
B. The nature of the duty bearers and their obligations (duties) corresponding to the rights of the rights holders; and
C. The nature of the agents of accountability, and the procedures through which they ensure that the duty bearers meet their obligations to the rights holders. The accountability mechanisms include, in particular, the remedies available to the rights holders themselves.

Rights imply entitlements, which are claims to specific goods or services. Rights are, or are supposed to be, *enforceable* claims. There must be some sort of institutional authority to which rights holders whose claims are not satisfied can appeal to have the situation corrected. Enforceability means that the duty bearers, those who are to fulfill entitlements, must be obligated to do so, and they must be held accountable for their performance.

If we agree that these ABCs are the key elements of rights systems, we can highlight these dimensions when exploring or assessing any concrete example. For example, we could study traditional rights system based on local culture to see how they identify the rights, duties, and accountability. Doing this would make it clear that rights involve much more than just norms or codes of ethics. Rights imply the existence of specific types of institutional arrangements.

The international human rights system, based on a series of international agreements, is one concrete manifestation of rights-based social systems. The term *human rights* is reserved for those rights that are universal and relate to human dignity. In principle, if one has a human right, one can make a claim that the government and others must do or desist from doing specific things to further human dignity. Human rights, by definition, are universal.

Although human rights are universal, they do allow latitude for differing interpretations, depending on local circumstances. They are mainly, but not exclusively, about the obligations of national governments to people living under their jurisdictions, as spelled out in international human rights law. All the international human rights agreements are available at the Website of the Office of the High Commissioner for Human Rights, at http://www.ohchr.org/EN/Pages/WelcomePage.aspx.

THE HUMAN RIGHT TO ADEQUATE FOOD

The human right to adequate food has come into focus at the global level through a steady decades-long process. It was articulated as early as 1963, when a Special Assembly on Man's Right to Freedom From Hunger met in Rome, and it has been mentioned at many subsequent global food conferences. As in other meetings, in November 1996, the World Food Summit concluded with the declaration supporting "the right to adequate food and the fundamental right of everyone to be free from hunger" (Food and Agriculture Organization of the United Nations [FAO], 1996, para. 1).

Up that point, talk about the right to food was mainly rhetorical, a nice flourish in global conferences, but little was said about what it implied. The 1996 summit was different, however, because its concluding *Plan of Action*, Objective 7.4 called upon:

> the UN High Commissioner for Human Rights, in consultation with relevant treaty bodies, and in collaboration with relevant special ized agencies and programmes of the UN system and appropriate inter-governmental mechanisms, to better define the rights related to food in Article 11 of the Covenant and to propose ways to implement and realize these rights. (FAO, 1996)

Several initiatives were taken to respond to this call, including supportive resolutions from the Commission on Human Rights; a Day of Discussion on Right to Food held by the UN Committee on Economic, Social and Cultural Rights; and Expert Consultations on the human right to adequate food held in Geneva, Rome, and Bonn. In April 1999, the United Nations System Standing Committee on Nutrition (then known as the United Nations Administrative Committee on Coordination/Sub-Committee on Nutrition) focused its annual meeting on the human right to adequate food.

In May 1999, the UN Committee on Economic, Social and Cultural Rights released its landmark *General Comment 12* on *The Right to Adequate*

Food (United Nations Economic and Social Council, 1999). It provides the most authoritative explanation of the sources the meaning of the human right to adequate food. Paragraph 6 presents the core definition:

> The right to adequate food is realized when every man, woman and child, alone or in community with others, has physical and economic access at all times to adequate food or means for its procurement.

The human right to adequate food in international human rights law arises in the context of the broader human right to an adequate standard of living. Article 25, paragraph 1 of the *Universal Declaration of Human Rights* of 1948 says:

> Everyone has the right to a standard of living adequate for the health and well-being of himself and of his family, including food, clothing, housing and medical care and necessary social services, and the right to security in the event of unemployment, sickness, disability, widowhood, old age or other lack of livelihood in circumstances beyond his control.

In the *International Covenant on Civil and Political Rights*, which came into force in 1976, the first article says, "In no case may a people be deprived of its own means of subsistence." In addition, Article 6 says, "Every human being has the inherent right to life." This clearly implies the right to adequate food and other necessities for sustaining life.

The right to an adequate standard of living was elaborated in Article 11 of the *International Covenant on Economic, Social and Cultural Rights*. Its first paragraph says:

> The States Parties to the present Covenant recognize the right of everyone to an adequate standard of living for himself and his family, including adequate food, clothing and housing, and to the continuous improvement of living conditions.

The article is explicit about food, clothing, and housing, but it also implies the right to other requirements that are addressed in other parts of the covenant and other human rights instruments. There is now a substantial literature on the human rights to health, education, housing, and other issues relating to an adequate standard of living. Food constitutes just one of the dimensions of adequate livelihood. It would be inappropriate to argue that it is more important than, say, housing or education. All aspects of livelihood should be kept in balance.

Thus, there is increasing recognition that adequate food is a human right under international human rights law. That right is discussed in General Comment 12 and many other documents (Eide, 1989; Eide, 1995; Eide & Kracht, 2005; FAO, 2005; Kent, 2005; 2008). A major landmark in the global effort to advance the right was the publication by the FAO of its five-volume *Methodological Toolbox on the Right to Food* in 2009:

1. Guide on Legislating for the Right to Food
2. Methods to Monitor the Human Right to Adequate Food (vols. I and II)
3. Guide to Conducting a Right to Food Assessment
4. Right to Food Curriculum Outline
5. Budget work to advance the right to food

The entire set can be accessed through http://www.fao.org/righttofood/publi_02_en.htm

OTHER RIGHTS TO FOOD

People can have rights to food in a local school, hospital, or prison that are not based on the human right to adequate food as formulated in international agreements. If everyone at a particular school agreed that all students should be entitled to, say, a piece of candy with every meal, and made arrangements to enforce that right, then that would become a right at that school. That would be a locally established right, and not a human right.

The U.S. government is one of the few in the world that opposes the idea of a human right to adequate food, based mainly on its long-standing opposition to the concept of economic rights (Kent, 2005, pp. 156–162). Nevertheless, within the United States, the Supplemental Nutrition Assistance Program (formerly known as the Food Stamps program); the school meals program, and the Special Supplemental Nutrition Program for Women, Infants, and Children (commonly known as the WIC program) establish clear entitlements for people who meet the programs' criteria for eligibility. They also have mechanisms of accountability, such as the Fair Hearings available to those who feel they are not getting what they are supposed to get. Thus we can say that in the United States there are rights to food, but these are not based on international human rights agreements.

Similarly, in India, there is a strong right to food law, but it was established based on national law, not the international law relating to the human right to adequate food (Kent, 2005, pp. 143–150). When the

Supreme Court of India specifies the entitlements of children to mid-day meals in detail, including minimum levels of calories and protein, this is based on national law, not international human rights law. Details on the right to food in India may be found at the Right to Food Campaign Website (http://www.righttofoodindia.org/index.html).

Often, the distinction between the universal right to food based on international agreements and rights of purely local origin is blurred because there is room for interpretation of international law. In addition, social service programs may be described as implementing international human rights even though they actually have local origins.

HUMAN RIGHTS AND HUMAN DIGNITY

Discussions of the human right to adequate food in terms of international human rights law and national law might suggest that rights come from above. However, there is a different perspective, described by a nongovernmental organization called *EqualinRights*:

> Equalinrights moves from an understanding that human rights are tools to protect human dignity, as defined by people themselves from within local social and cultural contexts. This means that local dialogue on the meaning, relevance and application of human rights-based strategies within these different contexts is a critical starting point. Human rights come from within, not from without. So for us, our support is about facilitating the internal learning and self-empowering process for people. Applied in this way, we believe that human rights can be a very powerful framework for bringing change to unequal power structures and relationships that perpetuate poverty. (Equalinrights, 2007)

The human rights that are set out in international law do not originate there. Rather, that law codifies rights claims that come up from a widespread moral consensus among ordinary people. Thus, local rights-based programs ought to be based at least in part on interpretations and assertions of rights that begin at the local level. They should include strong local components, with local people engaged as active participants not only in the implementation but also in the design of such programs.

Although the ABCs are the core of all rights-based social systems, *human* rights should not be interpreted in a mechanical way. They are not simply about the delivery of goods and services. Human rights should be based on clear recognition of and respect for human dignity.

Having rights enables us to "stand up like men," to look others in the eye, and to feel in some fundamental way the equal of anyone. To think of oneself as the holder of rights is not to be unduly but properly proud, to have that minimal self-respect that is necessary to be worthy of the love and esteem of others. Indeed, respect for persons . . . may simply be respect for their rights, so that there cannot be the one without the other. (Feinberg 1980, p. 151)

DIGNITY AND THE HUMAN RIGHT TO FOOD

The human right to food should not be understood simply as a matter of delivering specific quantities of nutrients to passive rights holders. Merely fulfilling individuals' biological nutritional needs through authoritarian measures is very different from fulfilling their human right to food. If people have no chance to influence what and how they are being fed, if they are fed prepackaged rations or capsules or are fed from a trough, their right to adequate food is not being met, even if they get all the nutrients their bodies need. Serving pork to a Muslim prisoner would violate his human rights, even if it contains the nutrients he needs.

The preamble of the Universal Declaration of Human Rights of 1948, the foundation document of the modern human rights system, begins by saying "recognition of the inherent dignity and of the equal and inalienable rights of all members of the human family is the foundation of freedom, justice and peace in the world . . ." The first article of the declaration begins by affirming, "All human beings are born free and equal in dignity and rights."

In the realms of nutrition and health, human rights are mainly about upholding human dignity, not about meeting physiological needs. Dignity does not come from being fed. It comes from providing for oneself. In any well-structured society, the objective should be to move toward conditions under which all people can provide for themselves. Strengthening dignity is understood to be a major objective of all human rights.

This understanding should influence the choice of means by which the right to food should be realized. People commonly ask how it will be possible to feed future generations. The question is deeply insulting. Why ask how people are to be fed, as if this had to be done by some external agent? Most people are motivated to provide for themselves, and only need decent opportunities to do that. Why is it that most people can be valued as competent persons, whereas the hungry are regarded as little more than passive gaping mouths? Who, when not deprived of the means, would not feed themselves (Kent, 1984, p. 148)?

International agencies often treat the hunger problem through large-scale interventions based on specially formulated foods brought in from the outside. They are sometimes criticized for taking a medical approach to the problems. That is inaccurate, because doctors generally talk with their patients. Theirs is actually more of a veterinary approach, with the beneficiaries not consulted at all, as if they were livestock in a feedlot.

The hunger problem is frequently addressed by the powerful in terms that are inherently humiliating. The issue needs to be handled not as one would approach livestock management, but rather as a partnership, based on genuine concern for the well-being of those who are hungry, and direct engagement with them.

One of the major critiques of humanitarian assistance programs has been that "Aid processes treat lives to be saved as bare life, not as lives with a political voice" (Edkins, 2000, xvi). One can ensure that people are treated like dignified human beings, rather than like animals on a feedlot, by their having some say on how they are being treated. This is why, in a human rights system, the people must have institutionalized remedies available to them that they can call on if they feel they are not being treated properly. There must be some meaningful action they can take if they feel their rights are not being acknowledged.

Just as the human right to adequate food must be seen in the context of the right to adequate livelihood, that cluster of rights, in turn, must be viewed in the broader context of all human rights. This refers not only to the quality of relationships between individuals and their governments but also to the quality of their relationships with one another. People must be recognized as social beings with the need and the right to share in determining not only their individual futures but also the futures of their communities.

At one level, human rights may appear to be individualistic, but the basis of the realization of individual human rights is the quality of our social relationships (Fields, 2003). Democracy is required for the realization of the human right to adequate food and all other human rights. A democratic social order is one in which individuals can play an active role in shaping the conditions under which they live.

USING THE RIGHT TO FOOD TO TEACH HUMAN RIGHTS

Teaching about rights should be done in a way that respects the learners' dignity, and does not treat them simply as passive containers to be filled with treaty law and court cases from distant places. There are ways to teach about rights through active engagement with rights-based systems in the local community. As illustrated in the following paragraphs, teaching/learning about rights in general and human rights in particular can be done through activities centered on the right to food.

Students can be actively engaged in creative rights work in many ways. For example, they could be asked to design a local food safety system that is based on the concept that ordinary people have specific rights to safe food; and that, if they suspect food is unsafe, they have clearly defined arrangements through which they can submit complaints (Rongguang & Kent, 2004).

Alternatively, in a local school meals program, students, teachers, and school administrators could work out rights that should to be applied in that program, and design arrangements to implement it.

Traditionally, well-meaning adults provide school meals to silent students who accept whatever is offered to them. The students are not encouraged to ask why they get what they get. The task of the rights approach to school meals would be to overcome the culture of silence, and to empower students by helping them to find their voice. Thus, establishing school meals as entitlements would apply the insight of the late Brazilian educator, Paulo Freire, to meal programs. Freire criticized schooling in which education "becomes an act of depositing, in which the students are the depositories and the teacher is the depositor" (Freire, 1993, p. 164; Kent, 1988). There is a striking analogy between this conventional "banking" education, designed only to fill passive students with information, and conventional feeding programs that are designed only to fill passive students with food.

School meals programs can be used to combine the best elements of human rights and critical pedagogy, in a setting in which "students and teachers struggle to make new meaning and develop cultural practices that are critical, transformative, and liberatory" (Leistyna & Woodrum, 1996, p. 5). Students' active, hands-on engagement with their schools' meal programs could turn out to have high educational value.

The discussion about what rights ought to be set in place could provide an important "teaching moment" for learning about nutrition and also about rules, guidelines, and laws that apply to the particular school. Students could learn how to make their voices count. They could learn about what rights contribute to enhancing human dignity.

In a rights-based school meals program, the duty bearers would include a broad range of people including cooks, servers, cleaners, the school principal, and government agencies that fund and oversee the school meals programs. Their duties should be plainly specified: who is to do what to ensure that the rights are realized?

Some people might assume that school feeding is intended primarily for children from poor families, but it is important to ensure quality school meals for all students. School meals are not necessarily free meals, just as the right to food in general does not necessarily mean free food. Where school meals are subsidized, there should be a discussion of who should subsidize it, and for how long, and why. There is a need for clarity on how outsiders are to support school meals programs not only in terms of money or food but also in terms of other kinds of support services such as technical advice. These issues should be discussed by all who are affected.

In many school meals programs, students passively accept the food they get. Some students may offer suggestions or complain from time to time, but they soon learn that their views have little impact. They may find that they don't get their meals, or meals of the quality they expect, but often they find there is not much they can do about it. Although these difficulties can never be totally eliminated, they will be reduced if school meals are organized as rights-based programs.

The content of rights would need to be plainly articulated. These rights could come to a school through its own creation, from subnational or national governments, or from human rights. Whether particular rights make sense (such as having each child entitled to a piece of candy at each meal) is entirely different from the question of whether there is an effective rights-based system in place to ensure that rights are realized.

The key to making the system truly rights based would be the mechanisms of accountability. The arrangements could be quite simple. For example, one parent or teacher could be appointed as the school meals ombudsman, responsible for taking complaints and passing them on to appropriate authorities. Or a small committee could be formed in each school to take complaints.

Older students could be involved not only in using rights-based school meals programs but also in designing, operating, and assessing them. Students could help to formulate the programs' rules of procedure, developing them incrementally over time. If they are well engaged in this process, and the teaching program supports it, students should be able to see that the principles of rights-based programming can be applied in the larger society outside their schools.

CONCLUSION

If students are treated liked potted plants, they will act like potted plants. Whether dealing with information or with food, students should be encouraged to become more critically involved as they mature. School meal programs provide an opportunity to support active engagement of students in helping to shape the world in which they live. Such programs could become an important point of entry for a liberating education for students, and, through that, for the culture as a whole. Students who learn to stand up for their rights in relation to school meals are more likely to stand up in the larger world.

Creating and living with rights and reflecting on how they work and fail to work would help students to grasp the deeper meaning of rights locally and in the larger world. If they learn to stand up for their local rights, they are then more likely to stand up in the world. In addition, even if they do not use the term, they would learn about dignity.

REFERENCES

Edkins, J. (2000). *Whose hunger? Concepts of famine, practices of aid.* Minneapolis: University of Minnesota Press.

Eide, A. (1989). *Right to adequate food as a human right.* New York: United Nations, Human Rights Study Series No. 1, Sales No. E.89.XIV.2.

Eide, A. (1995). The right to an adequate standard of living including the right to food. In A. Eide, C. Krause, & A. Rosas (Eds.), *Economic, social and cultural rights: A textbook.* Dordrecht, The Netherlands: Martinus Nijhoff.

Eide, W. B. & Kracht, U. (Eds.). (2005). Food and human rights in development (vols. I and II). *Legal and institutional dimensions and selected topics.* Antwerp, Belgium: Intersentia.

Equalinrights. (2007). *What is the human rights-based approach to development?* Retrieved August 31, 2010, from http://www.equalinrights.org/content/hrba_approach.html

Feinberg, J. (1980). *Rights, justice, and the bounds of liberty.* Princeton, NJ: Princeton University Press.

Fields, A. B. (2003). *Rethinking human rights for the new millennium.* New York: Palgrave Macmillan.

Food and Agriculture Organization of the United Nations. (1996). *Rome declaration on World Food Security and World Food Summit Plan of Action.* Rome: Author. Retrieved August 31, 2010, from http://www.fao.org/wfs/final/rd-e.htm

Food and Agriculture Organization of the United Nations. (2005). *Voluntary guidelines to support the progressive realization of the right to adequate food in the context of National Food Security.* Rome: Author. Retrieved August 31, 2010, from http://www.fao.org/docrep/meeting/009/y9825e/y9825e00.htm

Freire, P. (1993). *Pedagogy of the oppressed.* New revised 20th-anniversary edition. New York: Continuum.

Kent, G. (1984). *The political economy of hunger: The silent holocaust.* New York: Praeger.

Kent, G. (1988). Nutrition education as an instrument of empowerment. *Journal of Nutrition Education, 20*(4), 193–195. Retrieved August 31, 2010, from http://www2.hawaii.edu/~kent/NutEdGK.pdf

Kent, G. (2005). *Freedom from want: The human right to adequate food.* Washington, DC: Georgetown University Press.

Kent, G. (Ed.). (2008). *Global obligations for the right to food.* Lanham, MD: Rowman & Littlefield.

Leistyna, P., & Woodrum, A. (1996). Context and culture: What is critical pedagogy? In P. Leistyna, A. Woodrum, & S. A. Sherblom (Eds.), *Breaking free: The transformative power of critical pedagogy.* Cambridge, MA: Harvard Educational Review.

Rongguang, Z., & Kent, G. (2004). Human rights and the governance of food quality and safety in China. *Asia Pacific Journal of Clinical Nutrition, 12*(2) 178–183. Retrieved August 31, 2010, from http://www2.hawaii.edu/~kent/HUMAN%20RIGHTS%20AND%20THE%20GOVERNANCE.doc.pdf

United Nations Economic and Social Council. (1999). *Substantive issues arising in the implementation of the International Covenant on Economic, Social and Cultural Rights: General Comment 12 (20th Session, 1999) The Right to Adequate Food (art. 11)* Geneva: ECOSOC E/C.12/1999/5. Retrieved August 31, 2010, from http://www.unhchr.ch/tbs/doc.nsf/MasterFrameView/3d02758c707031d58025677f003b73b9?Opendocument

PART III

Rights-Based Approaches With Special Populations and Settings

CHAPTER 10

Human Rights and Women's Health

Padmini Murthy and Dhrubajyoti (Dru) Bhattacharya

INTRODUCTION

In spite of rapid advances in technology and shrinking of geographical barriers, women are still subject to discrimination. This is especially evident in the realm of health care, where women remain at a considerable disadvantage when compared to men. According to the World Health Organization (WHO, 2010), there is a strong correlation between health status and gender. *Gender risks* are often acquired, and usually result from women's greater exposure to poverty, as well as socioeconomic and political forms of discrimination. For example, Tarasiuk et al. (2006) concluded, "Low socioeconomic status (SES), regardless of the methodology used for determination, is inversely related to health and closely related to both mortality and morbidity from cardiovascular disease in women" (p. 767).

Some of the greatest threats to women's health worldwide stem from exposure to abuse, cultural practices such as female genital mutilation, child marriage, and human trafficking, to name a few. According to Murthy, Persaud, & Toda (2009), human trafficking is one of the biggest contributors to the rapid spread of sexually transmitted diseases including HIV/AIDS. Victims of trafficking are also prone to depressive disorders and have an increased risk of committing suicide and substance abuse. Unfortunately, most health care providers sadly lack the skills and awareness training on how to address these victims.

In the United States, gender discrimination remains an important, albeit tangential, theme in the ongoing debate on health care reform. Insurers frequently employ what is known as *gender rating*, whereby women are compelled to pay more than men do because women as a group allegedly use more medical services. One of the main reasons for this disparity is caused by the lack of adequate or no coverage for reproductive health services. This has also resulted in women paying up to 56% of the cost of prescriptive contraceptives. Hayden, in her article, "Gender Discrimination Within the Reproductive Health Care System: Viagra v. Birth Control," discusses the discrimination that women face from insurance carriers, many of which refuse coverage for contraceptives for women, but provide coverage of sildenafil citrate (Viagra) for men (Hayden, 1998).

International instruments and legal processes provide opportunities and challenges to secure women's health needs worldwide. For example, the Millennium Development Goals (MDGs), United Nations General Assembly resolutions, and numerous health-related treaties provide both aspirations and obligations on the part of governments to meet specific health needs and services for women. All of these will be examined within this chapter.

MILLENNIUM DEVELOPMENT GOALS AND WOMEN'S HEALTH

The MDGs are discussed in detail in chapter 5. Here, we will focus on three MDGs that have the most specific impact on women's health. Goal 3 entails the promotion of gender equality and empowerment of women; Goal 5 requires improvement of maternal health; and Goal 6 combats HIV/AIDS, malaria, and other diseases, which, although not exclusive to women, are extremely important owing to the disproportionate impact of HIV/AIDS on women in particular areas of the world.

Millenium Development Goal 3: Promote Gender Equality and Empower Women

Gender equality and female empowerment are essential to women's health. To be sure, health inequalities between the sexes may stem from biological, behavioral, and ecological determinants. Governmental action or inaction, however, may allow negative health trends to sustain. When duties are not upheld, and fundamental rights violated, inequalities become inequities that are otherwise avoidable. Examples include discrimination against women within extant laws, policies, and cultural norms that manifest in incidents of violence and physical abuse against women, mental health problems, and increased susceptibility to disease and other health risks.

Millenium Development Goal 5: Improve Maternal Health

Preventing maternal mortalities and prevention of mother-to-child transmission (PMTCT) should be prioritized. Hogan et al. (2010) recently estimated that approximately 342,900 women die annually because of pregnancy-related complications, many of which are preventable. Nonetheless, according to the WHO (2005), severe shortages of trained health workers means there are inadequate numbers of personnel who can oversee safe deliveries and postpartum care. PMTCT should also be prioritized. Newell, Brahmbhatt, and Ghys (2004) estimate that in Africa, approximately 60% of children infected with HIV/AIDS through their mothers die before their 5th birthday.

It is essential that advocates do not allow gender disparities to become subsumed in issues of universal import. Consider the right to clean water. Currently, in resource-poor settings, it is recommended that HIV-positive mothers breast-feed when substitute feeding is not viable; in such regions, the WHO (2003) recommends exclusive breast-feeding for the first months of life. Risk of diarrheal infection is high in areas with contaminated water, and diarrhea remains the second leading cause of death among infants, claiming 1.5 million lives each year (United Nations International Children's Emergency Fund, 2009). At first glance, the issue is merely reconciling the risk of morbidity and/or mortality associated with waterborne diarrheal infection from formula with the risk associated with possible mother-to-child transmission (MTCT) from breast-feeding.

In 2001, randomized clinical trials in four antenatal clinics in Nairobi, Kenya, found no significant difference in 2-year mortality rates between formula-fed and breast-fed infants, even when adjusted for HIV infection (Mbori-Ngacha et al., 2001). A 2-year follow-up study captured any potential adverse effects of formula feeding, but *not* the adverse effects of breast-feeding related to HIV transmission and mortality. In addition, formula-fed infants had a significantly higher HIV-free survival at 2 years. In conclusion, use of formula appeared to prevent up to 44% of HIV infections in an HIV-positive mother.

Evaluating this issue within a health and human rights framework would trivialize neither the findings nor their implications for women's health. It would assess the impact of water policies on women's rights, collect information from infected women (while considering privacy issues), take into account the scope of civic participation in the formulation of policies, and determine if, and how, the logistics of access (e.g., distance, cost) might affect utilization. The location of the aforesaid study is useful because Kenya affords numerous examples of discrimination against women, particularly inequality in rights to property, land access, and health (Federation of Women Lawyers–Kenya & International Women's Human Rights Clinic, 2008).

As such, the overarching issue may not be simply promoting access to particular goods or services or a particular practice such as breast-feeding, but addressing the inherent inequities women face within the social milieu. Improving maternal health should not be reduced to treatment-specific interventions, but should promote the social conditions that allow women to realize full physical, mental, and social well-being.

Millenium Development Goal 6: Combat HIV/AIDS, Malaria, and Other Diseases

Although HIV/AIDS poses a threat to both men and women, the latter are at heightened risk because of numerous social, economical, and cultural factors stemming from explicit violations of human rights, gender inequality, and inadequate forums to pursue legal redress.

The disproportionate impact of HIV/AIDS on women is startling. According to the WHO (2008), more than 60% of persons infected with HIV in sub-Saharan Africa are women; and females, aged 15–24, constitute 75% of persons afflicted with the virus. In fact, "male-to-female transmission during sex is about twice as likely to occur as female-to-male transmission, if no other sexually transmitted infections are present" (Joint United Nations Programme on HIV/AIDS [UNAIDS], 2004, p. 12).

These findings suggest the role of *structural violence* in HIV infection. The term was used by renowned physician-anthropologist Paul Farmer (2005) to explain how suffering is "structured by historically given (and often economically driven) processes and forces that conspire . . . to constrain agency" (p. 40). For example, lack of educational and employment opportunities coupled with restrictive property rights and other discriminatory practices may coerce women to remain in harmful relationships that increase their risk for HIV (Mukherjee, Farmer, & Farmer, 2009).

A recent UNAIDS (2008) report emphasizes the link between female education and substantial reduction in HIV risk and vulnerability. This affirms prior studies that found that girls who complete primary education are more than twice as likely to use condoms; those that go on to finish secondary education are 4–7 times more likely (Hargreaves & Boler, 2006).

Cultural norms may also increase women's susceptibility to infection. In Botswana, for example, it was found that individuals with "three or more discriminatory beliefs . . . were nearly three times more likely to have had unprotected sex with a nonmarital partner in the previous year than those without such beliefs" (UNAIDS, 2008, p. 67).

These examples illustrate the lack of power that women generally wield in relation to men. In the context of interpersonal relationships, this manifests in limited capacity to negotiate sexual practices, particularly the use of contraceptives. Moreover, the potential repercussions may silence women who otherwise know, but cannot voice, their health concerns. As a result, relationship dynamics preclude optimal female protection against the virus. It is imperative that advocates recognize the influence of social norms and practices on women's vulnerability to such health risks.

UNITED NATIONS HUMAN RIGHTS COUNCIL RESOLUTIONS AFFECTING WOMEN'S HEALTH

In 2006, the United Nations General Assembly created the United Nations Human Rights Council to address ongoing rights violations and make recommendations in response thereto. In 2009, the council considered several issues unique to women's health. Three resolutions were adopted regarding ongoing maternal mortality and morbidity, violence against women, and human trafficking. The resolution on maternal mortality is reviewed here to illustrate the benefits and challenges of using such measures to address such issues.

On June 17, 2009, the council adopted Resolution 11/8, Preventable Maternal Mortality and Morbidity and Human Rights (Human Rights Council, 2009). The resolution addressed the startling rates of maternal morbidity and mortality—WHO estimates that 529,000 maternal deaths occur annually (WHO, 2010)—and reiterated the need for urgent steps to combat this issue. Four particular aspects of the resolution exemplify the pressing challenges for human rights advocates and how the council sought to remedy them.

First, the council recognized the "leading role" of the WHO on maternal health, and particularly in relation to the monitoring of the achievement of health-related MDGs. Globalization has been accompanied by a proliferation of public and private organizations, obfuscating the presence (or perhaps need) of an authoritative voice on health-related matters. (This issue is addressed more thoroughly in chapter 6.) Still, the WHO Constitution grants the World Health Assembly the authority to "adopt regulations concerning" several pressing health issues, including sanitary and quarantine requirements, disease nomenclatures, standards of diagnostic procedures, and advertising and labeling of pharmaceutical products (International Health Conference, 1946, art. 21). The World Health Assembly also retains the "authority to adopt conventions or agreements with respect to any matters within the competence of the" WHO (International Health Conference, art. 19). These provisions provide an avenue to adopt legally binding measures to address emergent and nonemergent health issues.

Second, the council explicitly recognized that social determinants contributed maternal morbidity and mortality; they are "exacerbated by factors such as poverty, gender inequality, age and multiple forms of discrimination, as well as factors such as lack of access to adequate health facilities and technology, and lack of infrastructure" (Resolution 11/8, Preamble). This characterization is helpful in illustrating the need to adopt broad measures to go beyond the provision of health care delivery.

A third feature highlights the need to employ a combination of clinical and nonclinical interventions to prevent maternal deaths. Specific measures entail "promoting gender equality and empowering women," reiterating a commitment to the fifth Millennium Development Goal, including universal access to reproductive health (Resolution 11/8, Para. 3). The association between these latter rights and maternal health are not novel propositions, but are not prioritized within most health care interventions deemed necessary to secure women's health at the population level.

The fourth and final noteworthy aspect of the resolution was the council's request that the Office of the United Nations High Commissioner for Human Rights prepare a thematic study on preventable maternal mortality and morbidity and human rights. This effort would keep human rights as a central focus of future deliberations rather than narrow the debate to specific interventions. Such clinical measures are necessary but insufficient to adequately assess and determine the effect of human rights violations on maternal health.

The nonbinding nature of a resolution ought not to undermine its value in framing the issue, especially for legislators and even health care professionals unfamiliar with the multidimensional nature of maternal morbidity and mortality.

There has been progress in curbing maternal mortality rates worldwide. The 2005 Millennium Declaration resolved to reduce, by 2015, maternal mortality rates by three quarters (United Nations General Assembly, 2005). A recent study by Hogan et al. (2010) examined trends in 181 countries and found that approximately 342,900 women died in 2008 as a result of pregnancy-related complications, that is, 150,000 less deaths (or a 30% reduction) than previous estimates. Although much work remains to achieve a 75% reduction in maternal mortality rates, a concerted effort to advance human rights among women will only accelerate progress and yield positive health benefits.

THE CONVENTION ON THE ELIMINATION OF ALL FORMS OF DISCRIMINATION AGAINST WOMEN AND WOMEN'S HEALTH

The Charter of the United Nations (United Nations, 1945) was unique in espousing universality to the nature and scope of human rights. It also set forth obligations on the part of member states of the United Nations to "promote . . . human rights and fundamental freedoms," and "take joint and separate action . . . for the achievement of the purposes set forth" in the charter (U.N. Charter, Articles 55(c), 56). The subsequent Universal Declaration of Human Rights (UDHR) adopted by the United Nations General Assembly (1948) became the mechanism through which the charter could be realized. Since then, the UDHR has become the principal document of human rights advocates. However, the implementation of some rights within the document has been the source of ongoing controversy and deliberations (e.g., the right to health).

Nowhere was this controversy more evident than the successive adoption of two human rights covenants—the International Covenant on Civil and Political Rights (ICCPR) and the International Covenant on Economic, Social and Cultural Rights (ICESCR)—that impose different legal obligations on countries that have ratified them. Fulfilling the right to many of the economic, social, and cultural rights in the ICESCR may require more resources than establishing general parameters for governmental compliance with civil and political rights. To be sure, the (un)availability of resources does not necessarily undermine the necessity of securing such rights but does demand heightened consideration and collaboration to ensure their realization.

Although the rights espoused under ICCPR and ICESCR are essential to secure women's health, only the Convention on the Elimination of All

Forms of Discrimination Against Women (CEDAW) is devoted exclusively to promote women's rights. Apart from its focus on women, CEDAW is unique in two ways related to women's health in particular: first, it retains a health care provision that articulates services exclusively for women; and second, the treaty underscores the association between rights and health by promoting an array of civil, political, socioeconomic, and cultural rights.

CEDAW's health care provision provides that:

- States Parties shall take all appropriate measures to eliminate discrimination against women in the field of health care in order to ensure, on a basis of equality of men and women, access to health care services, including those related to family planning.
- Notwithstanding the provisions of paragraph 1 of this article, States Parties shall ensure to women appropriate services in connection with pregnancy, confinement and the post-natal period, granting free services where necessary, as well as adequate nutrition during pregnancy and lactation. (CEDAW, 1979, art. 12.)

Subsections (1) and (2) retains elements of both *formal* and *substantive* equality, respectively. Formal equality affords men and women the same rights, conditions, and opportunities. Substantive equality responds to the inadvertent disparities created by adhering to rigid standards of formal equality and requires programs that recognize the vulnerable status of women owing to biological, social, or other factors. Despite these provisions, outstanding issues abound. Under subsection (1), is emergency contraception "related to" family planning? Alternatively, under subsection (2), could abortion be considered an "appropriate service in connection with pregnancy. . .[?]" Several issues remain unresolved, but the health care provision affords advantages through explicit grants of services and conditions that were not available prior to its adoption.

CEDAW also illustrates the role of international law as a normative standard to analyze whether nations are respecting, promoting, and fulfilling their obligations. This is accomplished by monitoring and reviewing a country's progress on implementing the treaty, and issuing recommendations thereto. Under Article 18, states parties must submit a report within 1 year after "entry into force for the State concerned," (i.e., after ratifying the treaty), and "[t]hereafter at least every four years and further whenever the Committee so requests" (CEDAW, 1979, art. 18).

The report should also indicate the challenges affecting the country's inability to fulfill some, or all, of its requirements. In response, the CEDAW

Committee may issue "suggestions and general recommendations based on the examination of reports" (CEDAW, 1979, art. 21[1]).

Though legally nonbinding, these recommendations often form the basis of general recommendations that the CEDAW Committee may draft to facilitate adoption of specific programs and interventions. To date, the CEDAW Committee has issued more than 25 general recommendations.

OPTIONAL PROTOCOLS AND WOMEN'S HEALTH

In recent years, the adoption of treaties that authorize treaty-monitoring bodies to adjudicate claims brought by individuals against their governments marks a significant shift in international law. These treaties create opportunities to assess the kinds of health services that ought to be provided to women across the life span, as well as ways for individuals or organizations to challenge their governments when they fail to do so. Women who find that their domestic pleas for redress are futile may file a claim with an international body overseeing treaty implementation.

These treaties, dubbed *Optional Protocols*, empower individuals or organizations on their behalf to file a suit against a government for allegedly failing to comply with its treaty obligations. The ICCPR, ICESCR, and CEDAW all have Optional Protocols. Although there are some differences in their precise legal nature and scope, their similarities outweigh their differences in drawing some general conclusions about their potential impact on women's health.

Optional Protocols afford several substantive and procedural safeguards to protect alleged victims of human rights violations. The Optional Protocol to CEDAW, for example, empowers individuals alleging treaty violations to bring their claims before the CEDAW Committee. By ratifying the Optional Protocol, a state party "recognizes the competence of the [CEDAW] Committee to receive and consider communications" submitted by alleged victims (Optional Protocol to CEDAW, 1999, art. 1). After a decision has been issued, states parties shall submit "within six months . . . written explanations . . . clarifying the matter and the remedy," thereby indicating their actions taken in accordance with the CEDAW Committee's recommendations (Optional Protocol to CEDAW, art. 6). Additional safeguards include the CEDAW Committee's authority to impose "interim measures . . . to avoid irreparable damage to the victim" if circumstances so require (Optional Protocol to CEDAW, art. 5[1]).

To date, claims brought before the Human Rights Council and the CEDAW Committee, albeit limited in number, have met with success in articulating the explicit duties of governments in regard to providing access to reproductive health services and respecting a woman's decision-making autonomy. As examples, the cases of *Karen Noelia Llantoy Huamán v. Peru* and *A. S. v. Hungary* were landmark decisions that demonstrate the inextricable linkage between women's rights and women's health.

The Case of *K. L. v. Peru*

The case of *K. L. v. Peru*, which was filed under the Optional Protocol to the ICCPR, yielded a landmark decision in reproductive rights (*Karen Noelia Llantoy Huamán v. Peru*, 2005). The case involved a 17-year-old girl whose doctors refused to perform an abortion after she presented carrying an anencephalic fetus. She delivered the baby and was compelled to breast-feed until her baby died a few days later. She also suffered vulvitis and subsequently entered a severe state of depression. Peruvian law provided for a therapeutic exception, but imposed criminal liability on physicians who performed abortions. The Human Rights Council ruled in her favor and asserted the government's responsibility to ensure access to legal abortion services.

Although the international community provides a forum for scrutinizing governmental policies and reviewing individual claims, numerous challenges abound.

Scarce resources, the lack of political will, and cultural beliefs may all converge in governmental reluctance or even outright resistance to engage meaningful international scrutiny. In the case of *K. L. v. Peru*, the government of Peru refused to even engage the Human Rights Council by submitting a response to the official complaint. In practice, this type of resistance can be problematic for at least two reasons. First, it undermines the authority of the international body that interprets the claims; and second, it prevents an open deliberation on the merits of the claim, which may reveal different, though perhaps reasonable, interpretations of duties and rights. Governmental indifference to these processes thereby effectively prevents the development and review of policies and laws to secure women's health.

The Case of *A. S. v. Hungary*

The case of *A. S. v. Hungary* was brought under the Optional Protocol to CEDAW (*A. S. v. Hungary*, 2006). Here, a pregnant woman was rushed to a hospital after her amniotic fluid broke. Upon arrival, she was dizzy, bleeding heavily, and in a state of shock. The attending physician found that the fetus had died en route and informed her that he needed to perform a cesarean section to remove the dead fetus. She was then asked to sign a consent form for the C-section on an illegible note that actually authorized her sterilization (with the term for sterilization written in Latin rather than Hungarian). After later learning of what transpired, she brought suit charging a failure of informed consent. The CEDAW Committee agreed, and granted her relief, along with specific directives for the Hungarian government to update its law and policies related to informed consent.

These two cases reflect a nascent, but growing, jurisprudence related to women's health. Although several legal, political, and social issues abound, they present a hopeful shift in the role of international law that heretofore treated individuals as merely objects of governmental policies. Now, individuals are becoming empowered as subjects in control, however limited, of their rights and the opportunity to hold their governments accountable for their acts and omissions.

A fundamental challenge in using international law to promote women's health is fostering cooperation and collaboration among and within nations, as well as among public and private sector entities at all levels of governance. Their roles may entail a myriad of activities, such as providing technical assistance, distributing educational materials, securing financial aid, or delivering health care. To be effective, however, these entities must align their efforts toward the achievement of clearly defined objectives. This, in turn, would allow for the implementation of precise interventions.

CONCLUSION

Gender discrimination is pervasive throughout the world and permeates health systems in both developed and developing nations. Women face discrimination as patients and citizens, compounding the impact of human rights violations and their attendant health impact. Rectifying these disparities will require several activities, including a systematic assessment of how existent medical curricula address the role of gender in the delivery of health care. These efforts should constitute part of broader reform initiatives in laws, policies, and programs to ameliorate discrimination against women. Although international health-related resolutions and treaties abound, the availability of seeking redress for individual violations within an international forum marks a significant change in the women's rights movement. These developments are encouraging, but the stark disparities in health, wealth, and education demand a renewed effort across public and private sectors to forge new partnerships and secure women's health and human rights.

To address the issue of gender discrimination in health services and public health programs, a general audit of current policies and programs affecting women's health needs to be conducted. It is important to identify existent disparities in unmet needs and the delivery of care, particularly related to reproductive health and preventive services. It is important that the federal and state governments in all countries, including the United States, ratify CEDAW and its Optional Protocol and adopt policies that explicitly recognize women's rights, the duties of public health officials and health care providers as relates to the delivery of specific services, and the duties of legislators to ensure that related social determinants (e.g., education, socioeconomic status) are assessed and incorporated into determinations concerning whether existent laws and policies are adequately improving women's health.

REFERENCES

A. S. v. Hungary, Communication No. 4/2004, 36th Session (August 14, 2006).

Convention on the Elimination of All Forms of Discrimination Against Women. (1979). Art. 12. New York: United Nations.

Farmer, P. (2005). *Pathologies of power: Health, human rights, and the new war on the poor* ("On Suffering and Structural Violence," p. 40). Los Angeles: University of California Press.

Federation of Women Lawyers–Kenya, & International Women's Human Rights Clinic. (2008). *Kenyan laws and harmful customs curtail women's equal enjoyment of ICESCR rights.* Retrieved September 9, 2010, from http://www2.ohchr.org/english/bodies/cescr/docs/info-ngos/FIDAKenya41.pdf

Hargreaves, J. R., & Boler, T. (2006). *Girl power: Girls' education, sexual behaviour and AIDS in Africa.* Johannesburg, South Africa: ActionAid International.

Hayden, L. A., (1998). Gender discrimination within the reproductive health care system: Viagra v. birth control. *Journal of Law and Health, 13*(2), 171–198.

Hogan, M. C., Foreman, K. J., Naghavi, M., Ahn, S. Y., Wang, M., Makela, S. M., et al. (2010). Maternal mortality for 181 countries, 1980–2008: A systematic analysis of progress towards Millennium Development Goal 5. *Lancet, 375,* 1609–1623.

Human Rights Council. (2009). Preventable maternal mortality and morbidity and human rights (A/HRC/11/L.16). Retrieved September 9, 2010, from http://ap.ohchr.org/documents/E/HRC/resolutions/A_HRC_RES_11_8.pdf

International Health Conference. (1946). World Health Organization Constitution, Art. 21.

Karen Noelia Llantoy Huamán v. Peru, Communication No. 1153/2003, U.N. Doc. CCPR/C/85/D/1153/2003 (2005).

Mbori-Ngacha, D., Nduati, R., John, G., Reilly, M., Richardson, B., Mwatha, A., et al. (2001). Morbidity and mortality in breastfed and formula-fed infants of

HIV-1-infected women: A randomized clinical trial. *The Journal of the American Medical Association, 286*(19), 2413–2420.

Murthy, P., Persaud, R. D., & Toda, M. (2009). Human trafficking: A modern plague. In P. Murthy & L. Smith (Eds.), *Women's global health and human rights* (pp. 59–72). Sudbury, MA: Jones and Bartlett.

Mukherjee, J. S., Farmer, D. B., & Farmer, P. E. (2009). The AIDS pandemic and women's rights. In P. Murphy & L. Smith (Eds.), *Women's global health and human rights* (pp. 129–30). Sudbury, MA: Jones and Bartlett.

Newell, M. L., Brahmbhatt, H., & Ghys, P. D. (2004). Child mortality and HIV infection in Africa: A review. *AIDS, 18*(Suppl. 2), S27–S34.

Optional Protocol to the Convention on the Elimination of All Forms of Discrimination Against Women. (1999). Art. 2. Retrieved September 9, 2010, from http://www.un.org/womenwatch/daw/cedaw/protocol/text.htm

Tarasiuk, A., Greenberg-Dotan, S., Simon, T., Tal, A., Oksenberg, A., & Reuveni, H. (2006). Low socioeconomic status is a risk factor for cardiovascular disease among adult obstructive sleep apnea syndrome patients requiring treatment. *Chest, 130*(3), 766–773.

Joint United Nations Programme on HIV/AIDS. (2004). *Report on the global AIDS epidemic.* Geneva: Author.

Joint United Nations Programme on HIV/AIDS. (2008). Addressing societal causes of HIV risk and vulnerability. In UNAIDS, *Report on the global AIDS epidemic* (pp. 64–93). Geneva: Author.

United Nations International Children's Emergency Fund. (2009). *Diarrhoea: Why children are still dying and what can be done.* Geneva: World Health Organization.

United Nations. (1945). International economic and social cooperation. *United Nations Charter* (arts. 55[c], 56).

United Nations General Assembly. (1948). *Universal declaration of human rights* (art. 25).

United Nations General Assembly. (2005). UN Millenium Declaration 2005 (sec. 19, p. 5).

World Health Organization. (2003). *HIV and infant feeding: Guidelines for decision makers.* Geneva: Author.

World Health Organization. (2005). *The world health report 2005—Make every mother and child count* (p. 74). Geneva: Author.

World Health Organization. (2008). Gender inequalities and HIV. Retrieved September 9, 2010, from http://www.who.int/gender/hiv_aids/en/

World Health Organization. (2010). Social and gender inequalities in environment and health. Retrieved September 9, 2010, from http://www.euro.who.int/__data/assets/pdf_file/0010/76519/Parma_EH_Conf_pbl.pdf

World Health Organization. (2010). *WHO gender mainstreaming strategy.* Retrieved September 9, 2010, from http://www.who.int/gender/mainstreaming/strategy/en/

OTHER RESOURCES

America's Affordable Health Choices Act of 2009, H.R. 3200, 111th Cong., 1st Sess. (2009).

America's Healthy Future Act of 2009, S. 1796, 111th Cong. (2009).

Dinan, K. A. (2002). Trafficking in women from Thailand to Japan: Role of organized crime and governmental response. Harvard Asia Quarterly, 6(3): 4–13.

Human Rights Council. (2005). Accelerating efforts to eliminate all forms of violence against women (A/HRC/11/L.5). Retrieved August 7, 2010, from http://www.biceinternational.org/e_upload/pdf/un_hrc_accelerating_efforts_to _eliminate_all_forms_of_violence_against_women.pdf

Human Rights Council. (2005). Trafficking in persons, especially women and children (A/HRC/11/L.6).

Lockyear, P. L. B. (2004). Nutritional status of young women: Cultural differences: Socioeconomic status impact on health. *Medscape Ob/Gyn & Women's Health*, 9(1).

United Nations International Children's Emergency Fund. (2007). The state of the world's children 2007, women and children: The double dividend of gender equality.

CHAPTER 11

A Rights-Based Approach to Children's Health

Nichola Cadge

This chapter draws on and uses material from the following Save the Children publications[1]:

- Save the Children CRP-PEN. (2007). *Getting it right for children: A practitioners' guide to child rights programming.* London: International Save the Children Alliance.
- Save the Children CRP Coordinating Group. (2005). *Child rights programming: How to apply rights-based approaches to programming: A handbook for International Save the Children Alliance Members.* Save the Children Sweden.

INTRODUCTION

This chapter outlines the processes involved in a child rights program approach. It highlights the importance of analyzing the direct and underlying causes of rights violations to bring about legal, policy, and practice changes, which can make a sustained difference in children's lives. It outlines the steps required to plan, implement, and monitor health programs with the overall goal of improving child survival and development, and to ensure that children live in societies that acknowledge and respect their rights.

Each year, nearly million children die before the age of 5 years, largely from preventable causes (You, Wardlaw, Salama, & Jones, 2009). That is almost one child every 3 seconds. A total of 4 million of those within their first 28 days, including up to 2 million who die on their first day of life (Lawn, Cousens, & Zupan, 2005). Sixty-eight low- and middle-income countries account for 97% of all newborn and child deaths worldwide (United Nations International Children's Emergency Fund [UNICEF], 2008). Within these countries, children from the poorest families and most marginalized communities are at greatest risk of early death. Two thirds of child deaths could be prevented if those children could access good-quality health care services (Jones et al., 2003). The survival chances of children are intrinsically linked to the survival of their mothers yet 500,000 women still die through pregnancy-related causes each year—a figure that has not changed significantly for nearly 2 decades.

Health services are in a state of collapse in many developing countries; many children and their mothers do not have access to quality basic health services that are crucial to children's survival and development. There is growing recognition that stronger and more equitable health systems are a key policy response to child and maternal mortality (Save the Children, 2008). There is not only a clear moral imperative to redress this but also legal obligations enshrined in a series of human rights instruments.

CHILDREN'S RIGHTS

As described in earlier chapters, all governments have signed up to at least one international human rights instrument that obliges them to respect, protect, and fulfill the right to health (Save the Children, 2009) for their citizens. However, this obligation does not rest with governments alone; the international community is also obliged to support countries in this attainment.

Children's rights are also established through a series of international human rights and humanitarian law. The most significant of these is the United Nations Convention on the Rights of the Child (UNCRC, 1989). The UNCRC has been ratified[2] by more governments than any other human rights instrument; as of January 2009, it had been ratified by 192 out of 194 countries.[3] The UNCRC applies to all human beings younger than 18 years. It emphasizes that children are holders of rights,

FIGURE 11.1 The Four General Principles of the United Nations Convention on the Rights of the Child

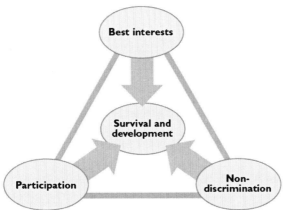

Note. From "Getting It Right for Children: A Practitioners' Guide to Child Rights Programming," by Save the Children, 2007. Reprinted with permission.

and their rights cover all aspects of their lives. It consists of 54 articles[4] and identifies four rights as general principles (see Figure 11.1):

- *Nondiscrimination (art. 2)*—All rights apply to all children *without* exception. The state itself has an obligation to put into place the means to ensure children are protected from any form of discrimination and to take positive action to promote their rights.
- *Best interests of the child (art. 3)*—This principle asserts that whenever decisions are made that affect children's lives, the impact of those decisions must be assessed to ensure that the best interests of children are the main consideration. The interests of others—such as parents, the community and the state—should not be the overriding concern, even though they may influence the final decision.
- *Rights to life, survival and development (art. 6)*—Although children's survival often relates directly to children's right to life, children's right to development must be interpreted in its broadest sense, encompassing the physical, psychological, emotional, social, and spiritual development of the child.
- *Child participation and the right to be heard (art. 12)*—Participation, as defined in the UNCRC, is about children and young people having the opportunity to express their views, influence decision making and achieve change in areas that affect their lives. Children's

participation is the *informed and willing involvement of children*, including the most marginalised and those of different ages and abilities, in all matters concerning them.

As with all human rights, these rights are universal, inalienable, indivisible, and interdependent.

Children's Right to Health and Health Care Services

A child's right to health is expressly covered by several articles in the UNCRC:

- **Article 6:** The inherent right to life, and the State's obligation to ensure the child's survival and development.
- **Article 24:** The right of the child to the enjoyment of the highest attainable standard of health and to facilities for the treatment of illness and rehabilitation to health.
- Reference to health and survival of the child is also made in CRC Articles 3, 17, 25, 27, 32, and 39.

Most other articles of the CRC also have bearing, directly or indirectly, on a child's health. This is important to appreciate, as many of the determinants of health lay outside the health sector. Likewise, it is important to have an understanding of the other rights treaties, conventions and consensus statements[5] that uphold both the right to health and the broader social, economic, political and cultural rights that impact on health and thus a child's right to health (see Figure 11.2).

Children's Rights and the Millennium Development Goals

In 2000, the attainment of several human rights was galvanized by the Millennium Development Goals (MDGs; see chapter 5): eight targets for poverty reduction and development. Although each of these are important and interrelated, four are particularly relevant to the survival prospects of children.[6] The MDGs have the added advantage of having specific targets, are time bound and, importantly, have the capacity to mobilize both domestic and international resources, national governments, and civil society toward a common cause. Despite some improvements, at current rates of progress, the goal of reducing under-5 mortality rate by two thirds will not be achieved globally by 2015. Clearly, national governments, civil

FIGURE 11.2 Linkages Between Health, Human Rights and Child Rights

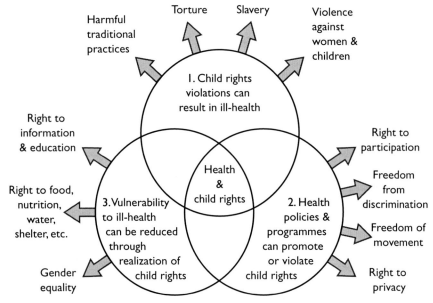

Note. From World Health Organization. Adapted with permission.

society, and the international community need to work together to acceler-ate progress on the health MDGs.

Figure 11.3 summarizes some of the language relevant to children's rights and health in various international documents.

Recognizing Distinctions in Childhood and Evolving Capacities

To work effectively with a child rights focus, you need to recognize and allow for the high level of diversity among children, including their age, culture, and contexts. The concept of "childhood" varies around the world. Children's needs and capacities also evolve during childhood in different ways: A 15-year-old girl in South Africa, for example, will have very differ-ent needs and capacities than a 6-month-old girl in Ethiopia. The concept of "evolving capacities" highlights the balance required between empow-erment and protection. This balance recognizes children as active agents in their own lives, entitled to be listened to, respected and granted increas-ing autonomy in the exercise of rights, while also being entitled to protec-tion in accordance with their relative immaturity and youth.

For workers in the health sector, this is particularly relevant when design-ing programs to address neonatal and child mortality. As already described,

FIGURE 11.3 Relevant Child Rights Language in International Instruments

UN Convention on the Rights of the Child

Article 6: The inherent right to life, and the State's obligation to ensure the child's survival and development.

Article 23: The right of the mentally or physically disabled child to special care . . . and to health care services. . . . State parties shall promote the exchange of information in the field of preventive health care and of medical, psychological and functional treatment of disabled children.

Article 24: The right of the child to the enjoyment of the highest attainable standard of health and to facilities for the treatment of illness and rehabilitation to health.

Reference to health and survival of the child is also made in CRC Articles 3, 17, 25, 27, 32, and 39.

International Covenant on Civil and Political Rights, Article 6
"The right to life and survival."

The Universal Declaration of Human Rights, Article 25
"Everyone has the right to a standard of living adequate for the health and well being of himself and his family, including food, clothing, housing and medical care and the right to security in the event of . . . sickness, disability . . ."

International Covenant on Economic, Social and Cultural Rights, Article 12 (1)
"The right of everyone to the enjoyment of the highest attainable standard of physical and mental health."

Convention on the Elimination of All Forms of Discrimination Against Women
Article 11(1)(f.) provides that state parties shall take all appropriate measures to eliminate discrimination against women in the enjoyment of "the right to protection of health and to safety in working conditions, including the safeguarding of the function of reproduction." Article 12 of the same convention provides that all appropriate measures should be taken by states parties to eliminate discrimination against women "in the field of health care in order to ensure on a basis of equality of men and women, access to health care services, including those related to family planning."

Convention on the Elimination of All Forms of Racial Discrimination
Article 5(e)(iv) provides that states parties undertake to prohibit and eliminate discrimination in the enjoyment of "the right to public health, medical care, social security and social services."

International Covenant on Civil and Political Rights, Article 17
"The right to decide freely the number and spacing of one's children"

World Health Organization Constitution (Preamble)
"The enjoyment of the highest attainable standard of health is one of the fundamental human rights of every human being without distinction of race, religion, political belief, economic or social conditions."

(Continued)

FIGURE 11.3 Relevant Child Rights Language in International
Instruments *Continued*

World Health Assembly Resolution 58.31
This resolution states what is needed to achieve the child, neonatal, and maternal
health Millennium Development Goals (MDGs). It includes calls in donors for
more resources, and policy changes such as moving away from user fees.

The UN Millennium Development Goals
Three of the eight MDGs are health specific; that is, by 2015:

Goal 4: Reduce child mortality
  • Reduce by two thirds the mortality rate among children younger than five

Goal 5: Improve maternal health
  • Reduce by three quarters the maternal mortality ratio

Goal 6: Combat HIV/AIDS, malaria, and other diseases
  • Halt and begin to reverse the spread of HIV/AIDS
  • Halt and begin to reverse the incidence of malaria and other major diseases

---

child survival is closely linked with maternal survival. This link becomes
even closer when the maternal age is younger than 20 years. Each year,
1 million babies are born to young mothers, 70,000 girls aged between 15 and
19 die as result of complications of childbirth, and a further 2 million are left
with chronic illness or disability that may lead to a lifelong cycle of stigma,
discrimination, and poverty (World Health Organization & United Nations
Population Fund, 2006). Infant mortality rates are significantly higher among
mothers younger than 20 years than mothers aged 20–29 years.

Developing an effective rights-based health sector response to this requires
not only the recognition that the availability, accessibility, and delivery of reproductive, maternal, neonatal, and child health services and information must be
addressed in an integrated way—from newborn into childhood through ado-
lescence and into safe motherhood, and from household to hospital[7]—but also
understanding the concept of evolving capacities and needs.

CHILD RIGHTS PROGRAMMING

Rights-based goals are only achieved when all people enjoy the right. To
realize such broad, ambitious, and long-term goals requires joint analysis,
common understanding of rights violations, gaps, and solutions, and common strategies to address them. A rights-based programming approach has
the potential for great impact (because influencing duty bearers supports

wider replication of effort) and greater sustainability (because it involves work at all levels of society to change policy and practice and continually hold the duty bearer to account).

For Save the Children, the UNCRC is the guiding framework and reference point for child rights programming (CRP). CRP brings together a range of ideas, concepts, and experiences related to child rights, child development, emergency response, and development work within one unifying framework.[8] The definition of CRP is as follows:

Child rights programming means using the principles of child rights to *design*, *implement*, and *monitor* programs with the overall goal of improving the position of children so that all boys and girls can fully enjoy their rights and can live in societies that acknowledge and respect children's rights.

Our role as child rights practitioners, therefore, is to support and empower children to claim their rights and to ensure that duty-bearers take seriously their responsibility to provide for these rights. States are the main duty-bearers and as such have the primary responsibility for realising children's rights, but they must also support others, especially parents and other primary care givers, to make the changes that are needed if children's rights are going to be upheld.

What Does Child Rights Programming Mean in Practice?

Using a CRP approach means adopting certain processes and methods (see Figure 11.4). These processes are grounded in human rights and child rights principles:

- Involving children at every stage of the program cycle
- Working with the most vulnerable children and countering discrimination
- Creating a rights climate through redressing power relations in favor of children and their rights
- Working in partnership
- Working with and enabling the state
- Empowering civil society and encouraging community involvement.

A CHILD RIGHTS SITUATION ANALYSIS

A Child Rights Situation Analysis (CRSA) is an analysis of the situation of children and their rights; the extent to which they have been realized and the obstacles to fulfilling them. The CRSA helps us to identify gaps and

FIGURE 11.4 Child Rights Programming Cycle

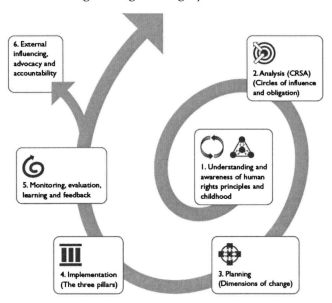

Note. From "Getting It Right for Children: A Practitioners' Guide to Child Rights Programming," by Save the Children, 2007. Reprinted with permission.

key areas for action. There are two levels of a CRSA: a countrywide general CRSA to help plan or review, which children's rights a particular country should be focusing on, in which sectors and which geographic locations; and a second, more in-depth thematic or sectoral CRSA. The following are the main areas covered in a health CRSA checklist (see Figure 11.5):

1. *Health situation of children and their caregivers:* What health rights are not realized for which children? What are the main causes of morbidity and mortality as well as the barriers preventing children and their caregivers from accessing quality health services? How many are in this situation, where are they, and what are their common characteristics? What are the trends? Sometimes primary data collection and research may be needed.

2. *The causes:* Why are children's health rights unrealized? What are the key political, economic, and social factors involved? How is the health system functioning and how are the services perceived and used by the target population groups? A causal analysis will review the immediate, intermediate, and structural causes of child health rights violations.

FIGURE 11.5 Child Rights Situation Analysis Checklists

1. DIRECT CAUSES OF MORTALITY AND MORBIDITY

   Identify the direct causes of preventable illness and death in program districts
   - Main direct causes of death among newborns (first 28 days of life)
   - Main direct causes of death (e.g., malaria, diarrhea) in children younger than 5 years and adolescents
   - Top 10 diseases in children younger than 5 years
   - Main direct causes of maternal deaths (related to pregnancy and its complications such as sepsis, hemorrhage, obstructed labor)
   - Main disease patterns including epidemics, trends over last 5–10 years, and seasonal variations

Note: If the general Child Rights Situation Analysis (CRSA) has not covered these points, you will need to look at the national situation as well as the situation in proposed program districts.

2. UNDERLYING CAUSES OF MORTALITY AND MORBIDITY

   A. Government Commitments, Policies, and Practice

   Health policy and strategies
   - Relevance to main health problems in the country
   - Emphasis on children, adolescents, and women of reproductive age
   - Commitment to rights and principles of equity
   - Main players influencing policy
   - Policy reforms (e.g., decentralization, contracting out to nongovernment providers)
   - Maternal and child health (MCH) roadmap for Millennium Development Goals (MDGs)
   - Reproductive and sexual health/HIV and AIDS strategies
   - Neonatal health strategies
   - Human Resources for Health (HRH) strategy/gap analysis

   Rights commitments
   - International covenants ratified and signed by the government
   - Monitoring and reporting on Convention on the Rights of the Child (CRC) and other covenants
   - Other declarations and consensus signed by the government (Alma-Ata, MDGs, World Health Assembly [WHA] resolutions, Beijing Platform for Action, International Conference on Population and Development [ICPD] Cairo)
   - National Constitution, government obligations for health
   - Health sector component of the Poverty Reduction Strategy Paper (PRSP)

   Health financing
   - Government expenditure on health per capita/per year (US$)
   - Health budget as proportion of total government budget for development

(Continued)

FIGURE 11.5 Child Rights Situation Analysis Checklists *Continued*

- Proportion of overall health expenditure from international agencies
- Out-of-pocket expenditure per capita per year
- Financing gap for health services
- National Health Account—conducted or not
- Public Expenditure Review—conducted or not
- Percentage of health budget allocated to children and women
- Distribution of health budget—urban/rural, primary/secondary/ tertiary care (be sure to identify discrepancies between budget allocation and what is actually disbursed)
- Health financing mechanisms such as sector-wide approach (SWAP) and budgetary support, trends over last 5 years and how they are functioning
- Policy and practice on user fees, revolving drug funds, health insurance, waiver and exemption systems
- Government, donor, and nongovernment organization (NGO) interest/ commitment to abolition of user fees at point of service in public sector
- Budget allocation for primary health care compared with hospital services
- Decentralization reforms for budget planning and management

Health sector coordination

- Coordination mechanisms and their effectiveness
- Opportunities for NGOs to engage on specific issues (e.g., Immunization Coordination Committees [ICCs] and Country Coordination Mechanisms [CCMs]) for the Global Fund to fight AIDS, TB, and Malaria

B. **Health System and Services**

Supply

Health system performance

- Immunization coverage rates (infants younger than 1 year fully immunized with six antigens)
- Percentage of deliveries by a skilled birth attendant (urban/rural)
- Average number of visits per person/per year for outpatient consultation
- Contraceptive prevalence rate
- Ratio of doctors and nurse-midwives/population (urban/rural)
- Percentage of population living within 5–10 km of a health facility (urban/rural)
- Percentage of health facilities fully staffed (urban/rural)
- Availability of essential drugs and vaccines
- Availability of basic and emergency obstetric care facilities
- Availability of adolescent friendly reproductive health services
- Availability of services for prevention of mother-to-child transmission (PMTCT) of HIV, voluntary counseling and testing (VCT), and antiretroviral therapy (ART). Availability of pediatric HIV/AIDS drugs at district level and below

(Continued)

FIGURE 11.5 **Child Rights Situation Analysis Checklists** *Continued*

Planning and management systems
- Financial planning and management capacity
- Health information management systems
- Supervision and support systems
- Transport management and logistics systems
- Human resource management and development
- Emergency preparedness and response capacity

Availability of health services
- Health facilities (hospitals, health centers, clinics)
- Trained personnel (doctors, nurses, midwives, pharmacists, other cadres)
- Goods (essential drugs, equipment and medical supplies)
- Major disparities, issues and gaps

Quality of services
- Essential drugs and vaccines supply and management
- Supervision and support system
- Standards for ensuring quality (e.g., rational use of essential drugs; universal precautions; protocols for management of labor and delivery)
- Attitudes and communication skills of health workers
- System of continued education of health workers
- Waste management systems
- Regulation and control of private and nongovernmental providers

Demand

Utilization of services
- Main users of the services
- Utilization data disaggregated by age groups, gender, socioeconomic status (ideally identifying those above or within the lowest quintile) and type of service (consultation, immunization, sexual and reproductive health services, antenatal, postnatal, deliveries, family planning, etc.)
- Average number of consultations per capita per year

Barriers to utilization of health services
- Physical—distance, roads, transport, climate
- Money and time/opportunity costs (including seasonal variability); fees for services (formal and informal), ineffective exemption systems
- Sociocultural factors (gender, traditional health beliefs and practices, who makes decisions in the home on health seeking behavior)

(Continued)

FIGURE 11.5 Child Rights Situation Analysis Checklists *Continued*

- Lack of health information and adequate understanding to make informed decisions about children's health: prevention and prompt treatment

Participation
- Extent to which children, adolescents, young people, women and men are involved in planning, monitoring, and evaluation of health services
- Awareness of rights to health by children, their carers, and communities
- Capacity of civil society to hold providers accountable

Child care practices in the home/community
- Care of the newborn
- Breastfeeding and weaning
- Hygiene practices
- Management of common illnesses (e.g., diarrhea, fever, cough) in those younger than 5 years
- Health seeking behavior

C. **Other Stakeholders and Actors**
   Who are the main players, what are their respective roles and their attitudes and commitments to children's rights to health? Who is influential, who holds power, and who decides how money is spent?

   Key groups to consider
   - International and Regional level aid agencies (UN agencies, World Bank, European Union [EU])
   - National level aid agencies (United States Agency for International Development [USAID], UK Department for International Development [DFID], Swedish International Development Cooperation Agency [Sida], Canadian International Development Agency [CIDA], Norwegian Agency for Development Cooperation [NORAD], etc.)
   - Joint Public-Private Initiatives (JPPIs; Global Alliance for Vaccines and Immunisation [GAVI], Global Fund to fight AIDS, Tuberculosis and Malaria - [GFATM], President's Malaria Initiative [PMI], etc.)
   - Private-for-profit and nonprofit providers (including NGOs, faith-based organizations, local and grassroots organizations)
   - Trade unions (nurses, midwives, doctors, pharmacists, etc.)
   - Global Health Workforce Alliance
   - Commonwealth Secretariat
   - Traditional practitioners and other nonformal health care providers
   - Civil society (parents, village leaders, religious leaders, People's Health Movement, etc.)

   Capacity of local civil society structures to influence government and other influential players regarding children's health

3. *The responsibilities:* Which people, groups, or organizations are responsible for realizing both health and child rights (known as "duty bearers" in human rights circles)? What are the obstacles and barriers to be overcome? What are the government commitments, policies, and practice to health and child rights?

4. *The solutions:* Which groups influence the duty bearers? What needs to be done or done differently to realize a child's right to health?

5. *Organizational capacity:* Internal strengths, weaknesses, and opportunities—this involves an honest strengths, weaknesses, opportunities, and constraints (SWOC) analysis of your own organization's current capacity to address the issues identified in the previous areas appraisal.

6. *Conclusions and recommendations:* Priority areas for action and programming.

The process should include duty bearer, stakeholder, and capacity analyses. It must be participatory—a CRSA is not a desktop exercise. The participation of children and their carers, duty bearers, and stakeholders are central—apart from informing the CRSA this also helps with later "buy-in" and support for your program strategy.

THE THREE PILLARS OF CHILD RIGHTS PROGRAMMING

The findings of the health CRSA are then used to inform a programmatic strategy using a framework of three defined, and mutually reinforcing, areas of activity: the three pillars of CRP (see Figure 11.6). The balance of activities between each of these pillars will depend on the context, as the program progresses and as the capacity of partners, the state, and other stakeholders change. Crucially however, Save the Children has found that it is possible to implement activities across the three pillars even in the most unpromising and difficult environments, such as in chronic conflict or poor governance countries. Moreover, achieving sustainable solutions effective realization of children's right to health requires achieving change within each of the three pillars and influencing decision makers at local, national, and international levels. The work in each pillar is informed by and reinforces work under the other two.

FIGURE 11.6 The Three Pillars of Child Rights Programming

Child Rights Situation Analysis		
PILLAR 1	**PILLAR 2**	**PILLAR 3**
Direct actions on violations of children's rights and gaps in provision	Strengthening the capacity of duty-bearers to meet their obligations (policies, practice and legislation)	Strengthening the understanding and capacity of children, their carers and civil society to claim rights and hold others to account
Organizational Capacity		

Note. "Getting It Right for Children: A Practitioners Guide to Child Rights Programming," by Save the Children, 2007. Reprinted with permission.

An Example From Save the Children United Kingdom

Save the Children United Kingdom's Right to Health objective is that "All children survive and grow up healthy." The ultimate aim of our health programs is to "Reduce preventable morbidity and mortality of children, adolescents and their carers." Based on CRP processes and tools the following areas for programming were identified as a guideline for country programs. Ultimately, however, the more detailed health program strategy in countries will be defined by both their general and thematic health CRSA. It is essential that in the planning cycle, attention is taken to ensuring monitoring, evaluation, learning, and feedback mechanisms are put in place. And that these mechanisms explicitly and actively engage the participation of children.

Supporting duty bearers to strengthen health systems that make quality healthcare accessible to all children and their carers, including the following:

- Improve the quality of health care provided
- Support the quality and retention of health workers
- Improve the quality and scale of health information systems ensuring that it captures marginalized and vulnerable groups

- Increase the amount, impact, and equitable allocation and distribution of health resources—including both domestic and international finance for health
- Support the Maternal Newborn and Child Health (MNCH) and the household to hospital continuums of care

In some situations (e.g., emergencies, fragile states), directly delivering services if the government is unwilling or unable to by:

- Empowering and strengthening the capacity of children and civil society, as rights holders, to understand and claim their health entitlements and hold duty bearers to account
- Increasing the participation of communities, particularly children, in the planning, monitoring, and evaluation of health services
- Reducing health inequity—ensuring that health services are accessible to the poorest and most marginalized
- Promoting a child rights focus in national health policy and strategic planning
- Demonstrating what works, why, and at what cost and using our programs and research to create enabling environments to deliver effective advocacy and changes in policy and practice

It is essential to use CRP in all stages of the program cycle including monitoring and evaluation to assess, to what extent, whether children's rights are better realized or no longer violated as a result of the program interventions. It will be necessary to assess changes in legislation, policy, structures, and practices and their impact on the realization of rights, changes in relation to equity and nondiscrimination, opportunities for participation and active citizenship of children, and other stakeholders, within their communities, and changes in civil society and community capacity. Children and their communities need to be actively engaged in the process of monitoring and evaluation. Their involvement both empowers them and improves the quality of the information. Framing your evaluation in these terms greatly facilitates the assessment and evaluation process and identification of results and outcomes to inform your next project cycle.

CONCLUSION

Adopting a child rights-based approach to health is the most effective way to bring about positive and lasting change for children, their families, and communities. It is not an easy process to embark on. It will take time, resources (both human and financial), and commitment, in both the short term and long term.

So where do you start? As explained earlier in this chapter, context is key; a situation analysis will always be your starting point. Review your program plans or outlines and ask yourself the following questions:

- What unfulfilled rights is this project addressing?
- What are the underlying causes for the rights not being fulfilled?
- Who is responsible for the fulfillment of rights?
- What action should be taken to improve the situation?
- What children are included in the target group of the project?
- Is the proposal gender sensitive?

Finally, what do you need to do to increase the impact of this project on the lives of children, and what work with partners you need to do to create an environment where children can fully enjoy their rights and live in societies that acknowledge and respect those rights?

You might need to change the way your organization works, its culture, structures, and management. You might also need to change the way you work with children, communities, partners, and donors. Nevertheless, your investment will reap huge rewards.

REFERENCES

Convention on the Rights of the Child. (1989, November 20) UN Doc GA 44/25. New York: United Nations.

Jones, G., Steketee, R. W., Black, R. E., Bhutta, Z. A., Morris, S. S., & Bellagio Child Survival Study Group. (2003). How many child deaths can we prevent this year? *Lancet, 362*(9377), 65–71.

Lawn, J. E., Cousens, S., & Zupan, J. (2005). Four million neonatal deaths: When? Where? Why? *Lancet, 365*, 1147–52

Save the Children. (2008). *Saving children's lives: Why equity matters.* Save the Children.

United Nations Children's Fund. (2008). *Countdown to 2015: Tracking progress in maternal, newborn, and child survival: The 2008 report.* UNICEF.

World Health Organization. (2002). *25 Question and Answers on Health and Human Rights.* Retrieved September 21, 2010, from http://whqlibdoc.who.int/hq/2002/9241545690.pdf

World Health Organization, & United Nations Population Fund. (2006). *Pregnant adolescents: Delivering on global promises of hope.* Geneva: WHO.

You, D., Wardlaw, T., Salama, P., & Jones, G. (2009). Levels and trends in under-5 mortality, 1990–2008. *The Lancet*, published online 10 September 2009, DOI: 10.1016/S0140-6736(09)61601-9.

NOTES

[1]Both publications are available on Save the Children Web site. Retrieved from http://www.savethechildren.org.uk/assets/php/library.php?Topic=Children%27s+rights

[2]Ratification of an international agreement (treaty, covenant, convention) represents the promise of a state to uphold it and adhere to the legal norms that it specifies. Ratification is an act of government or parliament that makes a treaty (covenant, convention) binding and enforceable in the state.

[3]Somalia and the United States of America have yet to ratify the convention.

[4]General measures of implementation (arts. 4, 41, 42, 44.6); definition of the child (art. 1); general principles (arts. 2, 3, 6, 12); civil rights and freedoms (arts. 7, 8, 13 - 17, 37); family environment and alternative care (arts. 5, 9–11, 18–21,25, 27, 39); basic health and welfare (arts. 6, 18, 23–24, 26–27); education, leisure, and cultural activities (arts. 28, 29, 31); special protection measures (arts. 22, 23, 30, 32–40).

[5]Such as the Universal Declaration of Human Rights (UDHR; 1948)—Article 25.1, International Covenant on Economics, Social and Cultural Rights (most detailed; Article 12.1 and 12.2), Convention on Elimination of All Forms of Discrimination Against Women (CEDAW), the Alma-Ata Declaration (Health for All), Millennium Development Goals (MDGs); Beijing Platform for Action, the International Conference on Population and Development and regional declarations such as the Abuja Declaration and the New Partnership for Africa's Development (NEPAD).

[6]MDG 1, 4, 5, and 6.

[7]These two concepts of the continuum of care are now used by many organizations working on child and maternal survival and is one of the guiding principles of the global Partnership for Maternal, Newborn, and Child Health (ref).

[8]Save the Children CRP Coordinating Group. (2005). *Child rights programming: How to apply rights-based approaches to programming: A handbook for International Save the Children Alliance Members.* Save the Children Sweden.

CHAPTER 12

Human Rights and HIV Prevention Among Drug Users

Salaam Semaan, Don C. Des Jarlais, Kasia Malinowska-Sempruch, Alexandra Kirby, and Tanya Telfair Sharpe

The HIV/AIDS epidemic brings human rights and public health together to address concerns that affect the lives of persons who use illicit drugs. The right to optimal health includes implementation of evidence-based public health strategies for prevention and treatment of substance use disorders (SUDs), for prevention and treatment of HIV infection, and for delivery of health care services to incarcerated persons with SUDs. Human rights protections include national and international responsibilities for health protection using evidence-based public health strategies.

This chapter focuses on how human rights considerations apply to the public health of persons who use illicit drugs and presents relevant examples from different countries. We examine three important aspects of illicit drug use: prevention and treatment of SUDs, prevention and control of HIV infection among persons who use illicit drugs, and drug use and incarceration. We recommend that evidence-based programs for preventing and treating SUDs and reducing HIV infection and transmission among persons with SUDs be universally adopted and that legislators and courts recognize addiction as an intractable mental health disorder rather than principally as a criminal activity.

INTRODUCTION

Human rights protections include societal responsibilities to respect and protect the health of people (Gruskin, Mills, & Tarantola, 2007). Citizens pledge their allegiance to their countries, and governments pledge to respect, protect, and ensure the human rights of their citizens. In commemoration of the 62nd anniversary of the 1948 United Nations Universal Declaration of Human Rights (United Nations General Assembly Resolution 217 A [III], 1948), we discuss the relationship between human rights and public health, and the protection of the health of people who use illicit drugs, presenting relevant examples from different countries. We use human rights as a framework to discuss how SUDs and how HIV infection should be prevented, controlled, and treated among persons who use illicit drugs. We focus on the human rights of persons who use illicit drugs in three public health situations: (a) the prevention and treatment of SUDs; (b) the prevention and control of HIV infection among persons who use illicit drugs; and (c) the prevention and treatment services for incarcerated persons with SUDs.

We believe in the interdependence of human rights and health. Health is a human rights matter, and upholding human rights is essential for everyone to attain the highest possible standard of health. Human rights are a determinant of health and affect the well-being of people (Mann, Gruskin, Grodin, & Annas, 1999). Protecting human rights is associated with good health, and implementing strategies that do not respect human rights can result in poor health (Hunt, 2005). People cannot be healthy when governments do not respect universal human rights and implement evidence-based health policies that would realize the rights of their citizens (Backman et al., 2008). SUDs, infection with HIV, and the incarceration of persons with SUDs are public health concerns associated with illicit drug use. Strategies to address these concerns can benefit from a combined focus on public health and human rights.

HUMAN RIGHTS AND HEALTH CARE

Human rights refer to provisions in international documents, including declarations and treaties issued under the auspices of the United Nations, and reflect a set of beliefs and values about the dignity and well-being of people (Office of the United Nations High Commissioner for Human Rights, 2009). More specifically, these documents include the Universal Declaration of Human Rights (issued in 1948), the International Covenant on Civil and Political Rights (issued in 1966), the International Covenant on Economic, Social and Cultural Rights (issued in 1966), and the Convention on the Elimination of All Forms of Discrimination Against Women (issued in 1979; Columbia University Center for the Study of Human Rights, 1994; United Nations Department of Public Information, 1996).

Ratification of a treaty places the treaty in force and binds the government to the terms of the treaty. Although ratifying human rights documents is a powerfully symbolic gesture, many countries, despite their ratification of several treaties, have not honored their treaty obligations by providing relevant interventions (Palmer et al., 2009). Conversely, the human rights records of countries can be favorable even if they have not ratified all treaties. For example, the United States has signed (agreed to by diplomats) and ratified (a two-thirds majority is required for the senate and the president's signature) the International Covenant on Civil and Political Rights. However, the United States has signed but not ratified the International Covenant on Economic, Social and Cultural Rights, the Convention on the Elimination of All Forms of Discrimination Against Women, and the International Convention on the Rights of the Child (Kinney, 2008). The status of treaty ratification alone is not a good indicator of the extent to which the right to health is realized, because financial resources are needed to support that realization (Palmer et al., 2009).

Human rights are often viewed as inspirational and aspirational because they are not commonly subject to close accountability (Fraser, Hopwood, Madden, & Treloar, 2009). The realization of human rights requires that governments invest resources to respect and protect their citizens and to acknowledge that human rights are endowed, not earned. Human rights can be described negatively and positively. Negative rights require that governments do not interfere with individual freedom. Positive rights require that governments engage in affirmative and obligatory actions that enhance the health and well-being of their citizens.

Provisions for human rights include the correlative right of everyone to attain the highest standards of physical and mental health. These provisions include the role of governments in preventing, treating, and controlling infection and disease, and the creation of conditions that ensure health and the delivery of medical services (World Health Organization [WHO], 2002). Provisions for human rights address the rights to health and to health care.

HUMAN RIGHTS AND THE PREVENTION AND TREATMENT OF SUBSTANCE USE DISORDERS

There are individual, social, and economic forces that lead people to use illicit drugs. Social and economic forces also influence responses of governments to prevent and treat SUDs (Galea & Vlahov, 2002; Gruskin,

Plafker, & Smith-Estelle, 2001; Moore & Elkavich, 2008; Pauly, 2008). The use of illicit drugs is not restricted to the poor; many middle-class and wealthy people use illicit drugs. Public health efforts aimed at preventing and controlling SUDs cannot succeed without addressing the social, economic, and personal determinants of illicit drug use.

During the past 30 years, illicit drug use has increased among women (Sharpe, 2005; Substance Abuse and Mental Health Services Administration, 2009). For many economically disadvantaged minority women, limited life opportunities provide a direct route to illicit drug use and sex work (Pinkham & Malinowska-Sempruch, 2008; Rockell, 2008; Sharpe, 2005). Neglecting women who use illicit drugs and the unique problems associated with motherhood can create future generations of marginalized people at risk for using illicit drugs (Sharpe, 2005).

Since the 1980s, the concept of biological determinism has resurged in influencing the debate on the notion of a permanent underclass (Gravlee, 2009; Murray, 1984). Biological determinists believe that some people are born inferior (intellectually and biologically) and are predisposed to socially unacceptable behaviors, such as illicit drug use and crime. Accordingly, the determinists consider assistance and support of struggling people to be a waste of time and money.

The ideology of biological determinism, which is not based on scientific evidence, divides people via an us-versus-them mentality that promotes fear of people who are labeled as social deviants (Akers, 2009). This divisiveness drives public opinion toward a polemical rather than a holistic approach to endorse strategies aimed at solving social problems. For example, although most persons who use illicit drugs in the United States are White, the media-created image of the illicit drug user is an ethnic minority image (Moore & Elkavich, 2008). Characterizing the illicit drug use problem as a racial or as an ethnic problem contributes to stigmatization and social marginalization of persons who use illicit drugs (Des Jarlais & Semaan, 2009). Stigmatizing forces isolate persons who use illicit drugs from the mainstream of society (Thomas, 2007). Stigma makes illicit drug use and prevention efforts more problematic and fuels a reluctance to support policies advocating comprehensive treatment for SUDs (Cleland et al., 2007; Sharpe, 2005).

The stigmatization ideology can justify limiting human rights of persons who use illicit drugs when they are described as the feared social deviants. To protect the human rights of persons who use illicit drugs, societal conditions and relevant public health interventions are needed to prevent or reduce illicit drug use and to provide treatment for those with SUDs.

Use of illicit drugs is not a problem specific to a certain country; it is a worldwide problem (Mathers et al., 2008). It is estimated that there are 16 million persons who inject illicit drugs in 148 countries worldwide; of whom, 10 million live in developing and transitional countries (Aceijas et al., 2006b; Mathers et al., 2008). Although achieving a world free of psychoactive drug use is an aspirational goal, it may not be realistic because use of illicit drugs continues to be reported in almost every country. In 1998, the United Nations Office on Drugs and Crime observed that a drug-free world was within reach (United Nations General Assembly, 1998), but more than 10 years later, achieving that goal is in question. Psychoactive drug use continues to be used for cultural, psychological, recreational, and medical reasons (Des Jarlais, 2000a). Different psychoactive drugs have been classified as legal or illegal in different countries and differently at different times within the same country. Determining which drugs should be classified as legal or as illegal and for which purpose is influenced by medical as well as societal realities and cultural influences. Criminal law by itself can be a very poor mechanism for regulating psychoactive drug use (Friedman et al., 2006). People do not forfeit their civil rights because of use of psychoactive drugs.

Rights-based public health efforts suggest the adoption of evidence-based strategies and interventions that prevent and treat SUDs and that respect people's dignity. However, countries vary in how they implement interventions to reduce, control, and treat SUDs (International Harm Reduction Development Program, 2008; Wiessing et al., 2009). Labor camps and forced detoxification programs, interrogating users of illicit drugs when they are in withdrawal, and imposing the death penalty for drug-related offenses are practices that do not respect the human rights of persons who use illicit drugs (Fraser et al., 2009; Hammett et al., 2007; Koester, 2009; Strathdee et al., 2010; Thanh, Moland, & Fylkesnes, 2009).

The declarations on human rights imply that treatment for SUDs must be voluntary, readily available, and accessible to persons who use illicit drugs. Treatment for SUDs should be voluntary to show respect for the human rights of persons who use illicit drugs (International Harm Reduction Development Program, 2008). Treatment of SUDs is based on the premise that such use is preventable and treatable (Cami & Farre, 2003).

Major public health organizations support the use of opioid substitution therapy to treat opioid dependence (WHO, United Nations Office on Drugs and Crime, & Joint United Nations Programme on HIV/AIDS, 2004). However, globally, this therapy is only available to 1 million injection drug users. Opioid injection drug users around the world need access to opioid substitution therapy (Mathers et al., 2008; Wiessing et al., 2009).

Methadone, a synthetic opiate medication, can be used to treat addiction to heroin. It blocks the effects of heroin for approximately 24 hours and eliminates withdrawal symptoms. Methadone has a proven record of success when prescribed at a high dose for people addicted to heroin (Coffin et al., 2006). Although methadone has appeared on the WHO's model list of essential medicines since 2005 (WHO, 2009), it remains classified as an illegal drug in many countries, including Russia and Kenya (Strathdee et al., 2010; Tkatchenko-Schmidt, Renton, Gevorgyan, Davydenko, & Atun, 2008; Wiessing et al., 2009).

Buprenorphine is another medicine that is used to treat heroin use (Carrieri et al., 2006). Buprenorphine differs from methadone because of its lower risk for an overdose. In addition, a combination of buprenorphine and naloxone, formulated for sublingual administration, is available to minimize abuse (Caldiero, Parran, Adelman, & Piche, 2006; Fischer et al., 2006; Kim, Irwin, & Khoshnood, 2009).

Treatment of SUDs tends to be more effective when combined with behavioral intervention strategies and social services (Farrell, Gowing, Marsden, Ling, & Ali, 2005; Prendergast, Urada, & Podus, 2001).

Behavioral approaches represent an effective strategy to treat SUDs. These approaches use outpatient and residential strategies. Treatment options include cognitive–behavioral interventions and contingency management therapy (Shroeder, Epstein, Umbricht, & Preston, 2006). Cognitive–behavioral interventions are designed to help modify the patient's thinking, expectations, and behaviors and to increase a person's skills at coping with various life stressors. Contingency management therapy uses a voucher-based system that allows patients to earn points for negative tests for illicit drug use and to exchange these points for items that encourage healthful living.

Therapeutic communities or residential programs with planned lengths of stay of 6–12 months offer another alternative to those in need of treatment for SUDs. These communities focus on the resocialization of persons with SUDs and can include on-site vocational rehabilitation and other support (Smith, Gates, & Foxcroft, 2006).

Prevention of initiation of illicit drug use remains an important strategy in reducing the harm experienced by persons with SUDs. Ensuring that persons who use illicit drugs have access to behavioral and biomedical interventions is an approach that represents a human-rights approach and an evidence-based approach for the treatment of SUDs.

RIGHTS-BASED APPROACHES FOR THE CONTROL OF HIV AMONG PERSONS WHO USE ILLICIT DRUGS

For more than a decade, research on treatment of SUDs has shown that such treatment reduces HIV risk behaviors and prevents HIV infection (Metzger & Navaline, 2003; Metzger, Navaline, & Woody, 1998). Many studies show that treatment for SUDs can decrease or eliminate HIV risk through reduction in risky injection practices and unsafe sex (Farrell et al., 2005; Prendergast et al., 2001; Prendergast, Podus, Finney, Greenwell, & Roll, 2006). Treatment for SUDs is part of a comprehensive strategy for HIV prevention (Donoghoe, 2006; Donoghoe, Verster, Pervilhac, & Williams, 2008; Sorensen & Copeland, 2000). Treatment programs for SUDs provide users with information on HIV/AIDS and other diseases, counseling and testing services, and referrals to medical and social services (Pollack, D'Aunno, & Lamar, 2006; Sullivan, Metzger, Fudala, & Fiellin, 2005).

Oral methadone treatment lowers the risk for HIV infection by decreasing rates of injection of illicit drugs (Gowing, Farrell, Bornemann, Sullivan, & Ali, 2008). However, information about the effectiveness of methadone for persons who inject illicit drugs is restricted in many countries (Parfitt, 2006; Strathdee et al., 2010). Restricting information can be deadly in countries where the HIV epidemic is fuelled by injection of illicit drugs (Grassly, Lowndes, & Rhodes, 2003).

The human rights of persons who use illicit drugs and who are infected with HIV must be respected. These persons should not be treated like the lepers of the 21st century and should not be denied health care (International Harm Reduction Development Program, 2008). Access to HIV antiretroviral treatment is often denied to persons who inject illicit drugs because of their SUDs, in spite of evidence that highly active antiretroviral therapy is as effective among those who use and those who do not use illicit drugs (Malta, Strathdee, Magnanini, & Bastos, 2008; Wood et al., 2008). At the end of 2004, less than 25% of HIV-infected persons who inject illicit drugs received antiretroviral therapy in developing and transitional countries (Aceijas et al., 2006a). Data show that persons who inject illicit drugs and who receive comprehensive services that include treatment for SUDs and psychosocial support adhere reasonably well to HIV antiretroviral therapy (Malta et al., 2008). Ensuring that HIV-infected persons who inject illicit drugs receive HIV treatment respects their human rights.

Racial and ethnic disparities in HIV infection rates are not explained completely by individual risk behaviors, but often by network-related and social variables, including network infection rates and availability of social support (Des Jarlais & Semaan, 2009). Failure to address the societal determinants and infrastructure that affect HIV risk does not respect the rights of persons who use illicit drugs (Poundstone, Strathdee, & Celentano, 2004; Rhodes, Singer, Bourgois, Friedman, & Strathdee, 2005; Strathdee et al., 2010).

Needle and syringe programs are services that provide persons who inject illicit drugs with sterile needles and syringes. Studies have shown the effectiveness of needle and syringe programs in preventing HIV transmission, without an increase in frequency or proportion of injection drug use (Vlahov & Junge, 1998; Wodak & McLeod, 2008). Needle and syringe programs have been associated with a reduction in needle reuse, sharing of syringes and other injection equipment, and in HIV seroconversion rates (Bluthenthal, Anderson, Flynn, & Kral, 2007; Des Jarlais et al., 1996; Des Jarlais, McKnight, Goldblatt, & Purchase, D, 2009; Des Jarlais et al., 2005; McKnight et al., 2007; Vlahov, 2000). Conversely, lack of access to sterile needles and syringes has been associated with an increase in injection-related risk behaviors (Broadhead, van Julst, & Heckathorn, 1999; Rich, Dickinson, & Liu, 1998).

Major reviews of needle and syringe programs in the United States include those by the U.S. National Commission on AIDS (National Commission on AIDS, 1991), a report from the Consensus Development Conference held by the National Institutes of Health (1997), a review by the National Academy of Sciences (Institute of Medicine, 1995), and a review by the Cochrane Collaboration (The Cochrane Collaborative Review Group on HIV Infection and AIDS, 2004). These reviews are in favor of needle and syringe programs.

In most developed countries, needle and syringe programs are a major component of HIV prevention under the philosophy of harm reduction or risk reduction (Wiessing et al., 2009; Wodak & Cooney, 2005). Harm-reduction programs are important because some users of illicit drugs are not able or are not willing to stop using or injecting illicit drugs. As another strategy in harm-reduction, pharmacy-based distribution programs allow for selling sterile needles and syringes to persons who inject illicit drugs. Access to sterile injection equipment from pharmacies has been associated with reduced rates of needle sharing and HIV transmission (Cooper, Bossak, Tempalski, Friedman, & Des Jarlais, 2009; Wodak & Cooney, 2005). Supervised injection facilities, which are spaces where persons who inject illicit drugs can inject preobtained illicit drugs under medical supervision, represent a recent effective strategy in harm reduction (Des Jarlais, Arasteh, Semaan, & Wood, 2009).

The overall scientific evidence shows that treatment for SUDs, needle and syringe programs, and HIV prevention and treatment programs reduce risk behavior and HIV infection among persons who use illicit drugs (Des Jarlais, 2000b; Vlahov et al., 2001). Despite the evidence of their effectiveness, harm-reduction interventions raise strong emotional responses and political controversy and they are not offered to persons who use illicit drugs in many parts of the world (Strathdee et al., 2010; Wiessing et al., 2009). Recently, the Joint United Nations Programme on HIV/AIDS provided information on a comprehensive package of HIV prevention services for persons who inject illicit drugs that includes nine interventions (Donoghoe et al., 2008). These interventions are needle and syringe programs; opioid substitution therapy; voluntary HIV counseling and testing; antiretroviral therapy for those who are HIV-infected; STD prevention and treatment; condom distribution; information and education for those who inject illicit drugs and for their partners; hepatitis diagnosis and treatment or vaccination; and TB prevention, diagnosis, and treatment.

Respecting human rights implies the need to provide effective and evidence-based strategies to prevent and treat HIV among persons who use illicit drugs.

ILLICIT DRUG USE AND INCARCERATION

A human rights–based approach to optimal health implies the need to consider the relationship between illicit drug use and incarceration and to provide prison-based services to treat SUDs and to prevent HIV transmission (Burris & Strathdee, 2006). Health-related policies and law enforcement policies that do not respect human rights and that treat use of illicit drugs principally as a criminal activity can increase susceptibility of persons who use illicit drugs to HIV infection. Such policies force persons who use illicit drugs underground and can hamper access to harm-reduction services for HIV prevention and treatment.

Incarceration of nonviolent users of illicit drugs has not proved to be an effective deterrent for illicit drug use. Such incarceration is counterproductive from both public health and human rights perspectives (Friedman et al., 2006). Although depriving persons who use illicit drugs of their freedom can be a convenient way to address a legal problem, it has proved to be an inadequate way to deal with a poorly understood and a much-feared social problem (Cottrell & Neuberg, 2005; Okie, 2007). In spite of the growth in the number of prisons around the world, prisons remain overcrowded, unhealthy, and dangerous places (Restum, 2005; Spaulding et al., 2009).

Since the United States declared a "war on drugs" in the early 1980s, the percentage of drug-related arrests has more than doubled (Abiona, Adefuye, Balogun, & Sloan, 2009; Golemkeski & Fullilove, 2005). Drug-related offenses rank near the top of prosecuted criminal activities in the United States (Golemkeski & Fullilove, 2005; Lee & Rasinski, 2006; United States Bureau of Justice Statistics, 2008). During the 1980s, the crack cocaine drug epidemic in poor neighborhoods in the United States contributed substantially to the rise in the prison population for both men and women (Golemkeski & Fullilove, 2005). In 1972, the national prison population was fewer than 200,000. By the middle of 2004, the number of inmates in U.S. prisons and jails had grown to more than 2.1 million; 1 in 138 Americans was incarcerated (Golemkeski & Fullilove, 2005; United States Bureau of Justice Statistics, 2008). A disproportionate number of inmates in the United States are Black, Hispanic, poor, less educated, or have mental and physical health challenges. Racial and ethnic minorities constitute most incarcerated people in many other countries around the world (Abiona et al., 2009; Bobrik, Danishevski, Eroshina, & McKee, 2005). Worldwide, opioid-dependent people are disproportionately represented in prisons. In the European Union, for example, prevalence of overuse of heroin among prisoners ranges from 5–66% (European Monitoring Centre for Drugs and Drug Addiction, 2004).

Illicit drug use in prison is inevitably accompanied by risky behavior, such as sharing injection equipment, because preventive measures such as provision and access to sterile needles and syringes are often prohibited (McLemore, 2008; Spaulding et al., 2002). High rates of HIV infection are reported among incarcerated users with SUDs. An estimated 30–40% of incarcerated users with SUDs in the United States are HIV-positive (Abiona et al., 2009; Baillargeon et al., 2009; Hennessy et al., 2008; MacGowan et al., 2009). The stigmatization and marginalization of persons who use illicit drugs and the use of incarceration as a punitive measure have exacerbated racial and ethnic disparities in HIV infection rates among persons who use illicit drugs. It has been recommended that drug treatment and sterile syringes and needles should be provided in prisons to reduce the harm associated with illicit drug use (Bruce & Schleifer, 2008; Jurgens, Ball, & Verster, 2009).

Users of illicit drugs who commit crimes to support their use of illicit drugs need drug treatment especially that SUD is a chronic, relapsing disease that requires treatment. Treating SUDs in prisons should be voluntary and based on sound medical and public health principles. In China, the duration of forced detoxification, used as an alternative to incarceration, has increased from 3 months to 2 years, although the detoxification process usually takes 1 week. Extended forced detoxification is a form of punishment in which persons who use illicit drugs are unwillingly isolated from their friends and families (Hammett et al., 2007). Poland offers drug-free rehabilitation centers; however, only 6% of persons who inject illicit drugs have access to these centers and use them (National Bureau for Drug Prevention, 2009). Ensuring that persons who use illicit drugs have access to treatment for SUDs shows respect for human rights.

Incarcerating nonviolent users of illicit drugs has enormous individual and social costs. Once incarcerated, persons who use illicit drugs are unable to work or take care of their families, placing the burden of the care for their families on society (Donohoe, 2006). Once incarcerated, persons who use illicit drugs find it difficult to secure employment after their release and they are frequently trapped in a vicious circle of poverty, illicit drug use, and incarceration. After release from prison, persons who inject illicit drugs face a high risk for a drug overdose (Kim et al., 2009). Alternatives to incarceration, such as drug courts and mandated drug treatment, are at the forefront of the human rights and drug policy debate. It is relevant that legislators and courts recognize addiction as an intractable mental health disorder rather than principally as a criminal activity. Decriminalizing the possession of small amounts of illicit drugs, for personal use, is another potential alternative, although it remains a controversial alternative. There are few data on decriminalization of the possession of illicit drugs for personal use. Portugal's recent experience has been evaluated as a positive experience; with no increase in proportion of drug use or in criminal activity, and with a substantial decline in new HIV infections and in drug-related mortality rates (Greenwald, 2009).

Alternatives to incarceration, providing treatment for SUDs, and providing HIV prevention and treatment services to incarcerated persons who use illicit drugs are important human rights-based public health strategies.

CONCLUSION

Human rights are a set of distinct values that are codified in international treaties ratified by most countries. Public health professionals are morally bound to focus their efforts to fulfill the right to health. Public health professionals in many countries, including the United States, are employed or supported by governments that are signatories to international treaties (Office of the United Nations High Commissioner for Human Rights, 2009). Thus, public health professionals are bound to respect, protect, and fulfill the rights outlined in those treaties. Some may construe the language of human rights to represent a Western, neoliberal philosophy;

however, self-determination, dignity, and the well-being of people represent intrinsic values embraced by different cultures.

The discourse on human rights and HIV prevention for persons who use illicit drugs is characterized by passionate conversations, policy debates, and a reliance on scientific data. The intricate interactions between human rights and public health are often manifested by agreement on global principles and disagreement on allocation of resources, social obligations, and specific strategies. As practitioners and policy makers evaluate and implement evidence-based public health strategies, they shape human rights and they act in an environment that is shaped by human rights. There is a need to reduce the gap that exists between the enunciation of human rights and their full realization, particularly that the international guidelines of the Joint United Nations Programme on HIV/AIDS call for enforcing and monitoring human rights.

Respecting human rights is at the basis of good public health policies. Advocating for evidence-based policies indicates that persons who use illicit drugs, including those who are HIV-positive, have the same human rights as anyone else. The human rights of people, including those who use illicit drugs, need to be respected if we are to live in fully democratic societies. By respecting the human rights of all people, we can take positive steps toward preventing and treating SUDs and toward controlling the HIV epidemic among persons who use illicit drugs. Undergirding the policies should be a fundamental understanding that risk behaviors for illicit drug use and for HIV infection do not exist in a vacuum. Social determinants of health, including poverty and lack of opportunities for education and employment, play a critical role in illicit drug use and in HIV transmission. Failure to address the societal determinants and the infrastructure that affect risk for illicit drug use and for HIV transmission does not respect the human rights of persons who use illicit drugs.

Engaging persons who use illicit drugs in the development of relevant interventions represents an acknowledgment of their human rights and shows respect for their autonomy for decision making and for their right to self-determination. Involving persons who use illicit drugs in discussions about relevant interventions has been instrumental in controlling the HIV/AIDS epidemic (Friedman et al., 2007). Persons who use illicit drugs are able to discuss and identify successful public health responses and to engage in participatory research and programs in different settings, including correctional settings.

The HIV/AIDS epidemic has played three major roles in bringing human rights and public health together. The HIV/AIDS epidemic among persons who use illicit drugs has been a catalyst highlighting the role of human rights in the prevention and treatment of SUDs and in the prevention and control of HIV infection among persons who use illicit drugs. The HIV/AIDS epidemic has also played a role in assessing incarceration as a response to illicit drug use and as a mechanism and a setting for HIV prevention and treatment.

Effective evidence-based public health strategies exist to treat and prevent SUDs and HIV infection among persons who use illicit drugs. Strategies and policies for HIV prevention among persons who use illicit drugs need to include evidence-based interventions that are in accord with human rights. There is also a need to implement the programs and services on a sufficient scale, rather than on a pilot scale, to reach all those who need these programs to ensure an effective response in the prevention and treatment of SUDs and in controlling the HIV/AIDS epidemic. Policy barriers should be removed to allow implementation of prevention and treatment programs for SUDs, HIV/AIDS, and for prison-based public health programs.

In conclusion, as we reflect on the 62nd anniversary of the Universal Declaration of Human Rights, we note that the global community, including government and civil society, has a responsibility to implement sufficiently scaled and evidence-based public health interventions that protect the health of persons who use illicit drugs and that show respect for their human rights. We recommend that evidence-based programs, which prevent and treat SUDs and reduce HIV transmission among persons who use illicit drug, be universally adopted and that legislators and courts recognize addiction as an intractable mental health disorder rather than principally as a criminal activity.

ACKNOWLEDGMENTS

The findings and conclusions in this chapter are those of the authors and do not necessarily represent the views of the Centers for Disease Control and Prevention.

REFERENCES

Abiona, T. C., Adefuye, A. S., Balogun, J. A., & Sloan, P. E. (2009). Relationship between incarceration frequency and human immunodeficiency virus risk behaviors of African American inmates. *Journal of the National Medical Association, 101,* 308–315.

Aceijas, C., Friedman, S. R., Cooper, H. L. F., Wiessing, L., Stimson, G. V., & Hickman, M. (2006b). Estimates of injecting drug users at the national and local level in developing and transitional countries, and gender and age distribution. *Sexually Transmitted Infections, 82,* iii10–iii17.

Aceijas, C., Oppenheimer, E., Stimson, G. V., Ashcroft, R. E., Matic, S., Hickman, M., et al. (2006a). Antiretroviral treatment for injecting drug users in developing and transitional countries 1 year before the end of the "Treating 3 million by 2005. Making it happen. The WHO strategy (3 by 5). *Addiction*, *101*,1246–1253.

Akers, T. A. L. M. M. (2009). "Epidemiological criminology": Coming full circle. *American Journal of Public Health*, *99*(3), 397–402.

Backman, G., Hunt, P., Khosla, R., Jaramillo-Strauss, C., Fikre, B. M., & Rumble, C. (2008). Health systems and the right to health: An assessment of 194 countries. *The Lancet*, *372*, 2047–2085.

Baillargeon, J., Giordano, T. P., Rich, J., Wu, Z. H., Wells, K., Pollock, B. H., et al. (2009). Accessing antiretroviral therapy following release from prison. *The Journal of American Medical Association*, *301*, 848–857.

Bluthenthal, R. N., Anderson, R., Flynn, N. M., & Kral, A. H. (2007). High syringe coverage is associated with lower odds of HIV risk and does not increase unsafe syringe disposal among syringe exchange program clients. *Drug and Alcohol Dependence*, *89*, 214–222.

Bobrik, A., Danishevski, K., Eroshina, K., & McKee, M. (2005). Prison health in Russia: The larger picture. *Journal of Public Health Policy*, *26*, 30–59.

Broadhead, R. S., van Julst, Y., & Heckathorn, D. D. (1999). The impact of a needle exchange's closure. *Public Health Reports*, *114*, 439–447.

Bruce, R. D., & Schleifer, R. A. (2008). Ethical and human rights imperatives to ensure medication-assisted treatment for opioid dependence in prisons and pre-trial detention. *International Journal of Drug Policy*, *19*, 17–23.

Burris, S., & Strathdee, S. A. (2006). To serve and protect? Toward a better relationship between drug control policy and public health. *AIDS*, *20*, 117-118.

Caldiero, R. M., Parran, T. V., Adelman, C. L., & Piche, B. (2006). Inpatient initiation of buprenorphine maintenance vs. detoxification: Can retention of opioid-dependent patients in outpatient counseling be improved? *The American Journal on Addictions*, *15*, 1–7.

Cami, J. & Farre, M. (2003). Drug addiction. *New England Journal of Medicine*, *349*, 975–986.

Carrieri, M. P., Amass, L., Lucas, G. M., Vlahov, D., Wodak, A., & Woody, G. E. (2006). Buprenorphine use: The international experience. *Clinical Infectious Diseases*, *43*, S197–S215.

Cleland, C. M., Des Jarlais, D. C., Perlis, T. E., Stimson, G., Poznyak, V., & and the WHO Phase II Drug Injection Collaborative Study Group. (2007). HIV risk behaviors among female IDUs in developing and transitional countries. *BMC Public Health*, *7*, 271–283.

The Cochrane Collaborative Review Group on HIV Infection and AIDS. (2004). Evidence assessment: Strategies for HIV/AIDS prevention, treatment and care. University of California, San Francisco, Institute for Global Health.

Coffin, P. O., Blaney, S., Fuller, C., Vadnai, L., Miller, S., & Vlahov, D. (2006). Support for buprenorphine and methadone prescription to heroin-dependent patients among New York City physicians. *American Journal of Drug & Alcohol Abuse, 32,* 1–6.

Columbia University Center for the Study of Human Rights. (1994). *Twenty-five human rights documents.* New York: Columbia University.

Cooper, H. L., Bossak, B. H., Tempalski, B., Friedman, S. R., & Des Jarlais, D. C. (2009). Temporal trends in spatial access to pharmacies that sell over-the-counter syringes in New York City health districts: Relationships to local racial/ethnic composition and need. *Journal of Urban Health, 86*(6), 929–945.

Cottrell, C. A., & Neuberg, S. L. (2005). Different emotional reactions to different groups: A sociofunctional threat-based approach to "prejudice." *Journal of Personality and Social Psychology, 88,* 770–789.

Des Jarlais, D. C. (2000a). Prospects for a public health perspective on psychoactive drug use. *American Journal of Public Health, 90,* 335–337.

Des Jarlais, D. C. (2000b). Research, politics and needle exchange. *American Journal of Public Health, 90,* 1392–1394.

Des Jarlais, D. C., Arasteh, K., Semaan, S., & Wood, E. (2009). HIV among injecting drug users: Current epidemiology, biologic factors, respondent-driven sampling, and supervised injection facilities. *Current Opinion in HIV and AIDS, 4,* 308–313.

Des Jarlais, D. C., Marmor, M., Paone, D.,Titus, S., Shi, Q., Perlis, T., et al. (1996). HIV incidence among injecting drug users in New York City syringe-exchange programmes. *The Lancet, 348,* 987–991.

Des Jarlais, D. C., McKnight, C., Goldblatt, C., & Purchase, D. (2009). Doing harm reduction better: syringe exchange in the United States. *Addiction, 104,* 1441–1446.

Des Jarlais, D. C., Perlis, T., Arasteh, K., Torian, L. V., Beatrice, S., Milliken, J., et al. (2005). HIV incidence among injection drug users in New York City, 1990 to 2002: Use of serologic test algorithm to assess expansion of HIV prevention services. *American Journal of Public Health, 95,* 1439–1444.

Des Jarlais, D. C. & Semaan, S. (2009). HIV prevention and psychoactive drug use: A research agenda. *Journal of Epidemiology and Community Health, 63,* 191–196.

Donoghoe, M. C. (2006). Injecting drug use, harm reduction, and HIV/AIDS. In S. Matic, J. V. Lazarus, & M. C. Donoghoe (Eds.), *HIV/AIDS in Europe: Moving from death sentence to chronic disease management* (pp. 43–66). Copenhagen, Denmark: World Health Organization.

Donoghoe, M. C., Verster, A., Pervilhac, C., & Williams, P. (2008). Setting targets for universal access to HIV prevention, treatment and care for injecting drug users (IDUs): Towards consensus and improved guidance. *The Internal Journal on Drug Policy, 19S,* S5–S14.

Donohoe, M. T. (2006). Incarceration Nation: Health and welfare in the prison system in the United States. *Ob/Gyn & Women's Health, 11.*

European Monitoring Centre for Drugs and Drug Addiction. (2004). Drug users in prison. Retrieved September 8, 2010, from http://ar2004.emcdda.europa.eu/en/page094-en.html

Farrell, M., Gowing, L., Marsden, J., Ling, W., & Ali, R. (2005). Effectiveness of drug dependence treatment in HIV prevention. *International Journal of Drug Policy, 16S*, S67–S75.

Fischer, G., Ortner, R., Rohrmeister, K., Jagsch, R., Baewert, A., Langer, M., et al. (2006). Methadone versus buprenorphine in pregnant addicts: A double-blind, double-dummy comparison study. *Addiction, 101*, 275–281.

Fraser, S., Hopwood, M., Madden, A., & Treloar, C. (2009). "Toward a global approach": An overview of harm reduction 2008: IHRA's 19th international conference. *International Journal of Drug Policy, 20*, 93–97.

Friedman, S. R., Cooper, H. L. F., Tempalski, B., Keem, M., Friedman, R., Flom, P. L. et al. (2006). Relationship of deterrence and law enforcement to drug-related harms among drug injectors in U.S. metropolitan cities. *AIDS, 20*, 93–99.

Friedman, S. R., de Jong, W., Rossi, D., Touze, G., Rockwell, R., Des Jarlais, D. C., et al. (2007). Harm reduction theory: Users' culture, micro-social indigenous harm reduction, and the self-organization and outside-organizing of users' groups. *International Journal of Drug Policy, 18*, 107–111.

Galea, S., & Vlahov, D. (2002). Social determinants and the health of drug users: Socioeconomic status, homelessness, and incarceration. *Public Health Reports, 117*, S135–S145.

Golemkeski, C., & Fullilove, R. (2005). Criminal (in)justice in the city and its associated health consequences. *American Journal of Public Health, 95*, 1701–1706.

Gowing, L., Farrell, M., Bornemann, R., Sullivan, L. E., & Ali, R. (2008). Substitution treatment of injecting opioid users for prevention of HIV infection. *Cochrane Database of Systemtic Reviews, 2*, DOI:10.1002/14651858.CD004145.pub3.

Grassly, N. C., Lowndes, C. M., & Rhodes, T. (2003). Modeling emerging HIV epidemics: The role of injection drug use and sexual transmission in the Russian Federation, China, and India. *International Journal of Drug Policy, 14*, 25–43.

Gravlee, C. C. (2009). How race becomes biology: Embodiment of social inequality. *American Journal of Physical Anthropology, 139*, 47–57.

Greenwald, G. (2009). *Drug decriminalization in Portugal. Lessons for creating fair and successful drug policies* Cato Institute.

Gruskin, S., Mills, E. J., & Tarantola, D. (2007). History, principles, and practice of health and human rights. *Lancet, 370*, 449–455.

Gruskin, S., Plafker, K., & Smith-Estelle, A. (2001). Understanding and responding to youth substance use: The contribution of a health and human rights framework. *American Journal of Public Health, 91*, 1954–1963.

Hammett, T. M., Wu, Z., Duc, T. T., Stephens, D., Sullivan, S., Liu, W., et al. (2007). "Social evils" and harm reduction: The evolving policy environment for human immunodeficiency virus prevention among injection drug users in China and Vietnam. *Addiction, 103*, 137–145.

Hennessy, K. A., Kim, A. A., Griffin, V., Collins, N. T., Weinbaum, C. M., & Sabin, K. (2008). Prevalence of infection with hepatitis B and C viruses and co-infection with HIV in three jails: A case for viral hepatitis prevention in jails in the United States. *Journal of Urban Health, 86*, 93–105.

Hunt, N. (2005). Public health or human rights? *International Journal of Drug Policy, 16,* 5–7.

Institute of Medicine. (1995). *Preventing HIV transmission: The role of sterile needles and bleach.* Washington, DC: National Academy Press.

International Harm Reduction Development Program. (2008). *Harm reduction developments 2008: Countries with injection-driven HIV epidemics.* New York: International Harm Reduction Development Program: Program of the Open Society Institute.

Jurgens, R., Ball, A., & Verster, A. (2009). Interventions to reduce HIV transmission related to injecting drug use in prisons. *Lancet, 9,* 57–66.

Kim, D., Irwin, K. S., & Khoshnood, K. (2009). Expanded access to naloxone: Options for critical response to the epidemic of opioid overdose mortality. *American Journal of Public Health, 99,* 402–407.

Kinney, E. D. (2008). Recognition of the international human right to health and health care in the United States. *Rutgers Law Review, 60,* 335–379.

Koester, S. (2009). The disconnect between China's public health and public security responses to injection drug use, and the consequences for human rights. *PLoS Medicine, 5,* e240-doi:10.137/journal.pmed.0050240.

Lee, R. D., & Rasinski, K. A. (2006). Five grams of coke: Racism, moralism and White public opinion on sanctions for the first time possession. *International Journal of Drug Policy, 17,* 183–191.

MacGowan, R., Margolis, A., Richardson-Moore, A., Wang, T., Lalota, M., French, P. T., et al. (2009). Voluntary rapid human immunodeficiency virus (HIV) testing in jails. *Sexually Transmitted Diseases, 36,* S9–S13.

Malta, M., Strathdee, S. A., Magnanini, M. M. F., & Bastos, F. I. (2008). Adherence to antiretroviral therapy for human immunodeficiency virus/acquired immune deficiency syndrome among drug users: A systematic review. *Addiction, 103,* 1242–1257.

Mann, J. M., Gruskin, S., Grodin, M. A., & Annas, G. J. (1999). *Health and human rights: A reader.* New York: Routledge.

Mathers, B. M., Degenhardt, L., Phillips, B., Wiessing, L., Hickman, M., Strathdee, S. A., et al. (2008). Global epidemiology of injecting drug use and HIV among people who inject drugs: A systematic review. *Lancet, 372,* 1733–1745.

McLemore, M. (2008). Access to condoms in U.S. prisons. *HIV/AIDS Policy and Law Review, 13,* 20–24.

McKnight, C. A., Des Jarlais, D. C., Perlis, T., Eigo, K., Krim, M., Ruiz, M., et al. (2007). Syringe exchange programs—United States, 2005. *Morbidity and Mortality Weekly Report, 56,* 1164–1167.

Metzger, D. S., & Navaline, H. (2003). Human immunodeficiency virus prevention and the potential for drug abuse treatment. *Clinical Infectious Diseases, 37,* S451–S456.

Metzger, D. S., Navaline, H., & Woody, G. E. (1998). Drug abuse treatment as HIV prevention. *Public Health Reports, 113,* 97–106.

Moore, L. D., & Elkavich, A. (2008). Who's using and who's doing time: Incarceration, the war on drugs, and public health. *American Journal of Public Health, 98,* 782–786.

Murray, C. (1984). *Losing ground: American social policy 1950–1980*. New York: Basic Books.

National Bureau for Drug Prevention. (2009). Substitution Patients' Register. Retrieved September 8, 2010, from http://www.whitehousedrugpolicy.gov/publications/policy/ndcs09/2009ndcs.pdf

National Commission on AIDS. (1991). *The twin epidemics of substance use and HIV: Full report*. Washington, DC: U.S. National Commission on AIDS.

National Institutes of Health (1997). *Interventions to prevent HIV risk behaviors* (Rep. No. 15 (2). Washington, DC: Author.

Okie, S. (2007). Sex, drugs, prisons, and HIV. *The New England Journal of Medicine, 356*, 105–108.

Office of the United Nations High Commissioner for Human Rights. (2009). Human rights instruments. Retrieved September 8, 2010, from http://www2.ohchr.org/english/law

Palmer, A., Tomkinson, J., Phung, C., Ford, N., Joffres, M., Fernandes, K. A., et al. (2009). Does ratification of human-rights treaties have effects on population health? *Lancet, 373*(9679), 1987–1992.

Parfitt, T. (2006). Vladimir Mendelevich: Fighting for drug substitution treatment. *Lancet, 368*, 279.

Pauly, B. (2008). Harm reduction through a social justice lens. *International Journal of Drug Policy, 19*, 4–10.

Pinkham, S., & Malinowska-Sempruch, K. (2008). Women, harm reduction, and HIV. *Reproductive Health Matters, 16*, 168–181.

Pollack, H. A., D'Aunno, T., & Lamar, B. (2006). Outpatient substance abuse treatment and HIV prevention: An update. *Journal of Substance Abuse Treatment, 30*, 39–47.

Poundstone, K. E., Strathdee, S. A., & Celentano, D. D. (2004). The social epidemiology of human immunodeficiency virus/acquired immunodeficiency syndrome. *Epidemiologic Reviews, 26*, 22–35.

Prendergast, M., Podus, D., Finney, J., Greenwell, L., & Roll, J. (2006). Contingency management for treatment of substance use disorders: A meta-analysis. *Addiction, 101*, 1546–1560.

Prendergast, M. L., Urada, D., & Podus, D. (2001). Meta-analysis of HIV risk-reduction interventions within drug abuse treatment programs. *Journal of Consulting and Clinical Psychology, 69*, 389–405.

Restum, Z. G. (2005). Public health implications of substandard correctional health care. *American Journal of Public Health, 95*, 1689–1691.

Rhodes, T., Singer, M., Bourgois, P., Friedman, S. R., & Strathdee, S. A. (2005). The social structural production of HIV risk among injection drug users. *Social Science and Medicine, 61*, 1026–1044.

Rich, J. D., Dickinson, B., & Liu, K. (1998). Strict syringe laws in Rhode Island are associated with high rates of reusing syringes and HIV risks among drug users. *Journal of Acquired Immune Deficiency Syndrome and Human Retrovirology, 18*, (Suppl. 1), S140–S141.

Rockell, B. (2008). *Women street hustlers: Who they are and how they survive.* Washington, DC: American Psychological Association.

Sharpe, T. T. (2005). *Behind the eight ball: Sex for crack cocaine exchange and poor black women.* The Haworth Press, Inc.

Shroeder, J. R., Epstein, D. H., Umbricht, A., & Preston, K. L. (2006). Changes in HIV risk behaviors among patients receiving combined pharmacological and behavioral interventions for heroin and cocaine dependence. *Addictive Behaviors, 31,* 868–879.

Smith, L. A., Gates, S., & Foxcroft, D. (2006). *Therapeutic communities for substance related disorder* (Rep. No. Issue 1). Art. No.: CD005338. DOI:10.1002/14651858 .CD005338.pub.2: Cochrane Database of Systematic Reviews.

Sorensen, J., & Copeland, A. (2000). Drug abuse treatment as an HIV prevention strategy: A review. *Drug and Alcohol Dependence, 59,* 17–31.

Spaulding, A., Stephenson, B., Macalino, G., Ruby, W., Clarke, J. G., & Flanigan, T. P. (2002). Human immunodeficiency virus in correctional facilities: A review. *Clinical Infectious Diseases, 35,* 305–312.

Spaulding, A. C., Seals, R. M., Page, M. J., Brzozowski, A. K., Rhodes, W., & Hammett, T. M. (2009). HIV/AIDS among inmates of and releases from U.S. correctional facilities, 2006: Declining share of epidemic but persistent public health opportunity. *PLoS ONE, 4,* e7558-doi;10.1371/journal.pone. 0007558.

Strathdee, S. A., Hallett, T. B., Bobrova, N., Rhodes, T., Booth, R., Abdool, R., et al. (2010). HIV and the risk environment among people who inject drugs: Past, present, and projections for the future. *Lancet, 375,*1014–1028.

Substance Abuse and Mental Health Services Administration. (2009). *Results from the 2008 National Survey on Drug Use and Health: National Findings* (Rep. No. NSDUH Series H-36, HHS Publication No. SMA 09-4434). Rockville, MD: SAMHSA, Office of Applied Studies.

Sullivan, L. E., Metzger, D. S., Fudala, P. J., & Fiellin, D. A. (2005). Decreasing international HIV transmission: The role of expanding access to opiod agnoist therapies for injection drug users. *Addiction, 100,* 150–158.

Thanh, D. C., Moland, K. M., & Fylkesnes, K. (2009). The context of HIV risk behaviors among HIV-positive injection drug users in Viet Nam: Moving toward effective harm reduction. *BMC Public Health, 9,* 98.

Thomas, Y. F. (2007). The social epidemiology of drug abuse. *American Journal of Preventive Medicine, 32,* S141–S146.

Tkatchenko-Schmidt, E., Renton, A., Gevorgyan, R., Davydenko, L., & Atun, R. (2008). Prevention of HIV/AIDS among injecting drug users in Russia: Opportunities and barriers to scaling-up of harm reduction programmes. *Health Policy, 85,* 162–171.

United Nations Department of Public Information. (1996). *The United Nations and human rights* (Rep. No. DPI/1774/HR). Retrieved August 9, 2010, from http:// www.un.org/rights/dpi1774e.htm

United Nations General Assembly. (1998). Retrieved September 8, 2010, from http://www2.ohchr.org/english/law

United Nations General Assembly Resolution 217 A (III). (1948). Universal Declaration of Human Rights. Retrieved August 9, 2010, from http://www.un-documents. net/a3r217a.htm

United States Bureau of Justice Statistics. (2008). Estimated arrests for drug abuse violations by age group, 1970-2007. Washington, DC: U.S. Department of Justice. Retrieved September 8, 2010, from http://bjs.ojp.usdoj.gov/content/ glance/tables/drugtab.cfm

Vlahov, D. (2000). The role of epidemiology in needle exchange programs. *American Journal of Public Health, 90,* 1390–1392.

Vlahov, D., Des Jarlais, D. C., Goosby, E., Hollinger, P. C., Lurie, P. G., Shriver, M. D., et al. (2001). Needle exchange programs for the prevention of human immunodeficiency virus infection: Epidemiology and policy. *American Journal of Epidemiology, 154,* S70–S77.

Vlahov, D., & Junge, B. (1998). The role of needle exchange programs in HIV prevention. *Public Health Reports, 113,* 75–80.

Wiessing, L., Likatavicius, G., Klempova, D., Hedrich, D., Nardone, A., & Griffiths, P. (2009). Associations between availability and coverage of HIV-prevention measures and subsequent incidence of diagnosed HIV infection among injection drug users. *American Journal of Public Health, 99,* 1049–1052.

Wodak, A., & Cooney, A. (2005). Effectiveness of sterile needle and syringe programmes. *International Journal of Drug Policy, 16S,* S31–S44.

Wodak, A. & McLeod, L. (2008). The role of harm reduction in controlling HIV among injecting drug users. *AIDS, 22,* S81–S92.

Wood, E., Hogg, R. S., Dias Lima, V., Kerr, T., Yip, B., Marshall, B. D. L. et al. (2008). Highly active antiretroviral therapy and survival in HIV-infected injection drug users. *Journal of the American Medical Association, 300,* 550–554.

World Health Organization. (2002). 25 questions and answers on health and human rights. Geneva, World Health Organization. Health and Human Rights Publication Series. 7-14-2009.

World Health Organization. (2009). WHO model list of essential medicines. Retrieved August 9, 2010, from http://www.who.int/medicines/publications/ essentialmedicines/en/index.html/

World Health Organization, United Nations Office on Drugs and Crime, & Joint United Nations Programme on HIV/AIDS. (2004). *Substitution maintenance therapy in the management of opioid dependence and HIV/AIDS prevention* (Rep. No. Position Paper). Geneva, Switzerland: World Health Organization.

CHAPTER 13

Rights-Based Approaches in Conflict-Affected Settings

Emily Waller, Andrew D. Pinto, Neil Arya, and Anthony B. Zwi

INTRODUCTION

Armed conflict has a significant impact on the health of populations. Injury, malnutrition, disease, disability, sexual and gender-based violence, and death are the most direct and visible manifestations of violence (Krug, Mercy, Dahlberg, & Zwi, 2002; The University of New South Wales Health and Conflict Project, 2004; Zwi, Garfield, & Loretti, 2002). Less visible are the indirect impacts to the health sector in conflict-affected settings, including the destruction of critical health facilities, severely disrupted health services, and voluntary or forced migration of health professionals to safer settings (Murray, King, Lopez, Tomijima, & Krug, 2002). Further, conflict disrupts access to other basic necessities including food, water, shelter, education, and the means to generate income (Krause, Muggah, & Wennmann, 2008). Underlying these manifestations of conflict and instability lie deeper roots of exclusion, inequalities, and persistent denial and deliberate violations of human rights, which evidence suggests can act as a catalyst of violence and feed into a longer term cycle of conflict (Galtung, 1969; Geiger, 2000; Krause et al.; Stewart, 2002).

In spite of the deterioration of health systems in conflict-affected settings, health professionals have historically played a critical role in the humanitarian response by protecting life, responding to medical emergencies, and alleviating suffering (International Committee of the Red

Cross, 1996). Although conflict and instability have significant public health dimensions, responding to the root causes of conflict, mitigating their effects, and assisting in broader postconflict recovery have not always been considered responsibilities of the public health community. Recently, however, there has been growing recognition of the potential health practitioner contributions to a broader role in fostering longer term peace, well beyond providing medical care and supporting large-scale public health interventions during the acute phase of a humanitarian response. The scope for health practitioners' meaningful contribution to a sustainable peace is far-reaching and may include building trust, supporting reconciliation, promoting social cohesion, addressing psychological responses to conflict, and creating healthier environments (Banatvala & Zwi, 2000; The University of New South Wales Health and Conflict Project, 2004).

Despite the increased recognition of the potential for health practitioner roles in peace building,[1] there are few methods and instruments to assist field-based work. This chapter provides a brief overview of the links between health, international law, human rights, conflict, and peace building, including historical perspectives on the health practitioner's contribution in achieving these goals. It then describes a field tool for health practitioners, The Health and Peacebuilding Filter (Peacebuilding Filter), which offers a framework for health practitioners to consider principles related to fostering peace building that is inclusive of many components of a rights-based approach (RBA). This practical tool, complemented by a more thorough RBA, could provide a more comprehensive framework for addressing the complex interconnections between conflict, human rights, peace building, and health in conflict-affected settings.

INTERNATIONAL LAW AND THE RIGHT TO HEALTH

The field of international law is vast, and there are many components applicable to a discussion on health, human rights, conflict, peace, and security. International law, in relation to conflict, constitutes such components, though not limited to the laws of war (such as the Hague Conventions of 1899 and 1907), humanitarian law (such as the Geneva Convention of 1949), war crimes and crimes against humanity including genocide (including for example the International Criminal Court and ad hoc Tribunals for the former Yugoslavia in 1991, and Rwanda in 1994), and human rights law (e.g., the Optional Protocol to the Convention on the Rights of the Child [United Nations, 2000a] on the involvement of children in armed conflict in 2000). Two distinct, yet complementary fields of international law are particularly relevant to conflict-affected settings: international humanitarian law (IHL) and international human rights law. This chapter does not intend to offer an extensive overview of these fields, as many others have done so (Fleck, 2008; Lubell, 2005; Steiner, Alston, & Goodman, 2008). However, it is important to note the overarching legal frameworks guiding the work of health practitioners in conflict-affected and postconflict settings.

International Humanitarian Law

Both IHL and international human rights law stem from discussions and debates anchored in underlying values of human rights following the end of World War II. IHL applies norms and standards, established by treaty or custom, which are specifically intended to characterize, prevent, and respond to humanitarian problems directly arising from international and noninternational armed conflicts. It protects persons and properties that are, or may be, affected by an armed conflict and sets boundaries to the legitimacy and the use of methods and means of warfare. IHL's main treaty sources applicable to international armed conflict is the Geneva Convention (1949) and its Additional Protocols (1977 and 2003). Beyond these core treaties, there are several other conventions and declarations, which guide IHL, related to refugees, genocide, criminal courts, treatment of prisoners, and torture, to name a few. IHL is the overarching legal framework applicable to conflict-affected settings and guides health practitioners working to provide humanitarian care and treatment.

International Human Rights Law

Although the Geneva Conventions were revised to include earlier conventions and readopted in 1949, another international legal framework was taking shape: international human rights law. Several legal documents under the international human rights law framework either explicitly or implicitly refer to health in conflict-affected settings as well as in times of peace. The foundation document is the Universal Declaration of Human Rights (United Nations, 1948). Although not legally binding, it laid the groundwork for legally binding treaties, such as the International Covenant on Civil and Political Rights (United Nations, 1976a), the International Covenant on Economic, Social and Cultural Rights (ICESCR; United Nations, 1976b), and their Optional Protocols. A broad array of legally binding treaties and nonlegally binding human rights declarations relevant to health in conflict-affected settings, such as the Declaration on the Protection of Women and Children in Emergency and Armed Conflict (1974), the Convention Against Torture and Other Cruel, Inhuman or Degrading Treatment or Punishment (United Nations, 1984), and the Convention on the Rights of the Child (United Nations, 1989) have also been developed.

The Right to Health

As the international human rights framework is applicable both in times of conflict and in peace (Lubell, 2005), there is increased recognition of the value of using human rights principles, norms, and standards to guide health work. Several authors have more thoroughly explored the links between health and human rights (see, for example, Gruskin & Tarantola, 2001; Mann, Gruskin, Grodin, & Annas, 1999; Tarantola, 2008). In the context of focusing on health practitioners' work in postconflict settings, the right to highest attainable standard of physical and mental health (here within referred to as the "right to health") is particularly applicable. The right to health, as stipulated in Article 12 of the ICESCR (United Nations, 1976b), recognizes that both health care and social conditions are important elements of the right to health (Hunt et al., 2009). Impediments to the right to health include factors such as gender and age discrimination, inequitable resource distribution, poor sanitary conditions, and events that may damage health such as violence and armed conflict.

Substantive issues related to the right to health are elucidated within General Comment 14, which elaborates on the interrelated and essential elements guiding its application, notably the concepts of *availability, accessibility, acceptability,* and *quality* of health facilities, goods, and services (United Nations, 2000b; see Figure 13.1). Of particular note, it acknowledges that a wider definition of health must be inclusive of the impact of violence and conflict and that states should be held to account for health-related impacts during armed conflicts in violation of IHL (sections 10 and 34, respectively). Applying the international human rights framework, including the right to health, in practice through an RBA to health is explored further in this chapter.

MEDICAL ETHICS AND HUMAN RIGHTS

Complementing the broader legal framework inclusive of international human rights law is the ethical framework that guides the work of health practitioners (Kass, 2009). This framework was founded on the spirit of the

FIGURE 13.1 Elements of the Right to Health

The right to health in all its forms and at all levels contains the following interrelated and essential elements, the precise application of which will depend on the conditions prevailing in a particular state party:	
Availability	Functioning public health and health care facilities, goods, and services, as well as programs, have to be available in sufficient quantity within the state party. The precise nature of the facilities, goods, and services will vary depending on numerous factors, including the state party's developmental level. They will include, however, the underlying determinants of health, such as safe and potable drinking water and adequate sanitation facilities, hospitals, clinics, and other health-related buildings; trained medical and professional personnel receiving domestically competitive salaries; and essential drugs, as defined by the World Health Organization Action Programme on Essential Drugs.
Accessibility	Health facilities, goods, and services have to be accessible to everyone without discrimination, within the jurisdiction of the state party. Accessibility has four overlapping dimensions:
	Nondiscrimination: Health facilities, goods, and services must be accessible to all, especially the most vulnerable or marginalized sections of the population, in law and in fact, without discrimination on any of the prohibited grounds.
	Physical accessibility: Health facilities, goods, and services must be within safe physical reach for all sections of the population, especially vulnerable or marginalized groups, such as ethnic minorities and indigenous populations, women, children, adolescents, older persons, persons with disabilities, and persons with HIV/AIDS. Accessibility also implies that medical services and underlying determinants of health, such as safe and potable water and adequate sanitation facilities, are within safe physical reach, including in rural areas. Accessibility further includes adequate access to buildings for persons with disabilities.
	Economic accessibility (affordability): Health facilities, goods, and services must be affordable for all. Payment for health care services, as well as services related to the underlying determinants of health, has to be based on the principle of equity, ensuring that these services, whether privately or publicly provided, are affordable for all, including socially disadvantaged groups. Equity demands that poorer households should not be disproportionately burdened with health expenses as compared to richer households.
	Information accessibility: Accessibility includes the right to seek, receive, and impart information and ideas concerning health issues. However, accessibility of information should not impair the right to have personal health data treated with confidentiality.

(Continued)

FIGURE 13.1 Elements of the Right to Health *Continued*

Acceptability	All health facilities, goods, and services must be respectful of medical ethics and culturally appropriate, that is, respectful of the culture of individuals, minorities, peoples, and communities, sensitive to gender and life-cycle requirements, as well as being designed to respect confidentiality and improve the health status of those concerned.
Quality	As well as being culturally acceptable, health facilities, goods, and services must also be scientifically and medically appropriate and of good quality. This requires, inter alia, skilled medical personnel, scientifically approved and unexpired drugs and hospital equipment, safe and potable water, and adequate sanitation.

Source: United Nations, 2000b.

Hippocratic oath. It was further elucidated with the World Medical Association's adoption of the Declaration of Helsinki (1964), which focused on research of human subjects, and later the Declaration of Tokyo (1975), which set out guidelines for medical practitioners concerning torture and other cruel, inhumane, and degrading treatment or punishment in relation to detention and imprisonment. These were complemented by the updated physician's oath, known as the International Code of Medical Ethics (World Medical Association, 2006), which is an amended version of the Declaration of Geneva (1948) and is central to the provision of health care and services. The Nuremberg Code (1947), which lays out a set of research ethical principles for human experimentation following the end of World War II and contributed to forming the basis for the Helsinki Declaration, is also of critical importance in relation to conflict and the role of the health practitioner.

Although it is beyond the scope of this chapter to link human rights and medical ethics, both historically and conceptually, some authors have noted the divergence of the paradigms of human rights ethics, in particular in relation to their origin, application, processes, and audience, as well as their convergence as they are bound by shared values, principles, and commitment to supporting the dignity of every individual (Gruskin & Dickens, 2006; Rubenstein, 2009). These ethics drive the work of health practitioners in conflict-affected settings.

Human Rights, Conflict, and the Role of the Health Practitioner

In conflict-affected settings, the human rights concerns involving health practitioners are multifaceted. On the one hand, the protection of health care professionals' own human rights is of paramount importance to ensure their safety and well-being and capacity to deliver services. In many conflict-affected settings, health workers may be explicitly targeted (Rubenstein & Bittle, 2010).

On the other hand, health care professionals are often witness to grave human rights abuses of populations including, although not limited to, injury, mutilation, rape, torture, enslavement, trafficking, and death. The latter evokes considerable debate in the field as to the duties and responsibilities of health care workers when witnessing such violations (Orbinski, Beyrer, & Singh, 2007). Some argue that health practitioners, whose professional and ethical values should align with realizing human rights, have a duty to intervene when bearing witness to human rights abuses, through documenting and measuring the health effects of denials of human rights and acting as advocates to denounce such violations (Hannibal & Lawrence, 1999). However, when confronting such atrocities, health service providers face dilemmas regarding their responsibility to bear witness or intervene in any other form, often at the perils of having to suspend health services to the population they are meant to serve, and compromising the safety of fellow health professionals and humanitarian workers (Fox, 1995; Gruskin, Mills, & Tarantola, 2007; Médecins Sans Frontières, 2006; Redfield, 2006; Terry, 2002).

Despite the complementarities of medical values and the advancement of human rights, health professionals' role can often be overstated as some practitioners place self-interest over ethics at the sacrifice of public health and, in some egregious scenarios, become complicit in rights violations (Rubenstein, 2009). It is well documented that health professionals have contributed to inhumane experimentation and torture, most recently in relation to interrogation techniques associated with the so-called "War on Terror" (Farberman & American Psychological Association, 2005; Hargreaves & Cunningham, 2004; "How Complicit," 2004; Miles, 2004; Lifton, 2004; Marks, 2005). In conflict-affected settings, "these deplorable violations exist alongside more subtle activities that also have severe and long-lasting effects on health and human rights such as the absence of basic health-care systems" (Gruskin, Mills, & Tarantola, 2007), recruitment of child soldiers, disruption of education systems, and violations of civil and political rights (Orbinski et al., 2007). Such human rights challenges are often not adequately addressed within health interventions in conflict-affected and postconflict settings. As health practitioners are forced to navigate increasingly complex situations, and as only few have the necessary training in human rights to respond appropriately and effectively, much more support is critically needed in this field (Hunt, 2007).

THE CONVERGENCE OF HEALTH AND PEACE BUILDING

The creation of the International Committee of the Red Cross and the Geneva Convention, and later the founding of such organizations as Amnesty International, Médecins Sans Frontières, Médecins du Monde, and Physicians for Human Rights, linked humanitarian emergencies and medical responses. However, the associations between peace and health are neither well developed nor well defined within the bodies of international law and ethics, described earlier in this chapter, despite the fact that many refer to armed conflict and health.

Nevertheless, several public health fora acknowledge the important links between health and peace, most notably the World Health Assembly resolution in 1981 stating that "the role of physicians and other health workers in the preservation and promotion of peace is the most significant factor for the attainment of health for all" (World Health Assembly, 1981), as well as the Ottawa Charter for Health Promotion (1986), which identifies that "peace" is the first fundamental prerequisite for health.

In practice, recent history has begun to delineate the different forms of connection that are present, and they have become more evident and better documented. Advocacy is evident in the actions of some practitioners who opposed the Vietnam War and later the wars in Iraq from a health perspective, and globally, physicians have opposed weapon systems, such as nuclear arms, landmines, and small arms because of their inherent inhumanity (Arya, 2002). Others have identified collaborative work on the ground, seeking to bring together opposing groups to address health issues of mutual concern. This approach became more developed, with some commentators crediting the Pan American Health Organization's (PAHO) initiative to promote transborder health system cooperation during conflict. The PAHO negotiated transborder mass immunization programs in Central America, which was viewed as a defining moment in history linking health and peace and contributing to the Health as a Bridge to Peace approach taken forward by the World Health Organization (WHO; de Quadros & Epstein, 2002). The WHO (2010) defined Health as a Bridge to Peace as:

> a multidimensional policy and planning framework which supports health workers in delivering health programs in conflict and post-conflict situations and at the same time contributes to peace building. It is defined as the integration of peace building concerns, concepts, strategies and practices into health relief and health sector development.

The premise for Health as a Bridge for Peace was based on the imperative of health as a shared human aspiration, which should transcend any political, cultural, or other divisions among nations or peoples. The concept seeks to integrate peace building concerns and strategies into health relief and health sector development in postconflict settings. Although many practical activities related to such initiatives focused on negotiating ceasefires for the provision of short-term public health interventions and humanitarian assistance, its scope expanded to include sectoral cooperation in countries such as Mozambique, Croatia, Bosnia, Sri Lanka, and Angola (WHO, 2009).

Although there was considerable enthusiasm by WHO, some key donors, and concerned health workers for this approach, there was also a critique that emerged from experiences of its application. For example, Large, Subilia, and Zwi (1998), in their evaluation of the WHO project in Eastern Slavonia, in the former Yugoslavia, found that there were somewhat overambitious targets of integrating the peace building components of health into health system development and program design with insufficient sensitivity to the experience of conflict and the different cultures of those affected, both health workers and clients. Health as a Bridge for Peace did, for a while, pave the way for larger scale integration of health interventions as a mode of promoting peace, but suffered some setbacks as more effective means of engaging at this interface were explored and evidence of effectiveness and impact was sought (Rushton & McInnes, 2006).

Although the Health as a Bridge for Peace approach highlights how government and international organization action can contribute to peace building, another movement, which highlights the importance of the role of the individual health worker, often working together, began to take shape (Arya, 2007; Arya & Santa Barbara, 2008; MacQueen, McCutcheon, & Santa Barbara, 1997; MacQueen, Santa Barbara, Neufeld, Yusuf, & Horton, 2001). The Peace Through Health movement can be simply defined as the theory and practice of how health workers and health perspectives can contribute to peace building and the reduction of violence (Arya, 2004). Peace Through Health was founded on five important ethical values and principles that, building on general medical ethics, provide the basis for connecting health work with peace work: conflict management, solidarity, strengthening the social fabric, dissent, and restricting the destructiveness of war (MacQueen & Santa Barbara, 2000; Santa Barbara & MacQueen, 2004). This work has largely centered on programs based in Croatia, Gaza, and Sri Lanka, documenting mental health consequences of war and the effects of prejudices largely on children (Chase et al., 1999; Miller, el-Masri,

Allodi, & Qouta, 1999; Santa Barbara, 2004; Woodside, Santa Barbara, & Benner, 1999). Although the underlying ethical values and core implementing principles of this approach are admirable, critical analysis of this work has focused on concerns regarding whether health workers necessarily play the positive roles they could play, whether the assumptions regarding respect for dignity and autonomy, acting honestly and with compassion, are necessarily present, and whether they do indeed have a lasting impact on either health outcomes or longer term peace (Grove & Zwi, 2008). If meaning to do well is not good enough, how can health practitioners approach health and peace building more systematically?

THE HEALTH AND PEACEBUILDING FILTER

There are several practical tools available to health practitioners in the field to assist in identifying gaps, designing and developing new programs, and providing monitoring and evaluation mechanisms. Many of the available tools, however, tend to focus on one domain, or at most, the intersection of two, from the fields of health, conflict, security, peace building, and human rights. Notable examples include the Health Impact Assessment (Harris, Harris-Roxas, Harris, & Kemp, 2007), Human Rights Impact Assessment (Human Rights Impact Assessment Resource Centre, 2009), Health and Human Rights Impact Assessment (Gay, 2008; Gostin & Mann, 1994; Tarantola et al., 2008), The Right to Health (Asher et al., 2007), Do No Harm (Anderson, 1999), Peace and Conflict Impact Assessment (Bush, 2005), Participatory Rights Assessment Methodologies (Department for International Development, 2000), United Nations International Children's Emergency Fund's Implementation Handbook on the Rights of the Child (Hodgkin & Newell, 2002), the Health and Peacebuilding Filter (Zwi, Bunde-Birouste, Grove, Waller, & Ritchie, 2006a), and many others. Despite the plethora of tools available, they may not be appropriate for the specific purpose at hand. In such instances, health practitioners may be required to adapt tools to suit their specific need.

In particular, although these tools provide guidance for several settings, issues, and outcomes, few provide health practitioners with an overview of the key issues to address when establishing or strengthening health services and systems in postconflict and peace building settings. The Health and Peacebuilding Filter (herein denoted as the Peacebuilding Filter) sought to fill this gap and to systematically address health, conflict, and peace building needs through a rapid assessment tool that could be used proactively for planning and programming (Zwi et al., 2006a).

The Peacebuilding Filter was designed to provide a rapid assessment of conflict prevention and peace building components of health initiatives in conflict-affected settings. The Peacebuilding Filter can be applied to new or existing health projects or programs to guide policy and program cycles so as to enhance conflict sensitivity and the health-related contributions to peace building (Bunde-Birouste & Ritchie, 2007; Bunde-Birouste & Zwi, 2008; Grove & Zwi, 2008). The Peacebuilding Filter is not prescriptive and can feed into an analysis of a project or program by (a) identifying project areas already applying peace building principles, seeking to reinforce these; (b) drawing attention to where health-related activities might make matters worse, seeking to refine these approaches and to do better; and (c) suggesting further actions and resources.

The Peacebuilding Filter is designed to assist practitioners to bring key values, ethics, and rights principles into their day-to-day practice. It complements and extends traditional modes of assessment and monitoring by ensuring attention to less quantifiable dimensions of project activity, shedding light on the relationships and processes underpinning health-related activities in fragile settings (Galtung, 1969; Grove & Zwi, 2008). In doing so, debate and response to issues such as building trust, promoting social cohesion and social justice, or assuring cultural, conflict and gender sensitivity are legitimized and enabled. The Peacebuilding Filter comprises of five core principles of health and peace building and 10 subcomponents, framed around 29 points of inquiry, which provide a structure for addressing whether a health project is effectively contributing to broader peace building goals (see Figure 13.2).

Although informed by human rights principles, during its development and application, these are implicit and not explicit within the Peacebuilding Filter. The tool focuses more specifically on drawing out key principles relevant to postconflict recovery and peace building, but provides a base that can be strongly complemented and deepened by a complementary application of RBAs.

RIGHTS-BASED APPROACH TO HEALTH IN CONFLICT-AFFECTED SETTINGS

Because many of the root causes and outcomes of conflicts are embedded in large-scale human rights abuses, it is important that responses toward creating and maintaining the peace embody and reflect a commitment to all human rights, including the right to health. A prominent approach to systematically applying and integrating international human rights norms, standards, and principles in policy and program planning, implementation, monitoring, and

FIGURE 13.2 Health and Peacebuilding Filter Principles and Components

Core Principles	Subcomponents	Key Elements Promoted Within the Tool
Cultural sensitivity	• Cultural sensitivity	• Promotes cultural sensitivity • Recognizes local capacities and responses to health • Respects cultural rituals and practice
Conflict sensitivity	• Conflict awareness • Trust	• Trains staff to conflict-sensitive approaches • Demonstrates sensitivity to the nature of the conflict • Promotes the building of trust among stakeholders and community groups
Social justice	• Equity and nondiscrimination • Gender	• Promotes tolerance and eliminate discrimination • Contributes to reducing inequalities within the community • Demonstrates sensitivity to gender issues and supports gender training for staff
Social cohesion	• Community cohesion • Psychosocial well-being	• Contributes to bridging the divide among different groups in the community • Supports and reinforces community reconciliation efforts • Demonstrates sensitivity to the community's psychosocial health and well-being and supports social recovery
Governance	• Capacity building and empowerment • Sustainability and coordination • Transparency and accountability	• Establishes mechanisms for genuine community participation • Promotes local ownership of the project • Includes mechanisms to coordinate with other service providers and build networks with communities • Encourages transparency and accountability of decision making to local communities • Strengthens the ability of community members to elicit greater accountability from service providers and government departments

Source: Zwi, et al., 2006a.

evaluation is the RBA (United Nations, 2003). An advantage of applying an RBA is that it offers a comprehensive framework inclusive of both guiding principles for analysis and a corresponding set of monitoring mechanisms and indicators (Gruskin & Tarantola, 2008; Tarantola, 2007). The value of bringing a human RBA to health in conflict-affected settings is that it links aid assistance to questions of obligation and responsibilities, rather than welfare or charity. It systemically shifts the approach to a human rights framework that considers survivors of war, conflict, and displacement as rights holders and state actors as duty bearers[2] of obligations under international treaties. By recognizing affected communities as rights holders, it is argued that they will be more empowered, and local capacity will be strengthened to address the broader public health issues during their postconflict recovery.

There is no single RBA, and many stakeholders have characterized the approach in different ways to suit their needs. The United Nations has developed a Statement of Common Understanding of an RBA to development cooperation as one means of identifying the core components of this approach (see Figure 13.3). Beyond the agreed common principles to an RBA, the right to health includes specific elements to guide policies and interventions: availability, accessibility, acceptability and quality of health structures, and goods and services (as depicted in Figure 13.1).

A RIGHTS-BASED APPROACH AND THE HEALTH AND PEACEBUILDING FILTER

This section examines the Peacebuilding Filter against the principles of an RBA. In particular, we consider the interdependence of rights including attention to the legal and policy context, participation, nondiscrimination, accountability, and elements of the right to health, including availability, accessibility, acceptability, and high quality of systems, services, care, and treatment (Gruskin, Ferguson, & Bogecho, 2007).

Interdependence

The RBA emphasizes the interdependence of rights and their mutual complementarities. No one right can be achieved without securing and promoting others. For example, a focus on health in conflict-affected settings will emphasize the right to health, although other rights, including rights to be free from violence, security, autonomy, physical integrity, information, education, food and nutrition, housing, and freedom of association, to name a few, also deserve due consideration (Tarantola et al., 2008).

FIGURE 13.3 UN Statement of Common Understanding on Human Rights-Based Approach to Development Cooperation

1. All programs of development cooperation, policies, and technical assistance should further the realization of human rights as laid down in the Universal Declaration of Human Rights and other international human rights instruments.	
A set of program activities that only incidentally contributes to the realization of human rights does not necessarily constitute an RBA to programming. In an RBA to programming and development cooperation, the aim of all activities is to contribute directly to the realization of one or several human rights.	
2. Human rights standards contained in, and principles derived from, the Universal Declaration of Human Rights, and other international human rights instruments guide all development cooperation and programming in all sectors and in all phases of the programming process.	
Human rights principles guide programming in all sectors, such as health, education, governance, nutrition, water and sanitation, HIV/AIDS, employment and labor relations, and social and economic security. This includes all development cooperation directed toward the achievement of the Millennium Development Goals and the Millennium Declaration. Consequently, human rights standards and principles guide both the Common Country Assessment and the UN Development Assistance Framework.	
Human rights principles guide all programming in all phases of the programming process, including assessment and analysis, program planning and design (including setting of goals, objectives, and strategies), implementation, monitoring, and evaluation.	
Among these human rights principles are universality and inalienability, indivisibility, and the following principles explained here:	

Interdependence	The realization of one right often depends, wholly or in part, on the realization of others. For instance, realization of the right to health may depend, in certain circumstances, on realization of the right to education or information.
Participation and inclusion	Every person and all people are entitled to active, free, and meaningful participation in, contribution to, and enjoyment of civil, economic, social, cultural, and political development in which human rights and fundamental freedoms can be realized.
Equality and nondiscrimination	All individuals are equal as human beings and by virtue of the inherent dignity of each human person. No one, therefore, should suffer discrimination based on race, color, ethnicity, gender, age, language, sexual orientation, religion, political or other opinion, national, social or geographical origin, disability, property, birth, or other status as established by human rights standards. In relation to health, facilities, goods, and services must be accessible to all, especially the most vulnerable.

(Continued)

FIGURE 13.3 UN Statement of Common Understanding on Human Rights-Based Approach to Development Cooperation *Continued*

Accountability and rule of law	States and other duty bearers are answerable for the observance of human rights. In this regard, they have to comply with the legal norms and standards enshrined in human rights instruments. Where they fail to do so, aggrieved rights holders are entitled to institute proceedings for appropriate redress before a competent court or other adjudicator in accordance with the rules and procedures provided by law.
3. Programs of development cooperation contribute to the development of the capacities of duty bearers to meet their obligations and of rights holders to claim their rights.	
In an RBA, human rights determine the relationship between individuals and groups with valid claims (rights holders) and state and nonstate actors with correlative obligations (duty bearers).	
It identifies rights holders (and their entitlements) and corresponding duty bearers (and their obligations) and works toward strengthening the capacities of rights holders to make their claims and of duty bearers to meet their obligations.	

Source: United Nations, 2003.

Although the Peacebuilding Filter does not emphasize and bring to the fore this interdependence, it does recognize that the different dimensions to promote peace are mutually supportive. Even though the tool is not specifically rights based, it was, in its development and potential application, rights informed, and highlights several principles (discussed later in this chapter) that illustrate these links. The language employed, however, is more focused on a social justice framework, resulting, in part, from field testing that suggested that the social justice framework might be less contentious and easier to advance in conflicted and highly politicized settings. In making this trade-off, some weaknesses may have resulted, although other elements might be stronger and more flexible than an RBA. Seeing both as valuable and being able to draw on appropriate tools and frameworks as required is of benefit but demands a more sophisticated analysis by the health or development worker on the ground.

Participation

Participation is a key component of an RBA because it allows for the process of decision making to be led by the community, especially those who are likely to be affected by the health intervention. Despite the centrality of promoting community participation, the reality can be challenging, especially in a conflict-affected setting where "communities are fragmented, people displaced, resources eroded, services undermined and tensions widespread" (Zwi, Bunde-Birouste, Grove, Waller, & Ritchie, 2006b). These challenges, however, are not insurmountable and facilitating widespread participation should be a priority for health service providers prior to, as well as during the development of, policies, programs, and/or interventions.

The Peacebuilding Filter explores the concept of participation under the principle of good governance and the community capacity building and empowerment indicators. The underlying value guiding participation is that community members should be recognized as decisive, rather than passive, actors. According to Zwi et al. (2006b),

> too often community participation has been merely a part of the rhetoric but not of the practice; participation occurs at a token level, consultation is seen as a means to ensure cooperation and agreement from communities is sought after key decision have already been made by project staff. (p. 26)

As such, the Peacebuilding Filter encourages users to consider whether the project or program has established mechanisms for genuine community participation in all phases, including monitoring and evaluation. For example, the Peacebuilding Filter reminds users that communities are not homogenous and that some members of the community may present themselves as speaking on behalf of all, when in fact many communities are divided and fragmented into groups with different interests and viewpoints. Health practitioners should ensure that there is a wide and meaningful representation of community members invited to participate in discussions, rather than a select few. Other issues to pursue include local ownership of the project, engaging with communities during all phases, and supporting community members and the project to demand appropriate levels of support at the national, district, and local level of government.

Closely related to participation is the concept of empowerment, which aims to give women, men, and young people the power, capacities, capabilities, and access to resources to enable them to change their own lives, improve their own communities, and influence their own destinies. In the Peacebuilding Filter, empowerment is viewed as an outcome of effective community capacity building, where community members feel confident in their ability to effect change, lead activities, and take decision-making roles. Empowerment is essential to peace building activities as it supports populations to regain a sense of control over their lives, which is central to the long-term healing and recovery process.

The Peacebuilding Filter addresses the issue of empowerment by first seeking to establish that there is local ownership of the health project. Do community members believe the project is theirs? Does the project provide opportunities to build and reinforce local structures (if they are positive for all community members) and to engage community members through involvement in planning and implementation? It should be noted that in the case of international health assistance, ownership should not simply apply at the community level, but should extend up to the national level. One Timor-Leste senior project officer noted,

> It is important that government representatives are present – not just at the start and the end but all the way through. For us, it is important that government is involved and seen to be involved, otherwise there is no ownership (Zwi et al., 2006b, p. 28).

Secondly, the Peacebuilding Filter prompts discussion around the idea that the project provides for the development of leadership and advocacy skills among staff and community members. Gaining agency and control, with community members as drivers and pacesetters, is especially important in communities emerging from periods of violence.

Nondiscrimination

Health programs have the opportunity to promote social justice, human rights, and dignity by respecting patients and health service users, and reducing inequalities (in service access, delivery, and staffing) and discrimination. Discrimination is the unfair treatment of individuals or communities on the basis of such attributes as race, color, gender, language, religion, political or other opinion, national or social origin, wealth, or other status (General Comment 20 – United Nations, 2009). Discrimination may perpetuate practices that precede or contribute to the conflict. The Peacebuilding Filter specifically highlights the need to promote, and wherever possible, ensure nondiscrimination as part of a health intervention. The tool forces one to consider existing tensions and forms of discrimination within the country or community and to consider how such discrimination manifests itself within health service provision. The Peacebuilding Filter promotes a commitment by the government and other actors in positions of power to provide transparent and fair grievance procedures for project personnel, patients, and the community in relation to public services.

A key component of nondiscrimination within an RBA is ensuring that specific attention is given to the most vulnerable groups. It is critical that work across all sectors in conflict-affected settings incorporates safeguards to protect the rights of marginalized persons, including, although not exhaustively, women and girls, minorities, indigenous populations, migrants, unaccompanied minors, child soldiers, survivors of sexual violence and/or torture, older persons, widowers, and those who have a physical and mental disability. Applying the RBA principles of participation and empowerment is a critical step in ensuring that vulnerable populations are included within the decision-making process, thus guarding against reinforcing existing power imbalances while meeting their specific needs.

The Peacebuilding Filter recognizes that particular attention must be paid to the most vulnerable communities and individuals, such as those with the fewest resources to protect and sustain themselves. The tool specifically prompts users to consider whether "the project promotes dignity and respect for beneficiaries, community members and all social subgroups, especially the most vulnerable groups" (Zwi et al., 2006b, p. 18). The Peacebuilding Filter encourages users to consider the special measures needed and/or taken to ensure health services reach vulnerable populations. In addition, the tool encourages health service providers to consider how the program or project assesses the access to services by vulnerable populations. Collecting and analyzing disaggregated data, such as by gender, age, and, where appropriate, ethnicity, is critical in ensuring that services are reaching all members of the population, especially the most vulnerable.

Accountability

Accountability is an important concept linked to human rights, and yet it is also one of the most difficult to implement (Organisation for Economic Co-operation and Development, 2005). Accountability enables rights holders to claim their rights and ensures that the state fulfills its obligation as duty bearer. With an RBA, states must be held to account against their obligations of treaties they have ratified. This component is important as it explicitly links an RBA to human rights legal documents. As indicated previously, the Peacebuilding Filter does not explicitly refer to legal mechanisms. Adapting the concept of accountability within the tool to consider these dimensions could add considerable value.

The Peacebuilding Filter views accountability from both the obligations that health service providers have to protect lives, promote health, and provide care and services, as well as refrain from perpetrating violations of rights. The Peacebuilding Filter states that health projects should strengthen the ability of community members to elicit greater accountability from central health service providers and government departments. It prompts greater public accountability by both state actors and nonstate actors alike, promoting availability and discussion of information on project achievements, limitations, and constraints. It also highlights the need to consider establishing a complaints procedure as a component of improving development practice. For example, in a remote Malaitan community in the Solomon Islands, community health centers had routinely requested medical and other related items, such as radios, from provincial and national health departments based in the capital, Honiara. Their requests had gone largely unheard, which frustrated the community. In the short term, a simple communication procedure could have provided the community with updates on the status of their requests, thus diffusing any potential tensions, but state services failed to do so. Making provisions to ensure accountability mechanisms are activated throughout the life of the health service delivery project enables it to better respond to community demands and contributes to building community capacity and social cohesion.

Availability, Accessibility, Acceptability, and Quality of Health Services, Care, and Treatment

In conflict-affected settings, health systems may be destroyed and services severely disrupted. As such, health service providers play an important role in (re)building these systems and providing services in postconflict settings. Applying an RBA to health includes ensuring health services, care, and treatment are *available, accessible, acceptable*, and of *good quality* (as indicated previously in General Comment 14; see Figure 13.1). These four elements of the right to health also include attention to physical, economic, and information accessibility, as well as reemphasizing the principle of nondiscrimination. Incorporating these elements into an RBA to health is critical.

The Peacebuilding Filter does make specific provisions for the consideration of two elements of an RBA to health: accessibility and acceptability, though the latter is not framed explicitly in this term. The tool specifically directs health practitioners to consider whether the project ensures that access (to health systems, services, care, and treatment) is not limited by economic or other barriers, including geographic and/or social factors. Examples of such barriers include service fees, lack of public transportation, travel distance and time, and discrimination based on ethnicity, gender, economic status, and other attributes (see earlier discussion under "Nondiscrimination"). The Peacebuilding Filter prompts consideration on the equitable access to health services when resources are severely constrained, particularly for the most vulnerable. In addition, the tool considers whether information is accessible by illiterate persons, various language groups, and other marginalized populations of society to fully benefit from the health program, service, or project.

The notion of "acceptability" of health services, care, and treatment is defined as

> all health facilities, goods and services must be respectful of medical ethics and culturally appropriate, that is respectful of the culture of individuals, minorities, peoples and communities, sensitive to gender and life-cycle requirements, as well as being designed to respect confidentiality and improve the health status of those concerned (United Nations, 2000b, par. 12.c.).

The Peacebuilding Filter implicitly refers to the acceptability of health services, care, and treatment by emphasizing cultural sensitivity and prompting users to ensure that there is local ownership of the project through genuine community participation in all phases of its development. The key challenge is translating these principles into practice. This is difficult in developed and developing countries alike, let alone in postconflict settings where tensions remain high, resources are scarce, and distrust is often rife. Although the Peacebuilding Filter does not offer specific solutions to address these issues, it does, however, allow health practitioners to reflect on them in relation to their work and determine how they could be better incorporated in practice.

There are elements of the right to health to which the Peacebuilding Filter does not implicitly or explicitly refer: *availability* and the *quality* of health structures, goods, and services. Adapting the Peacebuilding Filter to include these elements would add value to the tool. Assessing the available health care facilities, goods, and services should be done systematically (although even a crude picture could be useful) to identify gaps and place the particular health program or project in context of the greatest health needs. In addition, striving to provide the highest possible quality of services should be a guiding principle of health professionals. Noting that achieving a high quality of health care in conflict-affected settings is particularly challenging, applying the human rights principle of "progressive realization of rights" could be useful for health practitioners for this element of the right to health, as well as to the others (availability, accessibility, and acceptability). The principle of progressive realization is grounded in Article 2 of the ICESCR, which imposes on the state to "take steps . . . to the maximum of its available resources, with a view to achieving progressively the full realization of the rights recognized in the present Covenant by all appropriate means, including particularly the adoption of legislative measures" (United Nations, 1976b, Art. 2.1). The progressive realization of the right to health would require health practitioners to provide the highest quality of services within their means in the short term, while striving to work with governments and other actors, in particular nongovernmental organizations (NGOs), to improve the overall performance of health services as more resources become available from domestic or international sources. The Peacebuilding Filter acknowledges that there may be other important health, peace, and conflict issues associated with the program or project that need consideration and provides space within the tool to highlight these issues. Adapting the Peacebuilding Filter to include RBA principles that are currently not fully elaborated within the tool is an important step in creating a stronger synergy between the health and peace building tool and the RBA.

Adding Value to a Rights-Based Approach in Conflict-Affected Settings

Within the Peacebuilding Filter, there are several principles that build on an RBA in conflict-affected settings, including promoting conflict sensitivity, psychosocial well-being, project sustainability and coordination, gender, and trust. One issue, highlighted by many individuals and communities whose experiences fed into the development of the Peacebuilding Filter, can illustrate the benefit of these dimensions: trust.

In conflict-affected settings, the breakdown of the fabric of society, including networks, institutions, and governments spreads mistrust, suspicion, and may exacerbate tensions in situations prone to violence and instability. Violence and abuse experiences by members of different groups and perpetrated by somebody with a different background, may be generalized, at times exaggerated and fuelled by conflict "entrepreneurs," with a net result often of simmering collective distrust, exacerbated by further episodes of violence, between groups.

In the health sector, mistrust may be present especially when health workers are seen as reflecting (or representing) a particular group or authority structure, and may (sometimes unfairly) be thought to have political rather than professional motives for their work. Expatriate groups, from international NGOs, sometimes faith based, may also be distrusted. Although measuring and evaluating issues of trust is fraught with complications, the Peacebuilding Filter raises such questions for consideration: "Were health facilities a target of fighting, violence, or intimidation? Were health services perceived to be aligned with any of the groups involved in the tensions or conflict?" The Peacebuilding Filter highlights the issue of trust—promoting exploration of this "soft" issue (see Grove & Zwi, 2008) rather than the hard indicators usually measured in development projects—promoting an understanding of how it is eroded, and how it may be built up. As one project highlights: "It is difficult to measure the contribution of polio eradication to the final achievement of peace in that region, but, undoubtedly, the collaboration among all those working in health helped to raise the level of trust among people" (de Quadros & Epstein, 2002, p. 26). It is important for health practitioners to recognize fractures in trust, and incorporate mechanisms within their service delivery and projects to contribute to the rebuilding of trust within the community and between the community and health service providers.

In addition, it is worth noting that the Peacebuilding Filter makes explicit focus on gender issues as one of its subcomponents, whereas gender is implicit across an RBA. The issue of gender in relation to health and human rights, conflict, and peace building has been more thoroughly explored by other authors (Cook, 1999; Skjelsbæk & Smith, 2001), and thus the topic, though deeply warranted, remains outside the scope of this chapter. However, within the Peacebuilding Filter, it prompts users to be aware of the socially structured roles of women, men, and children and promotes a gender-sensitive perspective in delivering health services, programs, and projects. It also encourages the capacity building of staff members to raise their awareness of gender issues in relation to the provision of health service, care, and treatment. By explicitly naming gender as a central component to health and peace building, it ensures that the issue will be considered and encourages gender-sensitive action in the process of both delivering services and training of staff.

Highlighting additional issues, alongside the RBA in conflict-affected settings, may open the way for health practitioners to consider some of the specifics that characterize postconflict recovery and peace building. The Peacebuilding Filter not only provides a framework that promotes some human rights principles but also takes into consideration the complex network of factors that influence the day-to-day work of health practitioners and highlights issues that would benefit from more sensitive attention.

CONCLUSION

In conflict-affected and postconflict settings, the need to promote human rights and their achievement in practice is evident. Realizing these rights will be progressive, requiring attention, education, time, and both human and financial resources. Health practitioners have an important role to play in ensuring the key human rights principles, norms, and standards inform their day-to-day work. Given the lack of human rights training within medical and public health curriculum, and despite the fact that this field is growing and becoming more "practical" in its guidance to practitioners, making available useful tools to assist practitioners is of value. Although there may be a vacuum of such tools at their disposal, health practitioners should be cognizant of the key principles of an RBA to health to adapt existing tools.

Although the perfect tool for realizing the right to health during peace building may not exist, and work on this is ongoing, this chapter highlights the Peacebuilding Filter. This tool has been developed and is being used in a range of different settings, consistently with RBAs, which it can reinforce in these fragile settings. Enabling health practitioners to reflect on the synergy of health, peace, and human rights, while ensuring sensitive design of systems and ongoing delivery of services that will promote health and human rights into the future, is key: The Peacebuilding Filter, alongside human RBAs, will help apply best public health practice and build peace in postconflict settings.

ACKNOWLEDGEMENTS

Daniel Tarantola provided valuable and insightful comments on an earlier draft. He was also part of a larger team that contributed to develop the Peacebuilding Filter. A team led by Anthony Zwi and including Anne Bunde-Birouste, Natalie Grove, Emily Waller, and Jan Ritchie undertook the development of the Health and Peacebuilding Filter. The Australian Agency for International Development (AusAID) funded this project.

REFERENCES

Anderson, M. (1999). *Do No Harm: How aid can support peace—or war.* London: Lynne Rienner Publishers.

Arya, N. (2002). Confronting the small arms pandemic: Unrestricted access should be viewed as a public health disaster. *British Medical Journal*, 324(7344), 990–991.

Arya, N. (2004). Peace Through Health II: A framework for medical student education. *Medicine Conflict and Survival*, 20(3), 258–262.

Arya, N. (2007). Peace Through Health. In C. Webel & J. Galtung (Eds.), *Handbook of peace and conflict studies* (pp. 367–396). New York: Routledge.

Arya, N., & Santa Barbara, J. (Eds.). (2008). *Peace Through Health: How health professionals work for a less violent world.* Bloomfield, CT: Kumarian Press.

Asher, J., Hamm, D., Sheather, J., British Medical Association, Commonwealth Medical Trust, & International Federation of Health and Human Rights Organisations. (2007). *The Right to Health: A toolkit for health professionals.* London: British Medical Association.

Banatvala, N., & Zwi, A. B. (2000). Conflict and health. Public health and humanitarian interventions: Developing the evidence base. *British Medical Journal, 321*(7253), 101–105.

Bunde-Birouste, A., & Ritchie, J. E. (2007). Strengthening peace-building through health promotion: Development of a framework. In D. V. McQueen & C. M. Jones (Eds.), *Global perspectives on health promotion effectiveness* (pp.247–258). New York: Springer.

Bunde-Birouste, A., & Zwi, A. B. (2008). The peacebuilding filter. In N. Arya & J. Santa Barbara (Eds.), *Peace Through Health: How health professionals can work for a less violent world* (140–147). Bloomfield, CT: Kumarian Press.

Bush, K. (2005). *Peace and Conflict Impact Assessment handbook, version 2.2.* Retrieved November 15, 2009, from http://www.reliefweb.int/rw/lib.nsf/db900SID/RURI-6MBNLK/$FILE/PCIA%20Handbook.pdf?OpenElement

Chase, R., Doney, A., Sivayogan, S., Ariyaratne, V., Satkunanayagam, P., & Swaminathan, A . (1999). Mental health initiatives as peace initiatives in Sri Lankan schoolchildren affected by armed conflict. *Medicine, Conflict, and Survival, 15*(4), 379–390; discussion 391–393.

Cook, R. (1999). Gender, health, and human rights. In J. M. Mann, S. Gruskin, M. A. Grodin, & G. J. Annas (Eds.), *Health and human rights: A reader* (pp. 253–264). New York: Routledge.

de Quadros, C. A., & Epstein, D. (2002). Health as a bridge for peace: PAHO's experience. Pan American Health Organization. *Lancet, 360*(Suppl), s25–s26.

Declaration of Geneva. (1948). Adopted by the General Assembly of World Medical Association at Geneva, Switzerland, September 1948. Retrieved February 28, 2010, from http://www.wma.net/en/30publications/10policies/c8/index.html

Declaration of Helsinki—Ethical principles for medical research involving human subjects. (1964). Adopted by the 18th WMA General Assembly, Helsinki, Finland, June 1964. Retrieved February 28, 2010, from http://www.wma.net/en/30publications/10policies/b3/index.html

Declaration of Tokyo—Guidelines for physicians concerning torture and other cruel, inhuman or degrading treatment or punishment in relation to detention and imprisonment. (1975). Adopted by the 29th World Medical Assembly, Tokyo, Japan, October 1975. Retrieved February 28, 2010, from http://www.wma.net/en/30publications/10policies/c18/index.html

Declaration on the Protection of Women and Children in Emergency and Armed Conflict. (1974, December 14). Proclaimed by United Nations General Assembly resolution 3318 (XXIX). Retrieved February 15, 2010, from http://www2.ohchr.org/english/law/protectionwomen.htm

Department for International Development.(2000). *Realising human rights for poor people: Strategies for achieving the international development targets.* London: Author.

Farberman, R., & American Psychological Association. (2005). A stain on medical ethics. *Lancet, 366*(9487), 712.

Fleck, D. (Ed.). (2008). *The handbook of international humanitarian law* (2nd ed.). New York: Oxford University Press.

Forum on Early Warning and Early Response, & International Alert and Saferworld. (2003). *Conflict sensitive resource pack.* Retrieved May 22, 2009, from http://www.conflictsensitivity.org/resource_pack.html

Fox, R. C. (1995). Medical humanitarianism and human rights: Reflections on doctors without borders and doctors of the world. *Social Science & Medicine, 41*(12), 1607–1616.

Galtung, J. (1969). Violence, peace and peace research. *Journal of Peace Research, 6*(3), 167–191.

Gay, R. (2008). Mainstreaming wellbeing: An impact assessment for the right to health. *Australian Journal of Human Rights, 132*(2), 33–63.

Geiger, H. J. (2000). The impact of war on human rights. In B. S. Levy & V. W. Sidel (Eds.), *War and public health* (pp. 39–50). Washington, DC: American Public Health Association.

Gostin, L., & Mann, J. M. (1994). Towards the development of a human rights impact assessment for the formulation and evaluation of public health policies. *Health and Human Rights, 1*(1), 58–80.

Grove, N. J., & Zwi, A. B. (2008). Beyond the log frame: A new tool for examining health and peacebuilding initiatives. *Development in Practice, 18*(1), 66–81.

Gruskin, S., & Dickens, B. (2006). Human rights and ethics in public health. *American Journal of Public Health, 96*(11), 1903–1905.

Gruskin, S., Ferguson, L., & Bogecho, D. O. (2007). Beyond the numbers: Using rights-based perspectives to enhance antiretroviral treatment scale-up. *AIDS, 21*(Suppl. 5), S13–S19.

Gruskin, S., Mills, E. J., & Tarantola, D. (2007). History, principles, and practice of health and human rights. *Lancet, 370*(9585), 449–455.

Gruskin, S., & Tarantola, D. (2001). Health and human rights. In R. Detels & R. Beaglehole (Eds.), *Oxford textbook on public health* (pp. 311–335). New York: Oxford University Press.

Gruskin, S., & Tarantola, D. (2008). Health and human rights: Overview. In K. Heggenhougen & S. R. Quah (Eds.), *International encyclopedia of public health* (pp. 137–146.). New York: Elsevier.

Hannibal, K., & Lawrence, R. (1999). The health professional as human rights promoter: Ten years of physicians for human rights (USA). In J. M. Mann, S. Gruskin, M. A. Grodin, & G. J. Annas (Eds.), *Health and human rights: A reader* (pp. 404–416). New York: Routledge.

Hargreaves, S., & Cunningham, A. (2004). The politics of terror. *Lancet, 363*(9425), 1999–2000.

Harris, P., Harris-Roxas, B., Harris, E., & Kemp, L. (2007). *Health Impact Assessment: A practical guide.* Sydney, Australia: Centre for Health Equity Training, Research, and Evaluation, University of New South Wales.

Hodgkin, R., & Newell, P. (2002). *Implementation handbook for the convention on the rights of the child.* New York: United Nations Children's Fund.

How complicit are doctors in abuses of detainees? (2004). *Lancet, 364*(9435), 637–638.

Human Rights Impact Assessment Resource Centre. (2009). *Eight step approach to Human Rights Impact Assessment.* Retrieved November 15, 2009, from http://www.humanrightsimpact.org/hria-guide/steps/

Hunt, P. (2007). *Report of the UN Special Rapporteur on the right of everyone to the highest attainable standard of physical and mental health.* (UN Doc. A/HRC/4/28)

Hunt, P., Backman, G., Bueno de Mesquita, J., Finer, L., Khosla, R., Korljan, D., et al. (2009). The right to the highest attainable standard of health. In R. Detels, R. Beaglehole, M. A. Lansan, & M. Gulliford (Eds.), *Oxford textbook of public health* (5th ed.). New York: Oxford University Press.

International Committee of the Red Cross. (1996). *War and public health: A handbook.* Geneva: Author.

Kass, N. (2009). Ethical principles and ethical issues in public health. In R. Detels, R. Beaglehole, M. A. Lansan, & M. Gulliford (Eds.), *Oxford textbook of public health* (5th ed.). New York: Oxford University Press.

Krause, K., Muggah, R., & Wennmann, A. (Eds.). (2008). Global burden of armed violence. *Geneva Declaration Secretariat.* Retrieved December 15, 2009, from http://www.genevadeclaration.org/fileadmin/docs/Global-Burden-of-Armed-Violence-full-report.pdf

Krug, E. G., Mercy, J. A., Dahlberg, L. L., & Zwi, A. B. (2002). The world report on violence and health. *Lancet, 360*(9339), 1083–1088.

Large, J., Subilia, L., & Zwi, A. B. (1998). *Evaluation study: Post-war health sector transition in Eastern Slavonia (1995–1998).* Geneva, Switzerland: World Health Organization.

Lifton, R. J. (2004). Doctors and torture. *The New England Journal of Medicine, 351*(5), 415–416.

Lubell, N. (2005). Challenges in applying human rights law to armed conflict. *International Review of the Red Cross, 87*(860), 737–754.

MacQueen, G., McCutcheon, R., & Santa Barbara, J. (1997). Health initiatives to peace initiatives: The use of health initiatives as peace initiatives. *Peace and Change, 22*(2), 175–197.

MacQueen, G., & Santa Barbara, J. (2000). Peace building through health initiatives. *British Medical Journal, 321*(7256), 293–296.

MacQueen, G., Santa Barbara, J., Neufeld, V., Yusuf, S., & Horton, R. (2001). Health and peace: Time for a new discipline. *Lancet, 357*(9267), 1460–1461.

Mann, J. M., Gruskin, S., Grodin, M. A., & Annas, G. J. (Eds.). (1999). *Health and human rights: A reader.* New York: Routledge.

Marks, J. H. (2005, December 7). The silence of the doctors. *The Nation.* Retrieved June 3, 2007, from http://www.thenation.com/docprem.mhtml?i=20051226&s=marks [full article only available to subscribers]

Médecins Sans Frontières. (2006). *La Mancha agreement.* Adopted by the International Council of Médecins Sans Frontières in Athens, Greece on June 25.

Miles, S. H. (2004). Abu Ghraib: Its legacy for military medicine. *Lancet, 364*(9435), 725–729.

Miller, T., el-Masri, M., Allodi, F., & Qouta, S. (1999). Emotional and behavioural problems and trauma exposure of school-age Palestinian children in Gaza: Some preliminary findings. *Medicine, Conflict, and Survival, 15*(4), 368–378.

Murray, C. J., King, G., Lopez, A. D., Tomijima, N., & Krug, E. G. (2002). Armed conflict as a public health problem. *British Medical Journal, 324*(7333), 346–349.

Nuremberg Code. (1947). In *Trials of war criminals before the Nuremberg Military Tribunals under Control Council Law, 10*(2), 181–182. Washington, DC: U.S. Government Printing Office, 1949.

Orbinski, J., Beyrer, C., & Singh, S. (2007). Violations of human rights: Health practitioners as witnesses. *Lancet, 370*(9588), 698–704.

Organisation for Economic Co-operation and Development. (2005). *The Paris declaration on aid effectiveness.* Retrieved November 15, 2009, from http://www.oecd.org/dataoecd/11/41/34428351.pdf

Ottawa Charter for Health Promotion. (1986, November 21). The first International Conference on Health Promotion Ottawa. (WHO/HPR/HEP/95.1)

Redfield, P. (2006). A less modest witness: Collective advocacy and motivated truth in a medical humanitarian movement. *American Ethnologist, 33*(1), 2–26.

Rubenstein, L. (2009). Physicians and the right to health. In A. Clapham & M. Robinson (Eds.), *Realizing the right to health* (pp. 381–392). Zurich, Switzerland: Ruffer & Rub.

Rubenstein, L. S., & Bittle, M. D. (2010). Responsiblity for the protection of medical workers and facilities in armed conflict. *Lancet, 375*(9711), 329–340.

Rushton, S., & McInnes, C. (2006). The UK, health and peace-building: The mysterious disappearance of Health as a Bridge for Peace. *Medicine, Conflict, and Survival, 22*(2), 94–109.

Santa Barbara, J. (2004). The Butterfly Peace Garden. *Croatian Medical Journal, 45*(2), 232–233.

Santa Barbara, J., & MacQueen, G. (2004). Peace Through Health: Key concepts. *Lancet, 364*(9431), 384–386.

Skjelsbæk, I., & Smith, D. (Eds.). (2001). *Gender, peace and conflict.* London: Sage Publications.

Steiner, H. J., Alston, P., & Goodman, R. (Eds.). (2008). *International human rights in context: Law, politics, morals* (3rd ed.). New York: Oxford University Press.

Stewart, F. (2002). Root causes of violent conflict in developing countries. *British Medical Journal, 324*(7333), 342–345.

Tarantola, D. (2007). Global justice and human rights: Health and human rights in practice. *Global Justice: Theory, Practice, Rhetoric, 1,* 11–26.

Tarantola, D. (2008). A perspective on the history of health and human rights: From the Cold War to the Gold War. *Journal of Public Health Policy, 29*(1), 42–53.

Tarantola, D., Byrnes, A., Johnson, M., Kemp, L., Zwi, A. B., & Gruskin, S. (2008). Human rights, health and development. *Australian Journal of Human Rights, 13*(2), 1–32.

Terry, F. (2002). *Condemned to repeat? The paradox of humanitarian action.* Ithaca, NY: Cornell University Press.

United Nations. (1948). Universal Declaration of Human Rights. UN General Assembly Resolution 217 A (III). Paris: Author.

United Nations. (1976a). International Covenant on Civil and Political Rights. UN General Assembly resolution 2200A (XXI). New York: Author.

United Nations. (1976b). International Covenant on Economic, Social and Cultural Rights. UN General Assembly resolution 2200A (XXI). New York: Author.

United Nations. (1984). *Convention against Torture and Other Cruel, Inhuman or Degrading Treatment or Punishment.* UN General Assembly resolution 39/46. New York: Author.

United Nations. (1989). Convention on the Rights of the Child. UN General Assembly resolution 44/25. New York: Author.

United Nations. (2000a). *Optional Protocol to the Convention on the Rights of the Child on the involvement of children in armed conflict.* UN General Assembly resolution A/RES/54/263. New York: Author.

United Nations. (2000b). *The right to the highest attainable standard of health.* General Comment No. 14 (E/C.12/2000/4). Geneva, Switzerland: Economic and Social Council.

United Nations. (2003). *UN Statement of Common Understanding of the human rights-based approach to development.* Adopted by the United Nations Development Group (UNDG) in 2003. Retrieved February 28, 2010, from http://www.undg.org/ archive_docs/6959-The_Human_Rights_Based_Approach_to_Development_ Cooperation_Towards_a_Common_Understanding_among_UN.pdf

United Nations. (2009). *General comment no. 20: Non-discrimination in economic, social and cultural rights.* E/C.12/GC/20. Geneva, Switzerland: UN Committee on Economic, Social and Cultural Rights.

The University of New South Wales Health and Conflict Project. (2004). *Issues paper I: Health and peace-building: Securing the future.* AusAID, Canberra. Retrieved September 8, 2009, from http://www.med.unsw.edu.au/SPHCMWeb.nsf/ resources/AUSCAN_Issue_Paper_I.pdf/$file/AUSCAN_Issue_Paper_I.pdf

Woodside, D., Santa Barbara, J., & Benner, D. G. (1999). Psychological trauma and social healing in Croatia, *15*(4), 355–367.

World Health Assembly. (1981). *Resolution 34.38.* Geneva: World Health Organization.

World Health Organization. (2009). *Health as a bridge for peace.* Retrieved September 15, 2009, from http://www.who.int/hac/techguidance/hbp/en/index.html

World Health Organization. (2010). *What is health as a bridge for peace?* Retrieved September 15, 2010, from http://www.who.int/hac/techguidance/hbp/about/en/index.html

World Medical Association. (2006). *International code of medical ethics.* Retrieved February 28, 2010, from http://www.wma.net/en/30publications/10policies/c8/index.html

Zwi, A. B., Bunde-Birouste, A., Grove, N., Waller, E., & Ritchie, J. (2006a). *The health and peacebuilding filter: An assessment tool to determine how health projects or programs may contribute to peacebuilding in conflict-affected countries.* AusAID, Canberra. Retrieved September 8, 2009, from http://www.med.unsw.edu.au/SPHCMWeb.nsf/resources/AUSCAN_Filter.pdf/$file/AUSCAN_Filter.pdf

Zwi, A. B., Bunde-Birouste, A., Grove, N., Waller, E., & Ritchie, J. (2006b). *Companion Manual: The health and peacebuilding filter.* AusAID, Canberra. Retrieved September 8, 2009, from http://www.med.unsw.edu.au/SPHCMWeb.nsf/resources/AUSCAN_Comp_Manual.pdf

Zwi, A. B., Garfield, R., & Loretti, A. (2002). Collective violence. In E. G. Krug, L. L. Dahlberg, J. A. Mercy, A. B. Zwi, & R. Lozano (Eds.), *World report on violence and health.* Geneva, Switzerland: World Health Organization.

OTHER RESOURCES

Article Series on McMaster University's Health of Children in War Zones Project 1994–1996. (1999). *Medicine Conflict and Survival,* 15(4).

NOTES

[1]For the purpose of this chapter, we define peacebuilding in the context of development cooperation as "measures designed to consolidate peaceful relations and strengthen viable political, socioeconomic and cultural institutions capable of mediating conflict, as well as strengthen other mechanisms that will either create or support the creation of necessary conditions for a sustained peace" (Forum on Early Warning and Early Response, & International Alert and Saferworld, 2003). This definition of peacebuilding does not encompass broader peace mandates related to peacekeeping and/or peacemaking.

[2]Duty-bearer responsibilities also apply to surrogate authorities temporarily replacing the state as stipulated in the Geneva Convention's Additional Protocols, such as the UN-led transitional administrations in Cambodia (1992)—the first instance in which the United Nations had taken over the administration of an independent state, organized and ran an election, had its own radio station and jail, and been responsible for promoting and safeguarding human rights at the national level—as well as in Kosovo (1999), East Timor (1999), and Afghanistan (2001).

PART IV

Case Studies

Promoting Human Rights in Public Health Programs: Lessons Learned From HealthRight International

Vandana Tripathi, Mehlika Ozden Hoodbhoy, and Mila Rosenthal

INTRODUCTION

The rights-based promotion of health rests on a conceptual framework recognizing two crucial relationships: that health and human rights are inextricably linked; and that social exclusion exacerbates the relationship between human rights violations and negative health impacts.

The link between health and human rights was elucidated by the late health and human rights pioneer Dr. Jonathan Mann and reflects the bidirectional relationship between health and human rights—rights abuses lead to negative health impacts, such as epidemics and increased vulnerability to disease; they deprive children of healthy development and keep marginalized groups from the education and services needed to maintain health. Conversely, poor health limits individuals' ability to exercise their other rights, such as to education, work, and political participation.

Social exclusion can take many forms and often manifests in greater poverty for particular subgroups. These subgroups may be defined by geographic location; membership in a minority racial, ethnic, linguistic, religious, or sexual minority; disability; disease status; or other identity markers. Social exclusion may be the result or cause of a long history of political strife, including struggles over land, housing, and other resources.

Many excluded groups experience relative deprivation, high rates of illiteracy, and other markers of limited participation in society. They may also experience limited access to health information and services, which can result in higher mortality and morbidity than experienced by mainstream groups. Exclusion can be recognized as a relative indicator: even within poor communities and within least developed countries, excluded populations tend to have worse health outcomes than the majority; within more prosperous communities and nations, the disparities can be even more dramatic.

In some cases, limited access to health care is exacerbated by passive and active neglect on the part of the health system, ranging from the lack of availability of health information in a minority language, to discrimination by health care providers, to extreme violations of human rights such as forced sterilization. An example of the impact of social exclusion on health can be found in tuberculosis (TB). Greater vulnerability to TB is associated with poverty, via factors such as malnutrition, overcrowding, and labor migration.[1] Structural, social, political, and economic inequalities have been documented to lead to delays in TB diagnosis and treatment, which in turn lead to increased spread of TB among the same communities.

ESSENTIAL PRINCIPLES OF HEALTH AND HUMAN RIGHTS

Responding to these relationships between human rights violations, social exclusion, and worse public health outcomes requires attention to essential principles recognized in the World Health Organization's General Comment (GC) on the Right to Health and identified in documents of the international human rights framework. These include the following:

> *Progressive realization*—The United Nation's International Covenant on Economic, Social and Cultural Rights (ICESCR) requires states to "take steps . . . to achieve progressively" economic and social rights.[2] GC 3 emphasizes that, "even in times of severe resource constraint . . . vulnerable members of society can and indeed must be protected by . . . low-cost targeted programs" and that states must make "full use of the maximum available resources."[3] Even poor states must demonstrate progress and can be evaluated on treatment of marginalized members.

Nonretrogression—GC 14 prohibits backsliding on rights obligations through "deliberately retrogressive measures."[4]

Nondiscrimination—ICESCR requires that states "guarantee that the rights . . . will be exercised without discrimination"; both ICESCR and the International Covenant on Civil and Political Rights (ICCPR) note special protection for children regarding nondiscrimination.[5]

Availability, accessibility, acceptability, and quality—GC 14 specifies that health services must be available, accessible, acceptable, and medically appropriate and of high quality.[6]

In the context of this conceptual framework, external efforts by the international community, including donors and international organizations, can engage with national governments—the primary duty bearers for ensuring rights—in their obligations to respect, protect, and fulfill the right to health, by establishing health education and services through partnership with local government and civil society and by building local capacity to implement and sustain improvements. Interventions can both meet public health needs and promote the right to health recognized in the ICESCR.

The invocation of economic and social rights highlights how organizations working at the interface of public health and human rights face significant hurdles in internal debates within their respective fields. As described in chapter 1, the public health community has been slow to recognize the normative framework of human rights and to begin to shift from a caregiving model to one that recognizes the inalienability and indivisibility of rights, with the attendant demands of community participation, attention to individual liberties, principles of sustainability, and a genuine engagement with questions of impunity and accountability.

The Western-based international human rights movement has been equally slow to recognize the indivisibility of rights and the inalienability of economic and social rights, with the attendant demands of analyzing the linkages between abuses of civil and political rights and of economic and social rights; engaging with efforts to define concretely such principles as progressive realization and maximum available resources; and undertaking the complex analysis necessary to identify the responsibility of different actors for systemic abuses and apply appropriate measure of accountability and redress.

The long-standing Western resistance to recognizing economic and social rights as human rights has a deep political history in anticommunism and the Cold War.[7] Dr. Mann's recognition of the interplay between civil and political rights abuses on the one hand and economic and social rights abuses on the other, as early as HealthRight's founding in 1990, was a relatively early emergence of concerted efforts to reunify the two sets of rights and begin to overcome those hurdles.

This chapter follows the bold premise of this book, as laid out in chapter 1, that we are not constrained by the old debate of whether health is in fact a human right; it is appropriately taken as given. However, the elucidation of the right, and the question of how programmatically to engage with it, inevitably leads to engagement with the current politics that resulted from that history. We will revisit the challenges of this engagement at the close of this chapter, when we consider how to take forward the lessons learned from these early days of rights-based approaches.

THE HEALTH AND HUMAN RIGHTS EVALUATION

Although the preceding principles arise organically from the international human rights framework described in chapter 1, operationalizing and measuring them has been a challenge for nongovernmental organizations (NGOs) implementing public health programs. Although public health indicators and evaluation criteria are well established, less has been done to develop and apply human rights indicators in the context of public health.

To respond to this gap, HealthRight International conducted a Health and Human Rights Evaluation (HHRE) with two aims: (a) to assess the organization's capacity to implement health projects that positively impact the right to health as well as other human rights and (b) to identify questions that can be asked and tools that can be employed to strengthen the human rights impacts of public health programs.

HealthRight International (formerly known as Doctors of the World-USA) is a United States–based NGO founded in 1990 by Dr. Jonathan Mann and other U.S. physicians. HealthRight works with local partners to build lasting access to health information and services for excluded communities in the United States and around the world. The HHRE was led by Mehlika Hoodbhoy, an independent human rights expert, and Vandana Tripathi, then HealthRight's program director. The following are the HHRE findings as well as recommendations for strengthening the rights impacts of NGO-led public health programs.

The HHRE team evaluated completed, ongoing, and in-development HealthRight child health projects in Kosovo and Russia. The HHRE consultant reviewed program materials, literature on rights-based programming,[8] and international human rights documents. On-site evaluation included visits to service sites and interviews with policymakers, program staff, funders, civil society groups, health providers, and project beneficiaries.

For the HHRE, the term "rights-based" implied an explicit connection to normative documents in the field of international human rights. Thus, the HHRE was guided by UN human rights documents, particularly ICESCR and its General Comments 3 and 14 (GC 14).[9] A guiding principle was the obligation of states and non-state actors to respect, protect, and fulfill human rights.[10] While these documents guide states, they also create a framework for non-state actors and measuring whether and how their work affects human rights at individual, community, and system levels. For the purposes of this analysis, "system" refers to law, policy, and/or public resource allocation. The outcomes, recommendations, and practical tools resulting from the HHRE are described here, starting with a specific project case study. Table 14.1 lists human rights documents cited in the following analysis.

TABLE 14.1 Relevant Articles From UN Human Rights Documents

International Covenant on Economic, Social and Cultural Rights (1978)	Convention on the Rights of the Child (1990)
Article 11: Adequate Standard of Living (food, clothing, housing)	Article 2: Non-discrimination
Article 12: Right to Health	Article 3: Best Interests of the Child
Article 13: Right to Education	Article 6: Child Survival and Development
	Article 18: Assistance to Families
International Convention on the Elimination of All Forms of Racial Discrimination (1971)	Article 19: Violence Against and Abuse of Children
	Article 20: Social Assistance
Article 1: Definition of Racial Discrimination	Article 23: Disabled Children
	Article 24: Highest Attainable Standard of Health
International Covenant on Civil and Political Rights (1978)	Article 25: Periodic Review of Child's Treatment
Article 7: Freedom From Torture	Article 26: Social Assistance
	Article 27: Adequate Standard of Living
	Article 28: Education
	Article 33: Substance Abuse
	Article 34: Protection of Children from Sexual Exploitation and Abuse
	Article 35: Prohibition on the Sale and Trafficking of Children
	Article 36: Prohibition of All Forms of Exploitation
	Article 37: Prohibition of Torture

CASE STUDY
The Rights and Health of Children With Disabilities in Kosovo

HealthRight's Deinstitutionalization Project in Kosovo was implemented from 2000–2004. It was funded by the United States Agency for International Development, United Nations International Children's Emergency Fund (UNICEF), and the Canadian International Development Agency. The Deinstitutionalization Project serves as an example of whether and how NGOs can work with civil society, state, and multilateral actors to implement rights-based approaches in a setting where the fragility or transitional nature of the state creates ambiguities in the identify and nature of the duty bearer(s).

The Deinstitutionalization Project created services for and raised public awareness about children with physical and mental disabilities. The program responded to the *de facto* practice at the time of placing children with disabilities in adult institutions; HealthRight identified children confined in the state-run Shtime Special Institution (SSI) for adults, where they faced neglect and abuse. Deinstitutionalization Project partners built and staffed two facilities, in a majority and a minority area (Gracanica and Shtime, respectively), to serve as community-based children's homes, with provision of medical and other services for disabled children. Children were transferred from the SSI to these children's homes. HealthRight also surveyed families in surrounding communities who had children with disabilities, and formed parent support groups (PSGs) and community advisory boards (CABs) to enable parents to advise the project, find peer support, and advocate for local services for their children. At the end of the project, the Ministry of Labor and Social Work–Institutions Division (MLSW-ID) assumed financial and human resources responsibility for the children's homes.

At each level of HHRE, project activities were examined for their ability to promote principles or objectives identified in the international human rights instruments discussed previously, particularly the Convention on the Rights of the Child (CRC) and the ICESCR. The following project impacts are marked in parentheses with the specific human rights aim to which they can be linked. We also identified potential for retrogression at the community and system level.

INDIVIDUAL LEVEL

The first level of impact that the HHRE considered was the individual. In eastern Europe, the social exclusion of disabled people, including children, has often been dramatic, with many being segregated into

(Continued)

(Continued)

institutions.[11,12] By creating safe and nurturing Homes (ICESCR, art. 11 and providing health services (CRC, arts. 20, 24, 25) for ethnic Albanian and Serb (Convention on the Elimination of All Forms of Racial Discrimination [CERD], art. 1; CRC, art. 2) children with disabilities (CRC, art. 23) who were inmates of an institution, the Deinstitutionalization Project contributed to these children realizing numerous individual rights (CRC, art. 23). "A child with disabilities has the right to a full and decent life in conditions which ensure dignity and active participation in the community" (CRC, art. 23).

By removing children from SSI, the project addressed rights that had previously been violated—these are noted here with the specific prohibitions in human rights instruments they contravened. At SSI, children were subject to degrading treatment; when found, many were malnourished, some tied to their beds, and living amidst their own filth (ICCPR, art. 7; CRC, art. 34). Children at SSI had been sedated and confined and lacked specialized health care (ICESCR, art. 12; CRC, arts. 6, 24) and education to address their disabilities (ICESCR, art. 13; CRC, art. 28). The children wore dirty clothing (ICESCR, art. 11), were not sufficiently fed (ICESCR, art. 11), and lived in conditions inadequate for rehabilitation (ICESCR, art. 11).

When these children were relocated to HealthRight-built children's homes, these violations were reduced—living conditions improved and children received access to education, vocational training, and rehabilitative services to promote independence. During each step of the transition to new homes, children were told of what would happen next and given opportunities to visit the new residence before moving, in accordance with international standards of care. The homes were staffed by nurses and caretakers trained by HealthRight in rights- and inclusion-oriented rehabilitative care of children with disabilities. Physiotherapists and a speech therapist were hired to provide direct specialized services to children and to train house staff in complementing these through ongoing care. Where possible, children were supported to access mainstream public services. For example, staff negotiated with UN Interim Administration Mission in Kosovo (UNMIK) Department of Education authorities to obtain access for five children (whose disabilities did not prevent them from doing so) to public school education in Laplje Selo, near Gracanica.

Individualized rehabilitation plans were developed for all children based on evaluations by school staff and specialists; these were accompanied by daily activity plans that could be implemented by

(Continued)

house staff. Referral relationships were developed with the Gracanica and Shtime Health Houses for ongoing access to medical care.

The impacts of these processes were manifested in changes in the children's mental and physical health. As described in a Health-Right report to UNICEF:

> [At SSI] . . . the children had endured periods of malnutrition, and [at the community homes] all gained weight and many shot up in height. . . . Two children had been confined to their beds for the entirety of their lives. They can now walk with support and stand on their own. Another child has received prosthetic legs and is learning how to walk. . . . Two previously non-verbal children now speak. Although seven children remain largely non-verbal, all have developed the capacity to communicate readily with staff. . . . The large majority of the children can now dress, make their beds, bathe, brush their teeth, use the toilet, and eat by themselves. Only three are still in diapers.[13]

These changes demonstrate the tangible results of delivering services in a manner that respected and protected children's rights. Many of the most profound limitations experienced by the Deinstitutionalization Project's clients while at SSI were not the product of actual disability but of neglect and inhumane treatment.

COMMUNITY LEVEL

The next level the HHRE evaluated was that of the community, particularly its social norms and whether they created an environment of exclusion or inclusion. The Deinstitutionalization Project's creation of PSGs and CAB increased awareness about disability issues. Some parents of disabled children in Gracanica and Shtime brought them out of hiding (CRC, arts. 2, 3, 19, 20) and become aware of and sought access to now-available health services (CRC, arts. 18, 23). This increased visibility helped change social attitudes; the experiences of teachers and providers in caring for disabled children contributed to decreased discrimination among key community members.

Regarding the potential for retrogression, should CABs and PSGs disband, gains from individuals' engagement in disability issues would erode. However, few other civil society monitors exist to demand accountability for disabled children's rights or criticize retrogression in social stigma.

(Continued)

(Continued)

SYSTEM LEVEL

At the time of the analysis, Kosovo was not a state under international law and there was a debate within the international community about the extent to which it was explicitly bound by the full set of international human rights obligations. However, Kosovo did have public authorities and interim governance structures; system-level analysis refers to these. In 2004, MLSW-ID created a budget for monies to be disbursed among ministries assuming administration of children's homes, explicitly allocating public resources to services for this population.[14] Independently, a disability advisor was also designated by the World Bank to work with the MLSW-ID.

Regarding the potential for retrogression: Depending on MLSW-ID's capacity and commitment, children's homes could continue to be supportive environments, or they could devolve into the prior institutional model characterized by discrimination, abuse, and neglect. It is unclear whether there is sufficient understanding in MLSW-ID of the need to or process for taking a human rights approach to services for disabled children. Without monitoring from parent's groups or others, regression may not be criticized or even documented. Needs remain for building capacity in public sector authorities as well as for civil society monitoring.[15] To strengthen impacts at the system level, NGOs and other actors should strengthen PSG and CAB members' advocacy skills and rights knowledge, ensuring that the primary caretakers of disabled children living at home can influence policy, and community-based resources, including accessible schools, for disabled children living at home, so that all disabled children can access public services, in addition to those in the children's homes created by the Deinstitutionalization Project. However, given the provisional legal status of government actors and legal authorities, identifying the appropriate targets of advocacy was challenging.

SUMMARY OF FINDINGS

The HHRE showed that HealthRight's public health programs build bridges between excluded subpopulations and public services that fulfill these populations' right to health. For groups excluded from the health system, projects evaluated by the HHRE, including the Kosovo Deinstitutionalization

Project, have resulted in outcomes such as improved access to care (GC 14,12; GC 14,19), more acceptable options for care (GC 14,12), greater equality in standards for care, nondiscriminatory protection from hazardous circumstances (GC 14,12), protection of children's rights (CRC; GC 14,22–24), and allocation of government resources to serve groups facing discrimination (CERD; GC 14,18–19).

The HHRE illustrated that NGO-led public health programs can benefit individuals experiencing multiple rights violations; HealthRight programs examined advanced not only the right to health but also the right to adequate standard of living, education, liberty, and freedom from torture, among others.

For example, because of stigma against the disabled, disabled children in Kosovo were deprived of their liberty and denied the right to participation in community life. The Deinstitutionalization Project's efforts have assisted in beneficiaries realizing rights to health information and services (ICESCR, art. 12; GC 14; CRC, art. 24) and impacted the rights to education (ICESCR, art. 13), freedom from torture (ICCPR, art. 7; CRC, art. 37), adequate standard of living (ICESCR, art. 11), and freedom from economic (CRC, art. 32) and sexual exploitation (CRC, art. 34). At the community level, HealthRight has raised awareness about the rights of excluded groups. Outreach in Kosovo helped parents of disabled children bring them out of hiding, beginning social reintegration. In Kosovo, Ministry commitment of financial and human resources to serve disabled children was an important step toward systematic respect for and fulfillment of their rights.

However, despite progressive changes in the system outlined previously, the impacts of NGO public health programs at the system level can be far more fragile. The HHRE showed that HealthRight programs build local health capacity but not always human rights capacity, either in the state or in civil society to monitor the state. Potential for retrogression exists after handover of health activities to state partners, especially where advocacy capacity is weak. At the time of the HHRE report, the interim government of Kosovo had not provided adequate resources or systems to address the health needs of excluded children, specifically the disabled. Where resources have increased, state capacity to provide quality care has not necessarily increased. Kosovo traditionally had limited space or capacity for citizens to address social issues. In Kosovo, although MLSW assumed responsibility for children's homes, no mechanism exists to monitor services. Changes in home staff or ministry leadership may weaken children's access to quality care, causing retrogression at individual and system levels.

IMPLICATIONS FOR PUBLIC HEALTH NONGOVERNMENTAL ORGANIZATIONS

The HHRE identified several recommendations and challenges for public health NGOs that seek to promote human rights impacts and apply rights-based approaches to their programming. These are summarized here, with reference to the HealthRight experience where appropriate.

Recommendations

The implications of this HHRE are relevant to all public health organizations seeking to promote human rights, particularly those working with socially excluded subgroups within larger populations. To design and implement projects that create rights impacts, particularly at the system level, it is recommended that NGOs develop "rights threshold" criteria to determine whether conditions in proposed locations are conducive to such impacts. This requires expanding program assessments beyond health indicators to examining context (e.g., presence of civil society, structures for policy enforcement); channels to demand government accountability; and existence of local partners to take on follow-up—not only of service provision, which is frequently done, but also of monitoring quality of care and conducting sustained advocacy to address gaps. If these threshold criteria are not met at baseline, then NGOs should explicitly include strengthening local advocacy capacity as a program objective, in addition to health activities.

The HHRE highlighted the importance of developing indicators of rights impact to measure along with health indicators. Monitoring and evaluation should assess progressive realization or retrogression during the project, measured by changes in availability, accessibility, acceptability, and quality of services. Data collected for program monitoring should be disaggregated to measure decreases in disparity of care. Indicators can also be framed in human rights language (e.g., increases in the number of people accessing health commodities that reflect the right to benefit from scientific progress[16]). Indicators should measure improvements in state capacity to provide services and civil society capacity to monitor the state and track allocation of resources to a health problem or to disproportionately affected groups.

Challenges

The HHRE also identified challenges for public health NGOs in enabling rights impacts. These often arise from contrasts between traditional definitions of public health work and human rights work. First, much traditional public health work targets whole populations or communities (e.g., mass vaccination campaigns). In contrast, rights analysis often reveals those not reached by public systems, in both resource-rich and resource-poor settings. A rights analysis can suggest interventions that promote equity between groups; however, this may result in programs that target fewer beneficiaries and have a higher cost per beneficiary than a population-wide program. There can also be a tension between determining whether to focus on the law and policy level, as much traditional rights advocacy does, or on the *de facto* level, where real access to information, education, and services is controlled. Many of HealthRight's projects serve socially excluded groups whose rights may be guaranteed at the legal or constitutional level but are daily violated at the practical level, caused by discrimination and lack of mechanisms or resources to implement laws.

Another conflict may exist between mandates for NGOs to deliver services in place of a weak state and traditional rights approaches urging states to take responsibility for delivering services. Here, HealthRight's mission and approach suggest a partial resolution—training local providers, particularly within public systems, allows NGOs to provide services when necessary, but always progress toward state responsibility, ownership, and funding. Where the state is not a reliable partner (i.e., actively violating human rights), training civil society actors may be an interim substitute that creates system-level impacts. However, as highlighted earlier in this chapter, and as we return to this theme in conclusion, a rights-based approach still needs more development. We need to resolve the contradictions between working with the state on one hand to reduce discrimination and marginalization and improve delivery of services, and on the other hand, opposing human rights violations by the state and not undermining slowly developing national and international systems of accountability.

THE HEALTH AND HUMAN RIGHTS PLANNING PROTOCOL

The HHRE resulted in a tool to operationalize these recommendations and enable HealthRight and others to better achieve individual, community, and system-level human rights impacts through health projects. This tool, the Health and Human Rights Planning Protocol, is summarized in Table 14.2. The full protocol includes questions to ask at each step, annotated with human rights documents directly connecting rights principles and health activities. Questions help determine, which rights can be addressed by health projects and gauge projects' potential strengths and weaknesses from a rights perspective. For example, during

TABLE 14.2 Summary of Health and Human Rights Planning Protocol

Step 1: Needs Assessment (before determining health objectives and activities)	A: Government Capacity: Obtain a realistic assessment of present government interest and capacity from both a management and administrative perspective.
	B: Organizational Capacity: Assess the resources (human and financial) HealthRight brings and how the services it proposes to deliver will contribute to the realization of the right to health and other human rights.
	C: Human Rights Assessment: Ask three clusters of questions during preproject assessment missions: (a) Government Commitment to Human Rights; (b) Assessment Using Core Human Rights Principles; and (c) Law and Policy.[a]
Step 2: Human Rights Analysis (after determining potential health objectives and activities)	A: Human Rights Principles: Review applicable human rights framework documents to identify which specific human rights are addressed by the project.
	B: Accountability Through Public Education: Devise and plan project-related advocacy and media strategies. Government authorities are unlikely to change laws, policies, and resource allocation patterns independently, particularly regarding marginalized populations, who may be able to demand accountability.
	C: Principles Into Programs: Correlate planned project objectives and activities with the human rights issues identified in Part B, focusing on potential impact.
	D: Human Rights Indicators: Formulate indicators of how the proposed project meets requirements set forth in human rights documents, which specify that health services must be made available, accessible, acceptable, and medically appropriate and of high quality. Indicators should track and measure improvements in availability, accessibility, acceptability, and quality, disaggregating improvements by subgroup.

[a]These steps are explained in the full protocol and provide an opportunity to identify the human rights violations (health and others) manifested in the health needs and gaps, at both the *de facto* and *de jure* levels, that HealthRight is uncovering.

a project assessment, the protocol asks program leaders to consider, evaluate, and measure:

- *Legal and policy environment*—What laws and/or policies exist relevant to the specific health issue targeted by the project? Do these laws hinder or promote the ability of individuals to access related health information and services? Are some groups more affected by these laws/policies than others?

- *Exploitation*—Does the project's target population face economic and/or sexual exploitation that further compromises its health status? What indicators will the project use to document this?
- *Advocacy*—What is the strategy to use project-derived evidence to convince the government to change the way it provides health care to the target group?
- *Funding*—Where does the health field or issue addressed by the project fit into national health priorities? How is implementation funded in this specific area? What is the government contribution of financial and/or human resources to the proposed project? How will the project measure increased government investment throughout the project cycle?

The protocol applies the international human rights framework in shaping and understanding the objectives of health projects and makes linkages between health work and human rights impact more concrete.

CONCLUSION

For HealthRight International, applying rights-based approaches to public health programs has involved looking closely at the "Who" and "How" of its programs. The HHRE and other experiences have led HealthRight to codify a set of programming principles for rights-based approaches. These include the following:

- *Measure and seek to reduce disparities in access to health care*—for example, disaggregate data on community use of health services by wealth quintiles to understand who benefits from services introduced by NGO programs
- *Involve communities in program design*— for example, ensure that health services assessments and evaluations include the viewpoints of health service users as well as nonusers, in order to identify quality and access barriers as experienced by communities
- *Build capacity of local providers and organizations*—for example, introduce new health and social services into existing points of care rather than setting up parallel delivery mechanisms; orient, encourage, and support existing providers to reach underserved populations

- *Promote sustainability by building local ownership or funding of services*—for example, advocate for local government funding of health services that reach socially excluded groups and plan programs to include increased local co-funding each year
- *Support civil society groups and local advocacy*—for example, identify and train community groups to evaluate and report on quality of care

HealthRight International considers these steps to be fundamental for any organization approaching public health from a rights perspective. However, these are only the first steps toward bridging the gap between health and human rights. It remains a challenge for all stakeholders to help forge a movement of global to local civil society that goes beyond facilitation of the provision of services and cohesively addresses accountability. Ideal rights protection is preventive through systems such as the public health ones described here that reduce the chances of systemic violations but also through rule of law, including responding to violations in order to discourage future abuses. Access to justice for victims, the potential punishment of perpetrators, and the reduction of impunity are all elements of this prevention. The widespread impunity that now prevails for abuses of economic and social rights, the extremely limited toolbox of legal responses, and the difficulties surrounding their justiciability are all challenges that need to be faced together if long-term solutions are to be found.

These issues include both practical and conceptual challenges for public health practitioners working within a rights-based framework. One recent example of these challenges came in 2009, when the International Criminal Court issued an arrest warrant for Sudan's President Omar al-Bashir for war crimes and crimes against humanity in Darfur. In response, Sudan revoked the licenses of international aid organizations working in the country, including several organizations that explicitly embrace a rights-based framework, including Oxfam Great Britain, CARE International, and Save the Children UK. Aid organizations, working to address displacement, homeless, hunger, disease, and other results of extreme trauma suffered by victims of the conflict, faced immediate expulsion from the country and potential collapse of their life-saving services. Human rights organizations generally hailed the indictment as a positive step for international justice and against impunity for atrocities committed in Darfur. Thus the human rights and public health organizations involved, as well as the international community generally, faced an apparent contradiction between an international human rights mechanism to address abuses of civil and political rights in Darfur and efforts to ameliorate the economic and social rights abuses resulting from the conflict.

Such real-world challenges to the indivisibility of rights are a longstanding feature of international humanitarian aid and development work, and we are just beginning to identify ways to resolve them. Like Oxfam and Doctors Without Borders/ Médecins Sans Frontières (MSF), and a handful of other international NGOs, HealthRight International has been working to expand national and global advocacy on the right to health and the health and human rights link, beyond the borders of its own programs. Over the previous decade, international organizations have played an increasingly important role in promoting the right to health, through engagement on issues such as improving access to medicines, increasing state health budgets and eliminating user fees, reshaping donor strategies and reducing international debt burdens. These are crucial steps forward, and begin to map out a world where the indivisibility and inalienability of rights are more widely recognized, and the gap between health and human rights begins to close.

ACKNOWLEDGEMENTS

HealthRight is grateful for the support of the Oak Foundation, which has funded HealthRight's human rights capacity building activities including the HHRE. The authors express particular thanks to reviewers for their time and invaluable suggestions: Dr. Howard Minkoff, chairman of the Department of Obstetrics and Gynecology at Maimonides Medical Center and chair of the Program Committee of HealthRight's board of directors; Marta Schaaf, an independent consultant on health and human rights; and Thomas Dougherty, former HealthRight executive director. Key findings in this chapter were first presented at the conference, *Lessons Learned From Rights Based Approaches to Health*, convened by the Institute of Human Rights at Emory University and other collaborating partners in April 2005.

NOTES

[1] Equi-TB. Who is Most Vulnerable to TB and What Can We Do About It? Retrieved from http://www.equi-tb.org.uk/uploads/tb_vulnerable.pdf

[2] ICESCR, Article 2(1).

[3] The United Nations Economic and Social Council Committee on Economic, Social and Cultural Rights. The Nature of States Parties Obligations. UN doc E/C. 14/12/90, ICESCR GC 3 ¶ 12, 9.

[4] The United Nations Economic and Social Council Committee on Economic, Social and Cultural Rights. The Right to the Highest Attainable Standard of Health, UN Doc E/C.12/2004/4, ICESCR General Comment 14 (2000). ¶ 1.

[5] ICESCR 10, ICCPR 24.

[6]ICESCR GC 3 12a, 12b, 12c, 12d.

[7]See Anderson, C. (2003). *Eyes off the prize: The United Nations and the African American struggle for human rights, 1944–1955.* Cambridge: Cambridge University Press; Glendon, M. A. (2001). *A world made new: Eleanor Roosevelt and the Universal Declaration of Human Rights.* New York: Random House.

[8]See for example Save the Children-UK. (2001). An Introduction to Child Right's Programming: Concept and Application. Retrieved from www.savethechildren.org.uk; and United Nations International Children's Emergency Fund. (1998). A Human Rights Approach to UNICEF Programming for Children and Women: What it Is, and Some Changes it Will Bring. Retrieved from www.unicef.org.

[9]The United Nations Economic and Social Council Committee on Economic, Social and Cultural Rights. (2000). The Right to the Highest Attainable Standard of Health, UN Doc E/C.12/2004/4. ICESCR General Comment 14.

[10]GC 14 ¶ 33 summarizes these obligations as follows: The obligation to respect requires states to refrain from interfering directly or directly with the enjoyment of the right to health (see also GC 14 ¶ 34). The obligation to protect requires states to take measures that prevent third parties from interfering with article 12 guarantees (see also GC 14 ¶ 35). Finally, the obligation to fulfill requires States to adopt appropriate legislative, administrative, budgetary, judicial, promotional and other measures toward the full realization of the right to health (see also GC 14 ¶ 36–37).

[11]See Schaaf, M. (2003). *Failure to protect: The situation of the mentally disabled in UN-administered Kosovo.* Unpublished research paper December 2003, at 2–3 for a description of the Soviet model of "defectology."

[12]Hunt, K. (1998). *Abandoned to the state: Cruelty and neglect in Russian Orphanages.* New York: Human Rights Watch.

[13]HealthRight International. (2002). Final narrative report: Year one de-institutionalization of Kosovar children with special needs [internal document].

[14]GC 14 ¶ 33 specifically mentions budgetary measures as part of the obligation to fulfill the right to health.

[15]GC 14 ¶ 36–37 give several examples of the state capacity to fulfill the right to health.

[16]IESCR 15.

CHAPTER 15

Operationalizing Rights-Based Approaches to Health: The Case of CARE in Peru

Ariel Frisancho, Jay Goulden, and Helene D. Gayle

INTRODUCTION

Founded in the United States in 1945, sending "CARE Packages" to help survivors of World War II in Europe, the work of Cooperative for Assistance and Relief Everywhere (CARE) has since evolved to address both the causes and consequences of poverty in more than 70 countries in Africa, Asia, Latin America, the Middle East, and Eastern Europe. Its community-based and advocacy-focused programs aim to support the realization of rights to health, education, water and sanitation, food security, and access to financial resources. CARE's health programs cover the areas of maternal and child health, nutrition, sexual and reproductive health, water and sanitation, and HIV/AIDS and other infectious diseases, through some 350 health-related projects reaching more than 13 million people annually, 8 million of whom are women and girls. CARE's vision is for a world of hope, tolerance, and social justice, where poverty has been overcome and people live in dignity and security. Human rights and, in particular, the right to the highest attainable standard of health are, thus, at the heart of our work.

CARE's understanding is that people are often trapped in a cycle of poverty not mainly because of lack of assets and skills but because of systemic social exclusion, marginalization, and discrimination, set within a context of systems and structures that perpetuate poverty. Poverty stems from political, social, economic, and environmental factors at the community, regional (subnational), national, and global levels. Supporting the realization of the right to health for the poor requires not only direct actions to improve their health status but also addressing the underlying and systemic factors and power imbalances that impact on health, including ensuring changes in public policies. It requires working with both rights-holders—the poor and marginalized and their representative organizations—and duty-bearers, from the state (authorities, Congress, public officers and health workers) and private sector, including other cooperation agencies and key stakeholders (i.e., political parties).

This chapter illustrates how CARE is applying this approach in practice, with examples drawn mainly from our work in Peru, where two of the authors have been working over recent years. We start by outlining our framework for rights-based approaches, before then giving detailed examples of its application in our health program in Peru. We end with a review of evidence that a rights-based approach can lead to increased impact of work to tackle poverty and social exclusion, as well as some principal lessons learned and remaining challenges.

CARE'S RIGHTS-BASED PROGRAMMATIC PRINCIPLES

As mentioned in the previous section, CARE understands that poverty stems from political, social, economic, and environmental factors at both the community and global level. One way to understand the complex web of poverty is to envision a three-tiered hierarchy of causes: immediate, intermediate, and underlying. Immediate causes relate directly to life-and-death situations, such as maternal and neonatal emergencies and natural disasters. Intermediate causes relate to people's well-being and generally point to what people lack, such as access to basic services, skills, and productivity. Historically, most development efforts have been targeted at these two levels.

Underlying causes focus attention on *why* intermediate causes exist and speak to the structural underpinnings that govern societies, the "social determinants of health." For example, why do some people have access to services and others do not? Why do only a few groups control the majority of resources? What are the power inequities that define and determine the way public providers relate to poor people when they look for public (health, education) services? Why do women in danger when giving birth at their homes cannot decide by themselves to seek for emergency health care? Why do some husbands or partners prevent women from demanding modern family planning methods? Finding answers to these questions and ways to ensure social justice and equity are critical to helping eradicate extreme poverty. Therefore, CARE's work focuses on three primary ends:

1. Increasing opportunities for people to meet their basic needs and ensure that future generations will have these opportunities too;
2. Promoting people's efforts to overcome social inequity, so that people can live a life of dignity and enjoy their rights without discrimination and exclusion; and
3. Promoting sound and equitable governance systems and policies, to create a climate that promotes equity, justice, and livelihood security for all, with governments and other actors meeting their human rights obligations to respect, protect, and fulfill.

Figure 15.1 offers an illustration of the framework for CARE's approach. The circle labeled "human conditions" refers to efforts to ensure that people's basic needs are met and that they attain livelihood security. Addressing "social positions" means supporting people's efforts to take control of their lives and fulfill their rights, responsibilities, and aspirations, and supporting efforts to end inequality and discrimination. Facilitating a sound "enabling environment" means strengthening public, private, civil, and social institutions to better respond to and involve constituents, in order to foster just and equitable societies. CARE recognizes that there is considerable interaction between and across these three areas, and successfully addressing all three of them concomitantly is critical to eradicating poverty and ensuring social justice (Gayle & Sinho, 2009).

During the late 1990s, CARE was one of several nongovernment organizations (NGOs), donors, and UN agencies that developed frameworks and strategies to apply thinking and approaches from the world of human rights to their development work. A rights-based approach for CARE means deliberately and explicitly focusing on people achieving the basic conditions for living with *dignity* (i.e., achieving their human rights). It empowers people to claim and exercise their rights and fulfill their responsibilities. A rights-based approach recognizes poor, displaced, and war-affected people as having inherent rights essential to livelihood security—rights that are validated by international

FIGURE 15.1 Framework for CARE's Approach

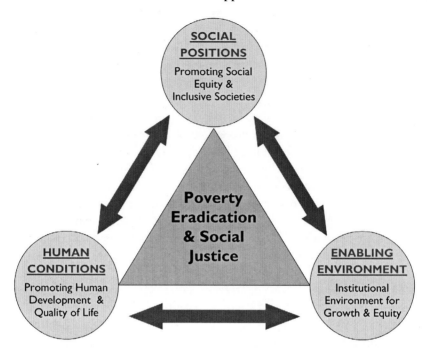

Note. CARE Health Strategy: 2005–2010.

law (Jones, 2001). CARE has chosen to operationalize this approach through six program principles (CARE International, 2003), developed out of an analysis of the organizational implications of a rights-based approach (CARE International UK, 2005). These six principles include the following: promote empowerment and more equal power relations; work in partnership with others; ensure accountability and promote responsibility; address discrimination; promote the nonviolent resolution of conflicts; seek sustainable results/including addressing underlying causes of poverty.

As can be seen in Table 15.1, these principles are similar to other main definitions of rights-based approaches to development, including those of the UK Department for International Development (DFID) and the United Nations. All stress principles of inclusion, participation, and fulfillment of obligation, and seek to tackle the underlying causes of poverty and disadvantage. There is a strong focus on working in partnership with a wide range of stakeholders to address these causes, both immediate and underlying.

TABLE 15.1 Principal Frameworks for Rights-Based Approaches

CARE (CARE International, 2003)	DFID (DFID, 2000)	UNITED NATIONS (Silva, 2003)
1. Promote empowerment and more equal power relations	• Participation	• Participation and inclusion
2. Work in partnership with others		• Strategic partnerships are developed and sustained
3. Ensure accountability and promote responsibility	• Fulfilling obligation	• Accountability and rule of law
4. Address discrimination	• Inclusion	• Equality and Nondiscrimination
5. Promote the nonviolent resolution of conflicts		
6. Seek sustainable results or including addressing underlying causes of poverty		• Assessment and analysis . . . [of] the immediate, underlying, and structural causes of the nonrealization of rights
		• Universality and inalienability
		• Indivisibility
		• Interdependence and Inter-relatedness

The main difference lies in CARE's stressing of the importance of addressing power imbalances as a core component of the implementation of a rights based approach. To do this, a series of processes are developed:

- The identification of those members of society with less power (e.g., rural and illiterate rural indigenous women) and those groups who have the power to determine the allocation of resources or make decisions (e.g., health or governmental authorities, health providers, mining companies);
- The implementation of strategies to promote better information and understanding of human rights amongst poor and excluded people;
- The facilitation of empowerment processes; and
- The provision of technical assistance and advocacy to support appropriate organizational environments for inclusion and participation of those traditionally excluded—or their genuine representatives—into the design, implementation, and assessment of social policies, in a way they could better claim and realize their rights.

Importantly, CARE also recognizes that such work to address power imbalances can lead to conflicts, and these therefore need to be identified, analyzed, and mitigated or transformed. On the other hand, if CARE succeeds in normalizing human rights standards where they are absent, and gaining more allies and key actors toward this purpose, changes in power structures could be less opposed.

APPLYING A RIGHTS-BASED APPROACH IN PRACTICE IN PERU

Despite its status as a middle-income country, Peru faces significant problems of poverty, discrimination, and inequity, including hugely different morbidity and mortality rates and a high prevalence of avoidable illnesses and deaths in people who are poor, people from indigenous populations, and people from excluded groups (Amnesty International, 2009; Frisancho & Goulden, 2008; Hunt, 2005; Yamin, 2007). In terms of under-5 mortality rate, Peru has the largest gap between the poorest and richest quintiles of all 58 countries with relevant data: a child born in the poorest quintile faces a risk of premature death more than 5 times (5.3) the rate faced by a child born in the top quintile (Vandemoortele, 2009).

As with many other countries, Peru has made insufficient success in reducing maternal mortality over recent years, and Millennium Development Goal (MDG) 5 (improve maternal health) is the least likely health goal to be achieved by 2015. Inadequate progress at national level also conceals huge internal disparities in the country. Estimated maternal mortality ratios in the poorer regions of the Andean Highlands, such as in Puno or Huancavelica, are far higher than the national average of 185 maternal deaths for every 100,000 live births: 361 and 302, respectively in 2000 (Watanabe Varas, 2002). Underlying the systemic failure to prevent maternal death is, depending on specific circumstances, the denial of the right to health, to equality and nondiscrimination, to reproductive self-determination, and to benefit of scientific progress (Frisancho, 2009; Yamin, 2007). A rights-based approach highlights the necessity of closing such gaps within countries, as well as to clarify the standards and criteria that are needed to eliminate these disparities.

Principle 1: Promoting Empowerment and Changing Power Relations

Over the past 5 years, CARE Peru's Health Rights Project partnered with ForoSalud (Health Forum), a major civil society network, which brings together more than 100 national, regional, and local organizations and movements and a wide and diverse range of citizens committed to the realization of health rights. As example of a North–South partnership focused on strengthening local actors, this collaboration between CARE and ForoSalud has sought to make health policies and institutions more responsive to the rights of poor and marginalized people. This work has contributed to a new vision of health policy, emphasizing health as a universal human right, against the backdrop of health sector reforms focused almost exclusively on efficiency and cost recovery. This human rights stance on health has had several implications: prioritization of quality health services that actually reach the most poor and excluded (an estimated 25% of the overall Peruvian population with no access to health services when they need them); establishing citizens' participation in policy decision-making at national and regional levels; and setting standards for social surveillance of health policies and public health services.

ForoSalud has gradually established itself as a major player in the national health sector. ForoSalud, CARE, and other organizations implemented participatory processes for generating health policy proposals. Training on health rights and developing capacities for collective action and advocacy brought the "voice of the poor" to regional and national policy dialogues through a bottom-up policy design process in 12 out of 24 regions. As a result, health policy proposals from all regions of Peru were widely discussed, and ForoSalud representatives have been elected as citizen representatives for the National Health Council and for 10 Regional Health Councils, getting some of ForoSalud policy proposals institutionalized. In ForoSalud's 2nd and 3rd National Health Conferences (2004 and 2006), nearly 2,000 nationwide delegates discussed and presented health policy proposals to the Peruvian minister of health (Potts, 2008b).

ForoSalud also worked together with a wide range of actors on the formulation of a legislative proposal on health service users' rights and responsibilities (Law on Health Services Users' Rights), which will ultimately help to hold the government accountable for service delivery quality and opportunity. ForoSalud collected more than 100,000 signatures of support for their legal proposal (2005), the first such example of a legislative proposal by citizens' petition, and engaged with the Health Commission of the Peruvian Congress to implement public audiences to be consulted on the contents of the law proposal during 2006–2007. In December 2008, the Health Services Users' Rights and Responsibilities Law was approved by all the political representatives in the Peruvian Congress, then observed by the Peruvian government and finally approved and officialized on October 2009.

In Participatory Mechanisms for Health Management

CARE's Health Rights Project has successfully supported the Peruvian Ministry of Health's (MoH) Shared Administration Program, through which citizens elected by the local community become members of the management committee of health facilities at the primary care level. From 2004–2007, CARE was part of a sustained advocacy effort and technical assistance process to the Health Commission of the Congress and MoH to press for the design and passing of the Health Co-Management and Citizen Participation Law (Law 29124), which included the realization of a series of six macroregional consultation workshops lead by the Health Commission. After the approval of the law, a participatory process of design of the law's regulations was put in place in diverse macroregional workshops, where a wide range of national and regional or local actors involved in the future development and implementation of the law had the opportunity to contribute with their final design (Arroyo, 2009).

In Analysis

Physicians for Human Rights conducted an investigation in 2007 to analyze the systemic and social factors that perpetuate the injustice of maternal mortality in Peru. Working in close collaboration with CARE Peru and using a rights-based approach to analyze maternal mortality in Peru, this groundbreaking study provides a "social X-ray of Peruvian society," illuminating the interactions of rural poverty and gender inequality, which disproportionately affect indigenous women and those who are illiterate and otherwise marginalized. The study also highlights the way in which the health system and political inadequate decisions and delays in decision making and prioritization exacerbate those patterns of exclusion (Yamin, 2007).

Principle 2: Working in Partnership

Working With ForoSalud

Instead of "developing" a new civil society organization, CARE sought to strengthen an existing civil society network (ForoSalud), with a clear commitment toward the realization of the right to health of the most poor and excluded, based on the principles of inclusion and informed citizen participation. ForoSalud was seen as an important social space for policy making, to help build consensus among the widely differing interests within Peruvian civil society in health. ForoSalud evolved from being a mostly professional-based, urban male organization, to be a gender-equitable, decentralized, umbrella organization, transforming itself into a social movement focused on health rights realization, including regional networks, community-based women's organizations and civil society coalitions, building increasing representation of the most poor and excluded in its own structures (Arroyo, 2007; Sandino, 2006).

Working With the Ministry of Health

Strengthening people's capacity to participate is essential. However, on its own, it is insufficient to ensure that their needs and views are incorporated into health policy decision making. That requires active engagement with the duty bearer, in support of their efforts to meet their responsibilities for the right to health, and so CARE's Health Rights Project also linked up with the Peruvian MoH, building on an early "window of opportunity" in 2004: the upcoming visit to Peru of the United Nations Special Rapporteur on the Right to Health and a newly appointed health minister. Both events allowed CARE to meaningfully address institutional shortcomings in cooperation with the MoH. Through a series of capacity building and cooperative meetings, cross-cutting principles of a rights-based approach were endorsed by the MoH. During the following years, positive change occurred within the MoH programs designed to promote inclusion and cultural appropriateness of health service provision became a priority. With the support of CARE Peru and others, a National Mobilization on Health Rights and Responsibilities was commenced and nationwide workshops and training on human rights and health and the promotion of citizen participation for regional health officers were conducted during 2004–2006 (MoH, 2006a). Additionally, the MoH created a technical unit concerned with the promotion of health rights, gender equity, and cultural appropriateness of health care. As a result, MoH institutionalized both a national technical document and a national directive on the definition and implementation of health rights, gender equity, and culture appropriateness in health, as reference for all Peruvian health services (Frisancho, 2007).

An important issue currently being addressed is the composition of the spaces for participation in the National Health Council and Regional Health Councils. Those are the unique policy dialogue spaces to discuss and analyze health policy design and implementation, though they still are more "formal" than effective: civil society and people representatives have only 1 seat of 11 in the council (made up of health providers and health worker organizations). In 2008, ForoSalud obtained the support of the minister of health for approval to its legal proposal to increase the presence of citizen's representatives within those "invited spaces." The proposal also includes the establishment of a national health congress, which would require the minister of health to present and discuss new government policy guidelines. The minister would also be required to account to the people for the implementation (both positive and negative) of national health policy in biannual national meetings (Potts, 2008b). Although approved, the implementation of ForoSalud's legal proposal is facing strong resistance from the MoH bureaucracy and other groups of interest, preventing a more equitable balance of power within the council's decision making.

Working With the Human Rights Ombudsperson

At regional and local levels in Peru, CARE's Participatory Voices Project has supported the development of citizen and civil society-based account-ability mechanisms, promoting citizen surveillance of health services. These initiatives have linked Quechua and Aymara women community leaders to regional offices of the human rights ombudsperson to monitor women's health rights, particularly their right to good quality and appro-priate maternal health services (Potts, 2008a).

Promoting Strategic Alliances for the Right to Health

CARE has engaged with a series of allies to promote health rights realiza-tion. In 2007, CARE collaborated with UN agencies on a National Alliance on Safe and Healthy Motherhood to advocate the MoH and Congress for increased resource allocation and adequate decision making to prevent maternal mortality, especially of poorest women. In 2008, CARE joined efforts with UN agencies and national NGOs to successfully advocate and provide technical assistance to the MoH for approval of specific national policies and a validated package of cost-effective interventions to improve neonatal health—a neglected health issue—nationwide.

Scaling Up Evidence-Based Models for Maternal Health for Vulnerable Populations

The Foundations to Enhance Management of Maternal Emergencies (FEMME) Project in Ayacucho, Peru, was a joint effort of CARE Peru, Columbia University's Averting Maternal Deaths and Disability Program, MoH, and the National Maternal and Perinatal Institute. Between 2000 and 2005, the project strengthened emergency obstetric care (EmOC) at the regional hospital of Ayacucho and four rural satellite health clinics in this region that has some of the highest levels of poverty in the country, was worst affected by the internal armed conflict, and is, not uncoincidentally, also a region where most people (63%) have Quechua as their mother tongue.

The principal objective of the project was to reduce maternal mortality through improvements in the availability, use, and quality of basic and comprehensive emergency obstetric care, improved technical capacity of healthcare personnel in internationally accepted evidence-based practices and protocols, strengthened management of healthcare services and the incorporation of rights-based approaches in the medical practice of health teams. As a result, CARE contributed to MoH efforts to reduce maternal mortality by 50% in Ayacucho region. An impact assessment conducted together by the MoH and CARE indicated that the success of the project, in comparison with efforts to reduce maternal mortality in a comparative, similar geographical region (Puno), was significantly higher. The MoH was interested in scaling up the strategies validated in Ayacucho region, incorporating some recent complementary MoH developments. CARE established a strategic alliance with the Peruvian MoH to carry out two studies to provide regional and local governments with a more realistic picture on how to address the reduction of maternal mortality: (a) a study to systematize and instrumentalize the eight strategies that comprise the FEMME model and (b) a study to determine the costs of implementing the eight strategies promoted through FEMME. As a result of this important joint work, in March 2009, MoH presented the "intervention model to improve the availability, quality and use of health facilities which provide emergency obstetric and neonatal care," based on FEMME's eight validated strategies, adding other national and regional interventions within health services in Ayacucho. MoH expects that the implementation of the intervention model will decisively contribute to the reduction of maternal mortality.

Principle 3: Promoting Responsibility and Accountability

Responsibility

To promote public accountability for health policy and development programs, CARE has supported several social reporting mechanisms working with a wide range of civil society allies. These have included the support to nearly 50 different national organizations for the participatory construction of a 2006 and 2008 civil society shadow report to the United Nations Special Rapporteur on the right to health, drawing on recommendations made by the Special Rapporteur to the Peruvian government following his mission in the country in 2004. CARE has also raised awareness on the situation of the right to health, through a nationwide report on the Enforceability of Sexual and Reproductive Rights and Access to HIV/AIDS Treatment, as well as the rights-based analysis on maternal mortality with Physicians for Human Rights mentioned earlier. These reports, altogether with a series of studies developed by national academic and research institutions, have been important for promoting specific issues in public debate and have provided important tools for advocacy and to hold the government accountable toward its obligations toward health rights (Bueno de Mesquita & Hunt, 2008).

Accountability

The International Initiative on Maternal Mortality and Human Rights is a collaboration of regional and national civil society organizations—including CARE, Center for Reproductive Rights, Averting Maternal Death and Disability Program, Family Care International, Physicians for Human Rights, and the former United Nations Special Rapporteur on the Right to the Highest Attainable Standard of Health (Paul Hunt)—committed to a comprehensive human rights approach to maternal mortality. This human rights approach includes a call for greater political will from governments and donors to take the necessary steps to reduce maternal mortality, as well as effective accountability mechanisms to realize women's right to maternal health.

Improving the health of the poor and marginalized in countries such as Peru will not be achieved through technical interventions and the provision of funding alone. Significant and sustainable change can only happen if the poor have a much greater involvement in shaping policies, practices, and programs, and by ensuring what is agreed to actually happens. A significant accountability mechanism, implemented through CARE's Participatory Voices Project, has been the strengthening of citizen monitoring of health services in the Piura and Puno regions of Peru. The main objective is to ensure there are social accountability mechanisms, which could effectively monitor implementation of the policies and at the same time promote the involvement of people. In the region of Puno, a strategic alliance between ForoSalud Puno, the regional ombudsperson's office, and networks of community Quechua and Aymara women leaders was established to implement citizen surveillance (monitoring) mechanisms on women's health rights, particularly their right to good quality, appropriate maternal health services. The women monitor health care, through direct observation and dialogue with service users and providers, and report their findings to the ombudsperson's office, who in turn reports the findings back, together with the women leaders, to the health facility managers and regional health authorities. The process has exposed obstacles to sexual and reproductive health, which have been addressed in public audiences (dialogues) between people's representatives and health authorities (Frisancho & Goulden, 2008; Potts, 2008a).

Principle 4: Addressing Discrimination

Focus on the Most Excluded

Working toward sustainable poverty reduction requires strategies to address the exclusionary power relations and ethnic discrimination that underlines Peru's inequality and inequities. CARE Peru's health interventions focuses on inclusive citizenship and rights realization through the strengthening of equitable relations between state and society and raising visibility on neglected groups (i.e., rural newborns, rural and poor women, sex workers, etc.), as CARE's Health Rights Project or Participatory Voices Project do (i.e., strengthening capacities amongst rural indigenous women who will both promote change and gender equity within their communities and allocate their best knowledge and learning to improve health services for their communities or raising national visibility and providing technical assistance to the MoH to implement evidence-based strategies to address rural newborns health, an issue historically neglected, as there were no specific neonatal health policies or interventions in place until late 2008).

Focus on Gender Discrimination

Women and children are too often denied the right to health. We have already highlighted previously the injustice of the largely avoidable deaths worldwide from complications of pregnancy and childbirth of one woman every minute, the vast majority in developing countries. CARE places a focus on working with women because they are disproportionately affected by poverty and inequity and because investing in them yields additional benefits for their families and communities. Gender equity and social inclusion are key leverage points for eradicating poverty and poor health. Development projects that fail to address these issues often miss the mark and do little to improve health conditions. The active citizenship displayed by indigenous women leaders in Puno in the health surveillance system mentioned earlier, or in regional and national ForoSalud advocacy work, are key examples of such work.

Principle 5: Conflict Resolution

Seeking to resolve and transform conflicts, CARE has focused on promoting more constructive, informed, and consensus-focused interactions between rights holders and duty bearers, building capacities on both sides to facilitate this process. CARE has also engaged with diverse governmental officers and ombudsperson regional officers to implement more effective, accessible, and transparent accountability mechanisms. This accountability approach does not intend to blame and punish governments or health professional teams—therefore, deepening the gap between rights holders and duty bearers—but rather facilitate understanding to resolve the health problems and needs of rural families, seeking to promote constructive citizen's participation in improvement of health service quality, something all actors can agree on as a goal.

Principle 6: Promoting Sustainable Results

Rights-based approaches focus on building capacities and competencies to understand, implement, and oversee development processes. Because of the focus on linking voice and response, rights-based programs concentrate on finding strategies to make this link possible and sustainable between and across different levels in society and on stretching from communities through to central government. They thus encourage local ownership of development and, because of the way that state and citizens are all encouraged to take up rights and responsibilities, dependency on state patronage decreases (although, of course, this does not lesson the obligation of the state). Their focus on the underlying causes of poverty, and the obligations of different actors, helps to establish and institutionalize capacities, systems, and mechanisms that are vital to ensuring that positive change is embedded and sustained. There is some evidence that skills learned and mechanisms established in such approaches are used and replicated beyond the project mandate (UK Interagency Group on Human Rights Based Approaches, 2007).

EVIDENCE OF CARE'S IMPACT

Ultimately, organizations such as CARE adopt approaches not simply to follow the latest development fad, but because they believe that these will lead to more significant and lasting impacts on poverty and social injustice. Our adoption of a rights-based approach was caused by our belief not only that it would change how we work and what we do—as has been illustrated in detail under "Applying a Rights-Based Approach in Practice in Peru"—but also that this would change the scale and quality of our impact.

Our monitoring and evaluation process for such rights-based programs focuses on a combination of process indicators, as well as quantitative and qualitative evidence. Through a performance monitoring and organizational learning system, we systematically analyze the incorporation of the six programmatic principles in the design, implementation, and assessment of all our interventions. Program and project logistical models determine project outputs and short-, medium-, and long-term outcomes, in terms of policy change and institutional capacities, as well as impacts on health outcomes, with indicators for each determined and evaluated throughout the project cycle. Impact assessments include both quantitative and qualitative evidence, using tools like the Most Significant Change method to promote a participatory analysis with our partners and key stakeholders of the real contribution of CARE's initiatives.

Globally, there have been few studies that have sought to show whether rights-based approaches lead to a differential level of impact, compared with interventions that do not adopt such approaches. Studies reviewing cases of rights based, and non–rights-based projects have concluded "rights based projects show a greater range and depth of positive impacts, and these are more likely to be sustained over time" (UK Interagency Group on Human Rights Based Approaches, 2007, p. 9); see also, Rand & Watson, 2008).

In Peru, the strongest evidence to date comes from the CARE/MoH jointly commissioned external final evaluation of the FEMME project (MoH, 2006b; Seclen et al., 2007), which included a section on rights-based and cross-cultural approaches. There was a clear positive difference between the project intervention area and the control region of Puno, both in terms of application of these approaches, as well as in use of and quality of EmOC services (but not on the availability of such services, in terms of human resources, equipment, and medicines, which was similar in both regions). The evaluation also shows a significant positive difference in impact on the registered maternal mortality between the two regions. Although the evaluation was not designed to prove the hypothesis that it was these rights-based interventions that made the difference, rather than solely upgrading EmOC skills of health professionals, it is clear from the qualitative part of the evaluation that they were critical in increasing acceptability of EmOC services and, therefore, their use by the largely indigenous women from the project area (see Figures 15.2 and 15.3).

FIGURE 15.2 Evidence of CARE's Impact: Changes in Obstetric Services

Changes in obstetric services	Intervention Group					Comparison Group				
	HRA	HCA	HSF	CSV	CST	HMNB	HHU	HAZ	HJU	HIL
Vertical delivery	✓		✓	✓	✓					
Maternal waiting home			✓	✓	✓	✓				✓
Mother can eat during labour	✓		✓	✓	✓	✓				✓
Liquids during labour	✓		✓	✓	✓	✓				✓
Give information on labour progress to pregnancy	✓		✓	✓	✓		✓			✓
Call women by their names	✓	✓	✓	✓	✓					
Allow companion during labour	✓	✓	✓	✓	✓	✓				✓
Husband presents during labour and birth	✓	✓	✓	✓	✓	✓				✓
Privacy during labour	✓	✓	✓	✓	✓	✓				✓
Active management of the third stage of labour (AMTSL)	✓	✓	✓	✓	✓	✓	✓			✓

CST, Centro de Salud Tambo-San Miguel (Tambo-San Miguel Health Center, Ayacucho); CSV, Centro de Salud Vilcashuamán (Vilcashuamán Health Center, Ayacucho); HAZ, Hospital de Apoyo Azángaro (Azángaro Support Hospital, Puno); HCA, Hospital de Apoyo Cangallo (Cangallo Support Hospital, Ayacucho); HHU, Hospital de Apoyo Huancané (Huancané Support Hospital, Puno); HIL, Hospital de Apoyo Ilave (Ilave Support Hospital, Puno); HJU, Hospital de Apoyo Juli (Juli Support Hospital, Puno); HMNB, Hospital Manuel Núñez Butrón (Manuel Núñez Butrón Hospital, Puno); HRA, Hospital Regional de Ayacucho (Ayacucho Regional Hospital, Ayacucho); HSF, Hospital San Francisco (San Francisco Hospital, Ayacucho)

FIGURE 15.3 Evidence of CARE's Impact: Changes in the Maternal Mortality Rates[a]

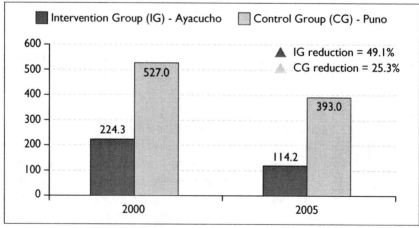

[a]Registered deaths, adjusted for underreporting.

CONCLUSION

CARE's experience in applying a rights-based approach to its work on health shows that such an approach is both feasible and practical to apply. Moving beyond a purely rhetorical level commitment or analysis, it has changed how we work and what we do. A relatively simple set of six principles, based on those outlined in the international human rights instruments, has been used to orient our work promoting the right to health of the poor, in different contexts. In this chapter, we have outlined in detail one particular case of our work in a highly unequal, middle income country such as Peru. But we could also have described work that applies this framework, in different ways to suit different contexts, in the Democratic Republic of Congo (United States Agency for International Development & CARE, 2007), Ethiopia (Rajadurai & Igras, 2005), India (Bailey, Usha Kiran, Babu, & Nalini, 2005), or Rwanda (Ruzindana & CARE International, 2007). Taken together, our global experiences shows that a rights-based approach to health makes a difference, not only in how you approach the work you do but also in what you do, who you do it with, and, with increasing surety, the nature and quality of the impacts achieved.

A core component of successfully applying a rights-based approach in our experience has been to work with both the supply side and the demand side to enable rights holders to be aware of and to claim their rights; to support the development of capacities of duty bearers to meet their obligations; and to be accountable for doing so. We have also learned that successful policy influence usually demands not only effective advocacy strategies to create the necessary political will but also technical assistance for "feeding the skills" of health authorities and providers, especially when engaging with new institutional approaches, such as incorporating right-based approaches within the institutional policies and practices of complex, hierarchical organizations as ministries of health. Therefore, while CARE prioritizes giving a voice to the poor and working with the communities and civil society organizations, it also strives to ensure that policy makers and public leaders have the tools and knowledge to respond.

We have also found a rights-based approach to offer important opportunities for new—and key—partnerships, as we have shown in the case of Peru with our work with more "traditional" human rights organizations, such as Physicians for Human Rights, the public human rights ombudsperson, Amnesty International, with their new global campaign on human dignity, or our collaboration with the United Nations Special Rapporteur on the right to the highest attainable standard of health

(2004–2008). The International Initiative on Maternal Mortality and Human Rights is just such a partnership at global level, bringing together development and human rights NGOs, from north and south. We believe that CARE's approach based around mainstreaming human rights principles can provide an important and useful complement to strategies focusing more on compliance of national and international standards, norms, and instruments.

National and local partnerships are all important, and so CARE needs to continue to identify local actors (i.e., civil society networks, indigenous movements, or women's grassroots organizations) that share our organizational vision and approach. We need to strengthen such organizations' capacities to develop their own agendas and be better positioned to influence public policies that affect them. Those local actors will sustainable keep the pace of all our joint efforts, once the "project cycle" is over.

Promoting *empowerment* amongst the poor and excluded also requires organizations as CARE downplaying its own power. It demands CARE to support the social movement agenda, with no intention on imposing the "aid agency" agenda ("trusting the locals").

Perhaps the largest challenge facing an NGO such as CARE in applying a rights-based approach to health comes from the project-based approach to development work that has been taken historically by NGOs and donors, based on relatively short time-frames (3–5 years) and quantifiable results to be reached in that period (e.g., "improve nutritional status of 3,000 children younger than 5 years"). CARE is now convinced that tackling the underlying causes of poverty or poor health and creating long-term change will require shifting from a project approach to a longer term approach that tackles underlying causes of poverty and promotes the realization of rights. This will involve a coherent set of activities, some specific short-term projects and some complementary initiatives, such as advocacy or research, undertaken by a group of stakeholders that over a period, contributes to lasting improvements in the health status of poor and marginalized people. Longer term programs need to include the six program principles, and be based on solid and holistic analysis of the underlying causes of poor health, focus on long-term impacts as well as immediate outcomes, and have clearly specified measurable goals. This approach requires a long-term commitment—generally 5–10 years—to demonstrate impact and build the networks and coalitions of change needed for sustainable success. Changing this model will involve a shift in the approach of both funders and implementers. In the case of Peru, through flexible and long-term funding, via CARE's partnership program agreement with DFID, which has funded the Peru Health Rights program, and through CARE's own funds and private donor funding to support its ongoing advocacy and technical support work on maternal health, we have been able to build such an approach over the last 5 years.

NGOs can bring a valuable perspective to addressing the immediate and underlying causes of poverty and poor health, drawing on strong ties with the most affected communities and with strong partner organizations, as well as constructive relations with local and national authorities. Sustaining a commitment as partners with those communities and stakeholders building their capacity; empowering women; sharing the projects' decision making with our partners and promoting their genuine participation in national, regional, or local spaces for decision making processes on public policies; opposing discrimination; promoting CARE's accountability to its partners and helping to create a culture of accountability amongst duty bearers; influencing policies and their implementation; and focusing on long-term impacts will help bring about greater health equity for the world's poorest and most vulnerable people. International agreements consistently affirm that all people have the right to health security; CARE's experiences provide many examples of ways to ensure that those rights are honored.

REFERENCES

Amnesty International. (2009). *Peru: Deadly inequalities: Maternal mortality in Peru.* Retrieved July 6, 2009, from http://www.amnesty.org/en/library/info/AMR46/002/2009/en

Arroyo, J. (2009). *The 2007 health co-management law and its regulation: The challenge of the sustainability of the CLAS.* Consultancy report, CARE Peru, Lima.

Arroyo, J. (2007). *ForoSalud: Memoria de una experiencia de construcción de sociedad civil* [ForoSalud: Report of an experience of building civil society]. Retrieved July 6, 2009, from http://www.care.org.pe/pdfs/cinfo/memoria/Memoria%20ForoSalud%20final.pdf

Bailey, L., Usha Kiran, T., Babu, S., & Nalini, N. V. N. (2005). *The IDEAS model for demonstration & replication: An experience from CARE India.* Retrieved July 6, 2009, from http://www.care.org/careswork/whatwedo/health/downloads/20050906_ideasmodel.pdf

Bueno de Mesquita, J., & Hunt, P. (2008). *International assistance and cooperation in sexual and reproductive health: A human rights responsibility for donors.* Retrieved October 2, 2010, from http://www.essex.ac.uk/human_rights_centre/research/rth/docs/Final_PDF_for_website.pdf

CARE International. (2003). *Programme principles.* Retrieved July 6, 2009, from http://www.care-international.org/Programme-Principles/

CARE International UK. (2005). *Principles into practice: Learning from innovative rights-based programmes.* Retrieved July 6, 2009, from http://www.careinternational.org.uk/download.php?id=140

Department for International Development. (2000). *Realising human rights for poor people.* Retrieved July 6, 2009, from http://www.dfid.gov.uk/Documents/publications/tsphuman.pdf

Frisancho, A (2007). The right to health in Peru. In S. Marks (Ed.), *Health and human rights: The right to health in comparative perspective.* François-Xavier Bagnoud Centre for Health and Human Rights. Unpublished manuscript. Harvard School of Public Health at Boston.

Frisancho, A. (2009). *Combating maternal mortality: Why bring human rights into the picture?* NGO Side-Event. 11th Session of the Human Rights Council. Retrieved August 8, 2010, from http://righttomaternalhealth.org/resource/HRC-panel-2009

Frisancho, A., & Goulden, J. (2008). *Rights-based approaches to improve people's health in Peru. The Lancet, 372,*(9655), 2007–2008. Retrieved July 6, 2009, from http://www.thelancet.com/journals/lancet/article/PIIS0140-6736(08)61785-7/fulltext

Gayle, H, & Sinho, S. (2009). CARE: The contribution of an international NGO to global health. In P. A. Gaist (Ed.), *Igniting the power of community: The role of CBOs and NGOs in global public health* (pp. 229–246). New York: Springer.

Hunt, P. (2005). *Report submitted by the Special Rapporteur on the right of everyone to the highest attainable standard of physical and mental health. Mission to Peru.* United Nations Human Rights Commission, Sixty-first Session. Retrieved July 6, 2009, from http://daccessdds.un.org/doc/UNDOC/GEN/G05/106/45/PDF/G0510645.pdf?OpenElement

Jones, A. (2001). *Incorporation of a rights-based approach into CARE's program cycle: A discussion paper for CARE's program staff.* Retrieved October 2, 2009, from http://pqdl.care.org/CuttingEdge/Incorporating%20RBA%20in%20CARE's%20Program%20Cycle.pdf

Ministry of Health. (2006a). *Ayacucho: Response to the health letter.* National crucade for citizens' rights and responsibilities in health. Lima, Peru.

Ministry of Health. (2006b). *Impact of the FEMME project in reducing maternal mortality and its significance for health policy in Peru.* Ministry of Health. Office of International Cooperation; CARE Peru. Lima, Peru. Retrieved July 6, 2009, from http://www.care.org.pe/pdfs/cinfo/libro/Evaluationofimpact_FEMME_2006_english.pdf

Ministry of Health. (2009) *Implementation Model to improve the Availability, Quality and Use of establishments providing Obstetric and Neonatal Functions.* Ministerial Resolution number 223-2009/MINSA.

Potts, H. (2008a). *Accountability and the right to the highest attainable standard of health.* Retrieved July 6, 2009, from http://www2.essex.ac.uk/human_rights_centre/rth/docs/HRC_Accountability_Mar08.pdf

Potts, H. (2008b). *Participation and the right to the highest attainable standard of health.* Retrieved August 8, 2010, from http://www.womensnet.org.za/node/1505

Rajadurai, H., & Igras, S. (2005). *At the intersection of health, social well-being and human rights: CARE's experiences working with communities toward abandonment of female genital cutting (FGC).* Retrieved July 6, 2009, from http://www.care.org/careswork/whatwedo/health/downloads/FGC_abandonment.pdf

Rand, J., & Watson, G. (2008). *Rights-based approaches: Learning project.* Oxfam America and CARE USA. Retrieved July 6, 2009, from http://www.hrea.org/index.php?base_id=104&language_id=1&erc_doc_id=5043&category_id=44&category_type=3

Ruzindana, R., & CARE International. (2007). *SNS final evaluation report.* Retrieved July 6, 2009, from http://expert.care.at/uploads/media/RWA084_Final_Evaluation_Report.pdf

Sandino, M. E. (2006). *Most significative change exercise with ForoSalud representatives.* Unpublished paper, CARE Peru.

Seclen, J., Esquiche, E., Bailey, P., Goulden, J., Kayongo, M., & Vega, M. (2007). Evaluation of the FEMME project: Outcomes and impact. In *Immpact Symposium: Delivering safe motherhood – sharing the evidence.* London. Retrieved July 6, 2009, from http://www.immpact-international.org/uploads/files/Session18_AMDD_Juan_Seclen.pdf

Silva, M. L. (2003). *The human rights based approach to development cooperation: Towards a common understanding among UN agencies.* Retrieved August 9, 2010, from http://www.hreoc.gov.au/social_justice/conference/engaging_communities/un_common_understanding_rba.pdf

UK Interagency Group on Human Rights Based Approaches. (2007). *The impact of rights-based approaches to development: Evaluation/learning process Bangladesh, Malawi and Peru.* Retrieved July 6, 2009, from http://www.crin.org/docs/Inter_Agency_rba.pdf

United States Agency for International Development, & CARE. (2007). *Voices from the Village: Improving lives through CARE's sexual and reproductive health programs: Meeting needs for reproductive health services in post-conflict environments: CARE's family planning project in the Democratic Republic of Congo.* Retrieved July 6, 2009, from http://www.care.org/careswork/whatwedo/health/downloads/vftv_drc.pdf

Watanabe Varas, T. (2002). *Tendencias, niveles y estructura de la mortalidad materna en el Perú, 1992–2000* [Trends, levels and structure of maternal mortality in Peru, 1992–2000]. Instituto Nacional de Estadística e Informática. Retrieved July 6, 2009, from http://www1.inei.gob.pe/web/InvestigacionDescarga.asp?file=4577.pdf

Yamin, A. (2007). *Deadly delays: Maternal mortality in Peru: A rights-based approach to safe motherhood.* Physicians for Human Rights. USA. Retrieved July 6, 2009, from http://physiciansforhumanrights.org/library/report-2007-11-28.html

Vandemoortele, J. (2009). *Taking the MDGs beyond 2015: Hasten slowly.* Retrieved July 6, 2009, from http://www.eadi.org/fileadmin/MDG_2015_Publications/Vandemoortele_PAPER.pdf

Liberation Medicine and Accompaniment in El Salvador: The Experience of Doctors for Global Health

Jennifer Kasper and Clyde Lanford (Lanny) Smith

INTRODUCTION

Doctors for Global Health (DGH) is a nongovernmental and an all-volunteer organization that affirms that every human being, regardless of geographic location, physical or mental disability, culture, age, or other attribute, has the right to a life of dignity, optimal health, and well-being. We consciously and conscientiously use health to promote human dignity and social justice with marginalized and vulnerable populations by *accompanying* communities while educating and inspiring others to action. *Accompaniment* refers to our practice: We respond to invitations, work side by side with our fellow human beings, and share risk and responsibility to create conditions that demand and facilitate social justice.

As Dr. Jack Geiger said in his keynote speech at the 2002 DGH General Assembly:

> What we are really saying to the people we work with is that their lives are as worthy as our own; that their lives are as worthy of life as everyone else's; that all life is equally valuable. And what we, by our presence and our work, demonstrate is a commitment to the idea of equity, not as an abstraction, but as something that has to do immediately and directly with the lives of the people we work with (Doctors for Global Health, 2002).

We amplify and empower the voices of marginalized communities as they advocate for their rights. We build long-term relationships and create learning partnerships that build local capacity so that those most affected are active protagonists in naming and prioritizing their needs and implementing effective solutions. We emphasize empathy, humility, and collaborative learning among our volunteers so that they work *with* our partner communities, rather than do things *to* or *for* them. In addition, we advocate in word and deed for nothing short of a transformation in existing social and economic power structures to create a more equitable world where all people can live healthier and dignified lives. A summary of our "principles of action" is provided in Table 16.1.

DGH practices *liberation medicine*: the "conscious and conscientious use of health to promote human dignity and social justice" (Smith, 2007, p. 132). Inspiration for this concept came from Ignacio Martin-Baro's *Writings for a Liberation Psychology* in the context of community and international solidarity in Morazán, El Salvador and the works of prominent liberation theologians, including Gustavo Gutierrez, assassinated Archbishop of El Salvador Oscar Arnulfo Romero, and Father Jon Sobrino. Their belief that heaven should be created on earth involved indefatigable human rights promotion and a preferential focus for the poor and oppressed. Rather than accept the economic status quo of rich elites and oppressed poor as something condoned by God, they spoke out about the abuses of the wealthy toward the poor and educated and radicalized the poor to not accept their lot in life, but rather fight for their rights, dignity, and equity.

The distinction between *liberation* and *development* is important to the work of DGH. Development has acquired a negative connotation in recent years because it usually implies a connection to groups that are closely tied to organizations and governments that control the world economy. Historically, therefore, many development initiatives have ensured that the interests of those organizations and governments in power are safeguarded, usually at the expense of true sustainable development initiatives that seek to benefit the poor by significantly raising their quality of life. As a result, poorer communities are realizing that the only way true "development" can come about is to break their ties with the dominant organizations and governments, and, thus, liberate themselves to be engines of their own change.

DGH employs liberation medicine so that the poor decide what they need and are empowered to explore different ways of achieving their goals. Once the poor are empowered, true development and liberation for health and healing can occur.

TABLE 16.1 Doctors for Global Health Principles of Action

DGH affirms that every human being regardless of race, gender, class, religion, sexual orientation, physical or mental disability, culture, age, or other attribute, has the right to a life of dignity, equal treatment, and social justice.

A. DGH works with those who are among the most poor, the most vulnerable, and the stigmatized of the world's population, amplifying their voices that they be heard.

B. DGH's approach is to accompany communities with small, community-oriented health initiatives that also promote human rights, encourage sustainability, and respect environmental concerns.

C. DGH sets an example for how medicine should be practiced by promoting Liberation Medicine: "The conscious, conscientious use of health to promote human dignity and social justice."

D. DGH promotes health equity as more basic and fundamental than private, corporate interests. Its mandate is to strive for the optimal health and well-being of all members of the human race regardless of ethnicity, sex, sexual preference, or religion.

E. DGH is committed to advocacy and working for social justice both locally and globally. It encourages its members to take action in their own communities and participate in the accompaniment of communities around the world.

F. DGH pledges to be active in the struggle to expose and confront the pervasive and destructive nature of racism and classism (personal and institutionalized, conscious or unconscious) and all other forms of discrimination, both within DGH and in the world at large.

G. DGH is a volunteer organization that invites and encourages those with a desire to help humanity by providing them with a vehicle to use their unique talents and skills in support of the DGH mission. Special efforts are made to reach out to youth, students of all ages, and people with the wisdom of experience.

H. DGH respects and invites those of all backgrounds and beliefs who agree with its mission and principles to join; proselytizing is contrary to the mission and principles.

I. DGH integrates artistic expression that promotes healing and celebrates all life into its activities. These expressions include literature, music, drama, painting, drawing, sculpture, and other art forms.

J. DGH is vigilant to ensure that its projects, programs, affiliations, and fund-raising efforts don't involve even subtle compromise of its values.

K. DGH participates only in investigations, publications, and/or research initiatives that are important to the work of DGH, ethically sound, benefit the involved communities, and are compatible with DGH's mission. Both the involved local communities and the board must approve these efforts.

HUMAN RIGHTS DOCUMENTS AND PRINCIPLES

The approach of DGH is deeply grounded in human rights principles, which were discussed in detail in Part I of this volume. We believe that every human being has the right to achieve an optimal state of health (Preamble to the World Health Organization [WHO] Constitution). We also know that the poor carry a disproportionate burden of disease. They consume the least in terms of material goods, and are consumed the most by the plagues of persistent poverty and illness. The poor are least likely to have their human rights respected and most likely to have their human rights violated (Farmer, 1999).

The WHO defines health as a "state of complete physical, mental, and social well-being and not merely the absence of disease or infirmity" (WHO, 1948, Pmbl.). According to this definition, a purely biomedical model of disease (one person, one illness, and one cure) is too narrow and does not capture the complexity of human health and the multitude of factors at play. The work of DGH incorporates the social and societal determinants that mitigate or exacerbate the risk of being ill and the risk of having the worst outcomes as a result of illness. Thus, food, clothing, shelter, safe water and sanitation, and family and community are equally important issues to consider when treating a person's illness and when attempting to prevent, reduce, or eliminate some illnesses (Universal Declaration of Human Rights [UDHR], 1948, art. 25).

Societal determinants of health encompass stable political, judicial and ecosystems, sustainable resources, and the equitable distribution of goods and services. With regard to access, the right to health (UN Committee on Economic, Social and Cultural Rights [CESCR], 2000, General Comment 14) encompasses the availability and accessibility of quality health facilities. There are significant disparities in access to health care. As the People's Health Movement Right to Health Campaign asserts, "those who are economically marginalized are also marginalized from accessing comprehensive health care."

DGH places special emphasis on the vulnerable and marginalized (e.g., children, women, elderly persons, the disabled, and indigenous persons). We strive to make operational the interdependence of human rights; to put economic, social, and cultural rights on equal footing with civil and political rights, with a strong focus on these social determinants of health.

People can and should be active protagonists for their health; they have a right and duty to participate individually and collectively in the planning and implementation of their health care (Declaration of Alma-Ata) and other activities that impact their health. The principles of nondiscrimination and participation by all so that all voices are heard – embodied, and codified in the articles of the UDHR, the International Covenant on Civil and Political Rights (ICCPR), International Covenant on Economic, Social and Cultural Rights (ICESCR), and the United Nations Convention on the Rights of the Child (UNCRC), are at the crux of our work.

PRINCIPLES OF COMMUNITY-ORIENTED PRIMARY CARE

DGH's work is informed by the principles of Community-Oriented Primary Care (COPC): a "continuous process by which primary health care is provided to a defined population on the basis of its defined health needs by the planned integration of public health with primary care practice" (Mullen & Epstein, 2002, p. 1750). DGH incorporates the five cardinal questions of community-oriented primary care into its discussions with communities (Epstein, Gofin, Gofin, & Neumark, 2002):

1. What is the community's state of health?
2. What are the factors responsible for this state of health?
3. What is being done about it?
4. What more can be done and what is the expected outcome?
5. What measures are needed to continue health surveillance of the community and to evaluate the effects of existing programs?

DGH applies the iterative COPC process (Epstein et al., 2002) into its work. This process follows seven steps:

1. Community diagnosis
2. Prioritization
3. Detailed problem assessment
4. Intervention planning
5. Implementation
6. Evaluation
7. Reassessment

COPC's focus on maximum community involvement and harnessing of collective energy is akin to DGH's focus on amplifying voices that are not normally heard so that decisions are taken and owned by the community. DGH also emphasizes that for COPC to be optimal, the community decides who to invite rather than outside groups (DGH included) inviting themselves. COPC's point that clinical practice is built on and responds to the communities' ongoing and new needs is in line with the responsive action mandate of liberation medicine.

ESTANCIA, EL SALVADOR

DGH works in partnership with communities in El Salvador, Guatemala, Mexico, Peru, Uganda, Burundi, and Sierra Leone. Estancia, El Salvador holds special significance because people who became founding members of DGH were invited in 1992 by the communities of Estancia to accompany them in addressing health as a human right and working to ameliorate and transform the fundamental causes of ill health plaguing their communities.

El Salvador has experienced human rights extremes: struggles for universal promotion of human rights by indigenous people, unions, teachers, students, intellectuals, Christian communities, and liberation theologians juxtaposed with flagrant human rights abuses by the Salvadoran government and military. This culminated in a brutal, repressive 12-year war from 1980–1992. "Drain the sea and catch the fish," "scorched earth policy," "free fire zones," "hammer and anvil operations" were code words for violations by Salvadoran government forces trained at the then U.S. Army School of the Americas (SOA, now known as the Western Hemisphere Institute for Security and Cooperation [WHINSEC]) in Columbus, Georgia. They murdered 75,000 people, disappeared innumerable others, and forced at least 1 million to flee as refugees. This had a devastating effect on the country's 6 million inhabitants (United Nations Security Council, 1993).

The indigenous communities of Estancia in the rural, mountainous province of Morazán in northeastern El Salvador were steeped in this struggle. It was one of the areas of the country most heavily devastated by the war; the inhabitants were tortured, killed, or lived as refugees in Honduras. The Salvadoran government's massive bombardment and use of napalm here caused severe deforestation and had a detrimental effect on humans.

Prior to the armed conflict, El Salvador had a mostly centralized health system, which made access to even the most rudimentary care difficult for isolated communities like the ones in Estancia. During the conflict, the health budget was cut in half and health posts located in areas believed to contain guerilla sympathizers were abandoned. Unmet health needs grew in Estancia.

Today, El Salvador, with a population of approximately 7.5 million, is the most densely populated country in Latin America. It has one of the highest income disparities in the world; the wealthiest 20% have 58% of the country's total income; the poorest 20% have 2.4%. Its economy, originally based in large part on a coffee oligarchy, has been replaced by a banking oligarchy; the top five banks have combined wealth 5 times greater than the government budget. Approximately one third of the populace works in the formal sector, earning an average salary of $154 per month. Half of the country lives on less than $2 per day. Approximately 2.5 million live and work in the United States and send $ 2 billion in remittances to their families in El Salvador. This accounts for 17% of gross domestic product (GDP), a significant portion of the Salvadoran economy. Many families throughout the country depend on this money for their economic survival. Currently, the number one export is people, and the number one import is remittances. The economic gains on a national scale overshadow the negative impact that migration may have on these transnational families; 40% of children grow up without one or both parents.

Human rights principles stress the importance of disaggregating data to understand the reality of vulnerable groups and communities and direct special attention and care to them. An analysis of El Salvador demonstrates this. Although country-level health and economic indicators give the impression that the populace lives a relatively secure, economically stable life, a closer examination of the communities of Estancia in Morazán reveals many stark disparities. One third of Morazán's population lives in extreme poverty (<$1/day). Small-scale agriculture, hammock and bag making, and remittances from abroad are the major sources of income. Migration to the United States has become the only option for impoverished families in Estancia, reflected in the increase in households headed by single women. Housing consists of one-room bamboo or adobe huts. Electricity, indoor plumbing, and running water are unavailable. Poor sanitation and lack of access to potable water continue to plague the area. Water for all uses is obtained from local rivers, with marked seasonal variations in quantity and quality; as a consequence, 60% of the population suffers from intestinal parasites. Most food comes from small plots of beans and corn. In the last 5 years, the cost of food in rural areas has increased by more than 30%. One third of the population does not have sufficient income to cover the cost of the basic food basket, and the rate of food insecurity is among the highest in the country. Morazán has the worst rate of adult illiteracy in the country (38%) and the lowest number of years of formal schooling (3.5 years).

The communities of Estancia remain relatively isolated to this day. Access to government-run public clinics is limited at best: The nearest Ministry of Health (MOH) clinic is one hour by 4×4 vehicle over a partially paved road; the nearest hospital is 1.5 hours away; and the only children's hospital is in the capital, San Salvador, an 8-hour drive. There is a public health system, but patients are seen on a first-come-first-served basis; wait times are long; and access to subspecialty care is inaccessible for the poor.

The private health care system is being touted as the solution, but its prices make it prohibitive to the majority of Salvadorans. El Salvador also has the highest priced medications in Latin America. The unhealthy environment and inadequate, largely inaccessible, and discriminatory health care system contribute to persistent ill health. Maternal mortality rate is 170/100,000 births; infant mortality rate is 22/1,000 (3 times the U.S. rate); and under-5 mortality rate is 24/1,000 (6 times the U.S. rate). Infants and children continue to die of neonatal causes (e.g., prematurity, low birth weight, infections, birth trauma, asphyxia), pneumonia, and diarrhea in large numbers. The fact that, nationally, 25% of households cannot afford the price of a basic food basket is writ large on the bodies of children: 10% of children younger than 5 years are underweight, and 19% are stunted; in Morazán, 45% of first graders are stunted (the fifth worst in the nation).

The *Alianza Republicana Nacionalista* (ARENA) political party dominated Salvadoran politics before, during, and after the civil conflict. Its focus on neoliberal policies, support of Central American Free Trade Agreement (CAFTA), and privatization of social services has had negative effects on the poor. Many subsistence farmers gave up their livelihoods and migrated to San Salvador to work in *maquilas* (sweatshops) or cities in the United States. Foreign businesses (Pizza Hut, Burger King, Blockbuster, Armani, Subway, Domino's Pizza, Payless ShoeSource, Texaco, and Shell stations) are visible on the streets. The country has no import/export taxes or property tax; it relies on 13% sales tax, which again disproportionately affects the poor. The government once put forth a program called *Plan Contra la Pobreza* (Plan Against Poverty, later renamed *Plan Oportunidades*). It proposed to give 20,000 families $15–20 per month annually (that works out to 10¢ per person per day for a family of five) to invest $100–300 for microenterprises and to invest $200 million to restart 100 MOH clinics. But money was never allocated for any of this.

In 2010, a seachange in Salvadoran politics took place: Mauricio Funes, of the Farabundo Martí National Liberation Front (FMLN), was elected president. His government has an ambitious plan for social, economic, and institutional reconstruction that includes increasing government transparency: creating 100,000 jobs; improving basic infrastructure, building 25,000 houses, providing educational grants and food programs for preschool and school-age children, nationalizing a curriculum for community health workers (CHWs) and incorporating them into the existing health care system, expanding health care to rural areas, and giving seeds to farmers. This is a tall order because the country has 1 billion USD in debt.

DOCTORS FOR GLOBAL HEALTH AND ITS RIGHTS-BASED APPROACHES IN ESTANCIA

On the heels of the conflict in 1992, the people of Estancia invited people who would later become the founders of DGH to create a health and human rights program entitled, "Building Health Where the Peace is New." These communities had suffered egregious violations of their civil and political rights; they asked these volunteers to help them focus on their economic, cultural, and social rights.

The rights-based approach practiced by the founders of DGH focused on the right to participation and the importance of primary care as a means of addressing the right to health. It involved participation by multiple actors—MOH, the Pan American Health Organization (PAHO), University of El Salvador, University of Central America, World Food Programme (WFP), health promoters, and community leaders—and use of community-oriented primary care principles. A cluster committee called the Committee for Health in Southeast Morazán (its acronym, CISOMOZ, means "yes we are," in Spanish) was formed and consisted of the MOH, local mayors of three municipalities, and local health workers of the three regions who made decisions and set local priorities. These pre-DGH volunteers also encouraged participatory investigation: each community, under the guidance of its elected and trained health promoter, explored its assets and problems and designed and implemented projects with the volunteers' assistance.

Health was our tool for reconciliation. Once the Peace Accords had been signed on 16 January 1992, most international nongovernmental organizations (NGOs) redirected their energies to other countries. However, these future founders of DGH felt that this was the most important time to be in El Salvador because physical and mental injuries were fresh, divisiveness was rampant, and the work of rebuilding was just getting started. And once DGH was formally incorporated as a 501c3 in the U.S. in 1995, it was in a unique position because it was one of very few international NGOs that chose to stay and work in this region of El Salvador. With the goal of improved health for all, people worked in a spirit of mutual respect. DGH recruited volunteers and raised funds in the United States and kept the eyes of the world on El Salvador during this vulnerable time.

ACTIVITIES REALIZED BY DOCTORS FOR GLOBAL HEALTH IN ITS ACCOMPANIMENT WORK

The people who would later become the founders of DGH initiated a CHW program in 1992, which continues to this day. Young and old, experienced and inexperienced were invited to participate and learn together as community regardless of gender, prior work, or political affiliation. The promoters were chosen by their communities and were required to pass an entrance test. Teachers for the health promoter training included people from the Salvadoran Red Cross, MOH, University of El Salvador, University of Central America, FUNDA SIDA (AIDS Foundation), and other groups. Themes included basic first aid; prevention, diagnosis, and treatment of common illnesses; human rights; and world geography, history, politics, and culture. An important aspect of the training was requiring all health promoters to complete their formal high school education program (many schools were closed during the armed conflict). The CHWs became well versed in how to use selected essential medications.

One of the first projects DGH embarked on with the communities was construction of a two-lane vehicular bridge across the *Rió Chiquito*. For years, the communities had asked the Salvadoran government to build one, but their request fell on deaf ears. In the meantime, more than 20 persons drowned while trying to cross it, including a Salvadoran pharmacy student who was volunteering with DGH at the time. With grants and elementary school cookie sales, coordination with the WFP and PAHO, a volunteer engineer from Spain, and participation and sweat equity from young and old community members, the Jaime Solorzano Bridge was completed in 1996.

In 1997, DGH helped construct and open *El Centro de Atención Integral para la Prevención y Educación en Salud* (CAIPES; The Center for Integrated Care for Prevention and Education in Health). This clinic is a lifeline to the communities. It is operated by locally trained community health promoters, accompanied by DGH physician or medical student volunteers, and supervised by the MOH physician for the municipality. The clinic, which initially had sporadic phone connection and no internet, now has internet, but it is slow and unreliable; the closest bus stop is 1-hour walk uphill, and the only emergency transportation is one pickup truck.

Its staff cares for children with malnutrition, respiratory and diarrheal diseases, skin infections, congenital malformations, and physical disabilities, whereas for adults with acute conditions such as respiratory diseases, gastritis, musculoskeletal problems, lacerations, dental abscesses, and chronic diseases such as diabetes, high blood pressure, glaucoma, and cataracts. The clinic serves an average of 300 patients per month, 20% of whom require further diagnostic and subspecialty follow-up.

Access to specialty care and diagnostic tests is extremely limited in this region. In January 2007, a survey of CAIPES patients revealed the major barriers to accessing emergency or specialty care were lack of financial resources and transportation; inability to take time off from work; fear of getting lost; and previous discriminatory treatment by governmental health system staff. The Access to Specialty Care project grew out of a demand for various services beyond primary care: emergency care for generally healthy patients (e.g., transportation to the nearest hospital for emergency appendectomy), specialty care for adults with chronic health problems (e.g., hypertension), and multidisciplinary pediatric care for children with disabilities. Leaders of *Asociación de Campesinos para el Desarrollo Humano* (Peasant Association for Human Development, CDH, described on the next page), community health promoters, and DGH volunteers created an electronic medical record (EMR) database to better organize and track socioeconomic and health data, identify patient needs and barriers to care, and overcome these to improve the quality of their healthcare. The DGH/CDH collaboration employs a triad of systematic advocacy (a CHW accompanies patients to their appointments), patient counseling and care coordination (e.g., phone calls to specialists and implementation of a custom-designed EMR), and modest financial assistance (for mostly medications and transportation). An initial evaluation revealed a modest impact: during the past year, 615 adult and pediatric referrals were made for emergency care, specialist consultation (gynecology, internal medicine, surgery and orthopedics for adults, speech, physical therapy, neurology, cardiology, ear/nose/throat, and orthopedics for children), and diagnostic testing. The reputation of the CAIPES clinic has spread; patients from far-flung communities seek care here and as a result, clinic volume has tripled. The project's goals fit within the framework of health as a human right and within the principles outlined in the Declaration of Alma-Ata in 1978: primary health care should be accessible to all people and "should be sustained by integrated, functional and mutually supportive referral systems, leading to the progressive improvement of comprehensive health care for all" (p. 2).

Another important accomplishment came at the request of Estancia's parents. During the civil conflict many people fled to Honduras as refugees. At the border, NGOs arranged pre-schools and regular schooling opportunities. When the people of Estancia returned home, they wanted to create something similar for their children. Hence, six *Centros de Integración Desarrollo Infantil* (CIDIs; Centers for Integrated Child Development) were created to serve children aged 2–7 years. In addition to teaching basic reading, writing, and math skills, the CIDIs were and are a place for children to play and socialize and learn a few words of the indigenous Lenkan language. The children receive the equivalent of school brunch prepared by their parents. In addition, community members, rather than leaving their families and communities to seek employment an hour-plus away (and risk exploitation) were trained to be teachers. A new program has sprung up out of the CIDIs: *Abriendo la Imaginación en Casa* (Opening the Imagination at Home, a global version of the U.S.-based Reach Out and Read Program). Here are two testimonials from participating mothers:

> Quiero agradecerle por este programa de libros. El leer juntos es un hábito que les da a los niños y a los padres. Les ayuda despertar el pensamiento. Los libros que recibimos y las memorias que creamos leyéndolos son regalos que tenemos para toda la vida.
>
> —María Santos Pérez

> [I want to thank you for this book program. Reading together is a habit that is given to children and their parents. It helps awaken the mind. The books we receive and the memories created reading them are gifts we have forever (for the rest of our lives).
>
> —María Santos Pérez]

> The books we receive through this program are so beautiful – they will stay with the kids. I, as an adult, really enjoy looking at the pictures in the books. The children get excited about them as well. They ask me, "When will it be time for us to get our next book?" Sometimes I sit with them to read and sometimes they read alone. When I have to make food, sometimes the three of them will gather around me as I make tortillas so we can read together.
>
> —Martina Pérez

Another vital project was Women's Health and Rights. It provided cervical cancer and STD screening, breast exams, and family planning and it facilitated women's groups and men's groups.

One of DGH's proudest moments of accompaniment was supporting Estancia's community members in the formation of *Asociación de Campesinos para el Desarrollo Humano* (CDH; Peasant Association for Human Development), a grassroots NGO officially founded in 2004. CDH has 42 members representing eight communities. It runs all of the health, education, nutrition, and environmental projects and programs, has a 15-member staff, operates a sizeable budget, and interfaces with the MOH at the local and national level.

Five years ago, CDH received a start-up grant from a Spanish NGO to initiate a microcredit project. The majority of the money goes to rural farmers who are unable to secure loans from local banks because of exorbitantly high interest rates. With a loan from CDH they can buy needed supplies for the yearly planting. It has been hugely successful and the extra monies are directed at CDH's health programs.

To address high rates of malnutrition, a community-based rehabilitation program was undertaken. The nutritional supplement (called *Siete Semillas*, Seven Grains) is community inspired and made from locally produced seeds and grains. The project involves intensive accompaniment and home visits by a CHW, and community participation is key to project success. Currently more than 100 children from nine communities participate and are gaining weight and height.

To address the right to education of adolescents, a high school scholarship program is in place. Recipients perform community service in return and have an opportunity to learn more about and become involved in CDH.

Environmental threats persist to this day: The World Bank has proposed constructing a dam on the river that runs through Estancia; if built, it would potentially flood the land (and CAIPES and the CIDIs). Community members are engaged and advocating for a halt to this. In all of these diverse activities, DGH consciously and conscientiously responds to the various social and societal factors that affected the health and well-being of the people of Estancia.

CONCLUSION

Estancia is exemplary of the way DGH takes a long view and puts the concept of liberation medicine to work in the field. In various ways, with small and large investments in human, material, and financial resources, DGH is committed to continuing this partnership and others in a responsive, flexible manner. Jonathan Mann, one of the foundational thinkers in human rights, spoke eloquently of the need for human dignity as a prerequisite for the realization of human rights and that loss of or damage to human dignity has negative health consequences (Mann et al, 1994). Poverty is an affront to human dignity. In all of its activities, in collaboration with affected communities, DGH strives to eliminate or mitigate poverty's ill effects and elevate every person's dignity.

DGH facilitates discussions to help ensure that all community voices are represented. This requires time, patience, and active listening. We debate, reflect, brainstorm, and redirect our energies to make our work complementary and responsive to the named priorities of the communities we accompany. We would like to create a measure for accompaniment that illustrates the value of human relationships in health. Rather than promoting a right to development we are challenged to promote a more expansive right to liberation. Regarding implementation costs, we offer two distinct perspectives: Our accompaniment work is cost-effective in that all DGH members are volunteers, no one receives salary, and all monies raised are directed at our projects; our ongoing partnerships are priceless.

The newly elected (2010) Salvadoran government and MOH have written several documents describing their goals and objectives for the coming years. Their plan includes creating a national curriculum for CHW and incorporating them into the national health care system, expanding comprehensive primary and subspecialty care to rural areas, and involving civil society in health decisions and directions. CDH has a unique opportunity to inform policymakers of its successes and challenges, to have more meaningful collaboration with MOH and other government structures to highlight and strengthen the existing model in Estancia and potentially replicate it in other rural areas of El Salvador. As these new developments unfold, DGH will define its role in establishing conditions for sustained, meaningful dialogue between rights holders (i.e., the people of Estancia) and other duty bearers (e.g., local, municipal, national leaders, health professionals, MOH) to advocate for a stronger, more comprehensive, equitable, and accessible health care system in El Salvador.

> Go with the people. Live with them. Learn from them. Love them. Start
> with what they know. Build with what they have. But of the best leaders,
> when the job is done, the task accomplished, the people will all say, we
> have done this ourselves. (Lao Tse, 700 BC)

REFERENCES

Declaration of Alma-Ata. (1978, September 6–12). Paper presented at the International Conference on Primary Health Care, Alma-Ata, USSR. Retrieved August 12, 2010, from http://www.who.int/hpr/NPH/docs/declaration_almaata.pdf

Doctors for Global Health. (2002). What we do and why we do it. Retrieved September 2, 2010, from http://www.dghonline.org/content/what-we-do-and-why-we-do-it

Epstein, L., Gofin, J., Gofin, R., & Neumark, Y. (2002). The Jerusalem experience: Three decades of service, research, and training in community-oriented primary care. *American Journal of Public Health, 92,* 1717–1721.

Farmer, P. (1999). Pathologies of power. *American Journal of Public Health, 89,* 1486–1496.

Geiger, H. J. (2002). Community-oriented primary care: A path to community development. *American Journal of Public Health, 92,* 1713–1716.

Gutierrez, G. (1988). *A theology of liberation: History, politics, and salvation.* New York: Orbis Books.

Hunt, P. (2004). Special rapporteur of the Commission on Human Rights. The right of everyone to the enjoyment of the highest attainable standard of physical and mental health. Submitted to UN General Assembly 59th Session, Agenda item 105(b), in accordance with Commission resolution 2004/27. A59/422

Ignacio Martin-Baro. (1995). *Toward a liberation psychology.* Cambridge: Harvard U. Press.

Mann, J. M., Gostin, L., Gruskin, S., Brennan, T., Lazzarini, Z., & Finberg, H. V. (1994). Health and human rights. *Health Human Rights, 1*(1), 1–13.

Mullen F., & Epstein L. (2002). Community-oriented primary care: new relevance in a changing world. *American Journal of Public Health, 92*(11), 1748-1755.

People's Health Movement. (2005). Proposal for a "Right to Health and Health Care Campaign" to be launched by the People's Health Movement. Retrieved August 12, 2010, from http://www.asnahome.org/peopleshealth/docs/righttohealth/global_phm_righttohealth_campaign_proposal.pdf

Smith, C. L. (2007). Building health where the peace is new in Near-Postwar El Salvador. *Development, 50*(2), 127–133.

UN Committee on Economic, Social and Cultural Rights. (2000). The right to the highest attainable standard of health. General Comment 14. E/C.12/2000/4. Retrieved September 3, 2010, from http://www.unhchr.ch/tbs/doc.nsf/%28Symbol%29/40d009901358b0e2c1256915005090be?Opendocument

United Nations Security Council. (1993). Annex, from madness to hope: The 12-year war in El Salvador: Report of the Commission on the Truth for El Salvador, S/25500, 1993, 5–8. Retrieved September 3, 2010, from http://www.usip.org/files/file/ElSalvador-Report.pdf

Universal Declaration of Human Rights. (1948). G.A. Res. 71, U.N. GAOR, 3d Sess., U.N. Doc A/810 (1948).

World Health Organization. (1948, April). Preamble to the Constitution of the World Health Organization (Official Records of the World Health Organization, no. 2, p. 100). Adopted by the International Health Conference, New York.

OTHER RESOURCES

Danner, M. (1993, December 6). The massacre at El Mozote: A parable of the Cold War. *The New Yorker.*

Declaration on the Right and Responsibility of Individuals, Groups and Organs of Society to Promote and Protect Universally Recognized Human Rights and Fundamental Freedoms. (1998). Adopted by General Assembly resolution 53/144 of 9 December 1998. Retrieved August 12, 2010, from http://www.unhchr.ch/huridocda/huridoca.nsf/%28symbol%29/a.res.53.144.en

Declaration on the Right of Peoples to Peace. (1984). Approved by General Assembly resolution 39/11 of 12 November 1984. Retrieved August 12, 2010, from http://www.wagingpeace.org/articles/0000/1984_declaration-people-peace.htm

Excerpts on peace, justice, poverty from final document. (1968, September). Paper presented at the Conference of Latin American Bishops, Medellin, Colombia. Retrieved September 3, 2010, from http://personal2.stthomas.edu/gwschlabach/docs/medellin.htm

El Salvador's decade of terror. (1991). Americas Watch, Human Rights Watch Books. Yale, University Press.

Facultad Latinoamericana de Ciencias Sociales. (2005). *Mapa de pobreza: Indica-dores para el manejo social del riesgo a nivel municipal.* El Salvador: Author.

Hayden, T. (2009, June 29). El Salvador Rising. *The Nation.* Retrieved August 12, 2010, from http://www.thenation.com/article/el-salvador-rising?page=0,2& comment_sort=ASC

Horton, R. (2004). Rediscovering human dignity. *Lancet, 364,*1081–1085.

Lenhart, A. (n.d.). Brief reflections on liberation medicine's roots in liberation theology. Retrieved August 12, 2010, from http://www.dghonline.org/content/ brief-reflections-liberation-medicines-roots-liberation-theology

Mullen, F., Focht, C., Gofin, J., Gofin, R., Neumark, Y., & Epstein, L. (1994). *Community-oriented primary care: An implementation guide.*

Myers, R. (1995). *The twelve who survive: Strengthening programmes of early childhood development in the Third World* (2nd ed.). Ypsilanti, MI: High/Scope Press.

North American Congress on Latin America Web site. www.nacla.org

People's Health Movement, Medact, Global Equity Gauge Alliance. (2005). *Global health watch 2005–2006: An alternative report.* Retrieved January 3, 2006, from www.ghwatch.org

Raine, F. (2006). Measuring human rights. *SUR—International Journal on Human Rights, 4*(3), 7–29.

United Nations Convention on the Rights of the Child. (1989). G.A. Res. 44/25, U.N. GAOR, 44th Sess., U.N.Doc A/44/736.

United Nations General Assembly, Declaration on the Right to Development. (1986). Adopted by resolution 41/128 of 4 December 1986.

United Nations International Covenant on Civil and Political Rights. Retrieved September 3, 2010, from http://www.hrweb.org/legal/cpr.html

United Nations Development Programme. (2008). *The human development index—Going beyond income.* Statistical Update for El Salvador. Retrieved September 3, 2010, from http://hdrstats.undp.org/en/countries/country_fact_sheets/ cty_fs_SLV.html

United Nations International Children's Emergency Fund. (2008). *State of the world's children.* Retrieved http://www.unicef.org/sowc/

United Nations International Children's Emergency Fund. <n.d.>. *At a glance: El Salvador.* http://www.unicef.org/infobycountry/elsalvador_statistics.html

United States Agency for International Development. (2009, December). USAID Country Health Statistical Report. Retrieved April 30, 2010, from www.usaid.gov

World Health Organization. (1986). *Constitution,* in *Basic Documents,* 36th ed. (Geneva, 1986). on, in *Basic Documents,* 36th ed. Geneva, Switzerland: Author.

World Health Organization. (1986). *Ottawa charter for health promotion: First international conference on health promotion: Report.* Ottawa, Canada: Author.

World Health Organization/Pan American Health Organization. (2000). *El Salvador statistics.* Retrieved September 3, 2010, from http://www.paho.org/English/ DD/AIS/cp_222.htm

World Food Programme. Retrieved September 4, 2010, from http://www.wfp.org/ countries/el-salvador

CHAPTER 17

The Right to Clean Air: The U.S. Clean Air Act's Approach

David P. Novello

INTRODUCTION

This chapter examines how parts of the U.S. Clean Air Act (CAA or the Act) can be viewed as providing a right to clean air—or more precisely, a right to clean *outdoor* air—in the United States. Although commentators do not generally describe the CAA as taking a rights-based approach, the sections of the Act requiring adherence to health-based air quality standards essentially do provide the public with a statutory right to breathe clean air. Other sections that call for the establishment of industry- or process-specific air emissions standards referred to as "technology-based" standards arguably do not. Still, the guarantees of protection from adverse health effects from a wide variety of air pollutants are broad. Moreover, even where the Act directs the U.S. Environmental Protection Agency (EPA) to set industry-specific, technology-based standards that do not necessarily guarantee such protection from substances identified as "hazardous air pollutants," (HAPs) EPA must later conduct a review to determine if a "residual risk" to human health remains. If EPA concludes that there is still a risk, and that the risk is unreasonable, the agency must require a further reduction in emissions.

Although many believe that people should have a *constitutional* right to clean air (and, more generally, to a clean environment), the U.S. Constitution does not confer such a right. In this way, the United States differs from several countries where the right to a clean environment is specifically stated in the constitution. (Of course, it is one thing to state such a right and another to provide citizens with a means to enforce it.) After briefly discussing the issue of a constitutional right to clean air—without taking a position on the matter—this chapter focuses on the federal *statutory* rights that the CAA provides.

LACK OF A FEDERAL CONSTITUTIONAL RIGHT TO CLEAN AIR

The U.S. Constitution, unlike the constitutions of several other countries, certainly does not provide an explicit right to clean air or a clean environment. Particularly in the 1970s, citizens and environmental groups argued in the courts that the federal constitution *implicitly* grants such a right. No court, however, has held that an implicit right exists.[1] As a result, there have been occasional calls to amend the U.S. Constitution to provide an express right. None of these efforts has made much headway.[2]

Several state constitutions, on the other hand, do explicitly guarantee the right to a clean and healthful environment—including the right to clean air. These constitutional provisions undoubtedly are of significant symbolic value. However, even where the state constitution provides the right, that right often has proved to be of little use. For example, in some states, the courts have held that the constitutional right is not "self-executing" and that it does not provide a "private right of action" allowing citizens to sue to enforce it. In addition, courts would be faced with the vexing question of exactly what constitutes a clean environment or clean/healthful air.[3]

Moreover, federal and state air pollution control legislation and regulations create comprehensive systems that aim to provide clean air meeting health-based standards. Vague constitutional guarantees of a right to a clean environment are not as useful as these legislative and regulatory regimes. Thus, we turn to the statutory regime that essentially does provide specific rights to clean air—the federal CAA and the associated state air pollution laws.

EXAMPLES OF CLEAN AIR ACT PROVISIONS THAT REQUIRE EMISSIONS REDUCTIONS BUT DO NOT PROVIDE A RIGHT TO CLEAN AIR

The CAA is a sprawling statute of hundreds of pages. It is really a smorgasbord of programs aimed at reducing different types of air pollution. The Act addresses pollutant emissions from a wide variety of sources, including "stationary sources" such as industrial facilities and electric generating plants, "mobile sources" such as motor vehicles, "nonroad" engines and fuels, and "area sources" such as consumer products.

Congress passed the original CAA in 1970, following the rising environmental consciousness in the 1960s. At that time, it was one of the most complex regulatory programs (and it remains so). A federal regulatory program was deemed necessary because efforts at the state level to control air pollution had proved unsuccessful; ambient concentrations of air pollutants had increased significantly in the previous decades. There have been a series of amendments enacted since 1970, with the principal ones—major overhauls to the air quality regulatory system—passed in 1977 and 1990.

The congressional purposes stated in the Act do not explicitly state a right to clean air. Rather, Congress' 1970 general statement concerning health is that a purpose of the CAA is "to protect and enhance the quality of the Nation's air resources so to as to *promote* [italics added] the public health and welfare and the productive capacity of its population."[4] Thus, promoting the country's "productive capacity" appears to be given no less weight than promoting the public health and welfare.

As noted previously, the CAA regulates only pollutant emissions to outdoor air. The Occupational Safety and Health Administration, rather than EPA, has jurisdiction over air pollution in the workplace, and for the most part, indoor air quality is not regulated even though pollutant concentrations inside houses and buildings often exceeds levels found outside.

The CAA is organized into six titles that contain a larger number of regulatory programs administered by EPA. Not all of these programs specifically aim to protect public health, even though reductions in pollutant emissions resulting from them can lead to ancillary health benefits. For example, the acid rain program, added in 1990 and found in Title IV of the Act, was designed to reduce deposition of sulfates and nitrates to the land and water, caused by emissions of sulfur dioxide and oxides of nitrogen. This deposition results in the acidification of water bodies, harm to trees and other vegetation, damage to buildings, and other environmental problems. But the sulfates and nitrates above certain levels in the air we breathe also cause health problems, so the acid rain program has provided secondary health benefits.

In other cases, it is difficult to establish a direct correlation between a decrease in pollutant emissions and health benefits *in the United States*. Title VI of the Act, which in part implements the international agreement known as the Montreal Protocol on Substances that Deplete the Ozone Layer, has resulted in very significant reductions in emissions of ozone-depleting chemicals. Reduction of ozone levels in the stratosphere results in increased ultraviolet radiation striking the earth, thus increasing the incidence of skin cancer and cataracts. But this is a global problem, with emissions of substances from a particular area generally leading to overall global depletion of ozone in the stratosphere, rather than in the stratosphere above that particular area.

Other sections of the CAA by themselves do not provide a right to clean air. For example, CAA Section 111 directs EPA to establish industry-specific "new source performance standards," known as NSPS. These are classic "technology-based standards," in which the benefit of emissions reductions is balanced with the feasibility and "cost of achieving such reduction—the standards must be 'achievable.'"[5] The consideration of cost and feasibility arguably means that this provision does not reflect a rights-based approach; public health might need to be sacrificed to make meeting the standard achievable. Furthermore, nothing in this type of technology-based standard guarantees that air quality near the regulated industrial process will be safe. The standards usually are expressed as a rate; for example, a certain mass of pollutant emissions per number of widgets produced. A facility producing a large number of widgets might emit pollutants at very high levels. In addition, several facilities might locate in the same area. In each case, if there were not an overlay of ambient limits (which the CAA does in fact provide), pollution concentrations in the ambient air could be much higher than levels considered safe. Background pollutant concentrations could also be relatively high; thus additional emission produced by the regulated facility could increase those concentrations above safe levels.

Thus, in countries with only these types of technology-based standards— often the easiest to develop and implement—the air quality regulatory regime does not provide a right to healthful air. This is not to disparage such standards, for they do require companies to employ clean processes and/or available air pollution control technology; it is just that to guarantee clean air, they must be coupled with health-based standards.

The same limitations apply to "tailpipe standards" and fuel standards that regulate emissions from motor vehicles and other "mobile sources."[6] Tailpipe standards have become much more stringent since the early 1970s, and fuels today are much cleaner than in the past. At the same time, however, total vehicle miles traveled has increased significantly. Total mobile source emissions certainly have declined in the past 4 decades, but much less than if vehicle miles traveled had remained relatively stable.

DEVELOPMENT OF NATIONAL AMBIENT AIR QUALITY STANDARDS

Probably the only true way to guarantee a right to healthful air is to establish "health-based standards" that the government determines to provide air that will not cause harm—and then to require that pollutant concentrations do not exceed those standards. This approach is at the core of the CAA. Sections 108 and 109 of the Act require EPA to set primary national ambient air quality standards (NAAQS) protective of human health, whereas various provisions (summarized in the next section) mandate adherence with those standards.[7] The NAAQS specify maximum pollutant concentrations in the ambient air for six substances that are referred to as "criteria pollutants"—pollutants that EPA has determined to be the most widespread and to be emitted by numerous sources. These six criteria pollutants—so named because the standards for these substances are based on scientific criteria developed by EPA—are particulate matter, carbon monoxide, sulfur dioxide, nitrogen dioxide, lead, and ozone (although beneficial in the stratosphere, ground-level ozone that we breathe is harmful).

The "primary" NAAQS are the most important. EPA must set them at levels that, in its judgment, and "allowing an adequate margin of safety, are requisite to protect the public health."[8] The Act also directs EPA to set "secondary" standards to protect the "public welfare" from such adverse effects as impairment of visibility and damage to crops, although EPA often has simply made the secondary NAAQS the same as the primary standards.[9] Although the statute requires EPA to use the latest scientific studies to review (and if necessary, revise) the NAAQS for a pollutant every 5 years,[10] in practice, the agency has done so less frequently (and usually only in response to lawsuits brought by environmental groups). There is an elaborate process for scientific review of health studies by an EPA advisory committee and the publication of an assessment during this review process. Next, EPA formally proposes the standards, reviews public comments on the proposal, and then issues the final NAAQS.

As commentators have noted, EPA's methodology for setting the primary NAAQS suggests a rights-based approach.[11] The agency consistently has taken the position that it may consider only health effects (i.e., and not the cost of compliance) in setting the primary standards. Industry challenged EPA's position, and in 2001, the U.S. Supreme Court unanimously ruled (as the U.S. Court of Appeals for the D.C. Circuit had on several occasions beforehand) that the CAA forbids the consideration of compliance costs in setting the primary NAAQS.[12]

The report of the committee that wrote the Senate bill for the 1970 CAA (the Environment and Public Works committee) stated that the purpose of the "adequate margin of safety" language in Section 109(b)(1) was to protect "sensitive groups" such as "bronchial asthmatics and emphysematics who in the normal course of daily activity are exposed to the ambient environment."[13] In addition, EPA has explained that:

> [i]n addressing the requirement for an adequate margin of safety, EPA considers such factors as the nature and severity of the health effects involved, the size of sensitive population(s) at risk, and the kind and degree of the uncertainties that must be addressed.[14]

EPA does not, however, set the primary standards at levels that ensure protection for the *most sensitive* individuals. This position finds support in the same 1970 Senate committee report noted previously, which goes on to state:

> In establishing an ambient standard necessary to protect the health of these persons, reference would be made to a representative sample of persons comprising the sensitive group rather than to a single person in such a group. Ambient air quality is sufficient to protect the health of such persons whenever there is an absence of adverse effect on the health of a statistically related sample of persons in sensitive groups from exposure to ambient air.[15]

IMPLEMENTATION OF THE NATIONAL AMBIENT AIR QUALITY STANDARDS

The existence of a safe, concentration-based ambient air quality standard does little more than inform the public of the nature of the air it breathes unless the standard is coupled with an implementation regime to reduce pollutant levels in the ambient air to that concentration—and to maintain the standard. The CAA state implementation plan (SIP) system provides the right to clean air (at least in regard to the criteria pollutants). Although the EPA sets the NAAQS, the states must develop implementation plans to meet those standards and ensure that they will continue to be met even with growth in the area. (EPA approves the requirements of these plans into the Code of Federal Regulations, so they may be enforced by both state or local agencies and EPA.) Given the repeated failures to meet some of the standards in populated areas, the implementation regime has grown more detailed and prescriptive since 1970. Air quality generally has improved during this time despite population growth, but standards are still exceeded in many areas.[16]

The SIP system has become enormously complex over the years (especially for areas exceeding the standards), so only the most basic elements are described here.[17] The program is often referred to as reflecting a federal–state partnership ("cooperative federalism") because although the states and local governments develop the plans (and Congress wanted them to have primary responsibility in controlling air pollution), EPA must approve them. It is not unusual for state and local governments to submit deficient SIPs, particularly when there is political opposition to costly controls. If EPA determines that a plan is not adequate to ensure attainment and maintenance of a NAAQS, EPA must disapprove the SIP and impose specified sanctions on the state. If doing so fails to prod the state into developing and submitting an acceptable plan, the CAA requires EPA to step in and develop its own "federal implementation plan." In practice, however, both sanctions and federal plans have proved to be extremely unpopular at the state level. As a result, EPA generally strives to avoid taking either of these measures unless necessary (and sometimes, only if compelled to do so by a lawsuit). Thus, one can argue that the CAA creates a right to clean air but the implementing agencies are not sufficiently rigorous in enforcing that right—or, as some have written, that it is simply politically infeasible to do so when control costs are high and inconvenience to the public (as with rules restricting driving) is great.[18]

States designate areas that are meeting the standards as "attainment areas," and those that are not as "nonattainment areas." For attainment areas, the SIP must include (among other things) pollution reduction measures and a "maintenance demonstration" that the area will continue to meet the standards. CAA section 110(a)(2)(A) states that these reduction measures are to include:

> enforceable emission limitations and other control measures, means, or techniques (including economic incentives such as fees, marketable permits, and auctions of emissions rights), as well as schedules and timetables for compliance, as may be necessary or appropriate to meet the applicable requirements of this Act.[19]

For nonattainment areas, the measures are overlaid with far more detailed requirements (often expressed on a pollutant-specific basis) that Congress has added since 1977. (The 1970 CAA called for SIPs requiring all areas to attain the NAAQS by the mid-1970s—an expectation that, in hindsight, was incredibly optimistic.) These prescriptive mandates, which go on for scores of pages in Title I, Part D of the Act,[20] reflect Congress' frustration with repeated failures to attain the standards. EPA had attempted to require several of these measures previously and has added additional ones. Thus, the federal–state partnership mentioned earlier began to tilt toward federally prescribed programs known to reduce air pollution. At the same time, in 1990, Congress gave areas more time to attain the standards, based on the severity of the pollution. State and local governments were required not only to provide a computer modeling "attainment demonstration" that they would meet the standards by the required dates and maintain those standards afterward, but also to demonstrate that they would achieve "reasonable further progress" toward attainment in the years prior to the deadline. This reasonable further progress mandate usually requires a linear reduction in emissions from the date the state adopts the SIP until the attainment date. If an area does not meet milestones toward attaining a NAAQS, the state or local government must adopt additional measures. Thus, for the criteria pollutants, the CAA can be said to provide a right to improved air quality in the years before an area is deemed able to attain the standards, as well as an ultimate right to clean air.

A HYBRID APPROACH TO REGULATION
OF HAZARDOUS AIR POLLUTANTS

The preceding discussion describes how health-based standards (when enforced) can be considered to reflect a rights-based approach, whereas technology-based standards—although often effective in reducing pollution—do not. The provision of the Act governing regulation of what are termed HAPs (or "air toxics") from stationary sources adopts a hybrid of these two approaches. HAPs are less widespread than the criteria pollutants and are usually more toxic. For example, many of these are carcinogens and neurotoxins.

Until 1990, CAA Section 112[21] provided that EPA was to set standards that protect human health at a level that "provides an ample margin of safety." This proved very difficult for EPA, in part, because the general view was that exposure to even minute amounts of a carcinogen can cause cancer—and EPA did not wish to issue standards that would shut down entire industries. As a result, EPA was able to issue only seven standards in 20 years.[22] Given this near total failure to obtain reductions from sources other than motor vehicles, a consensus developed in the late 1980s that it would be preferable for EPA to set technology-based standards for various industries. Congress adopted this approach in 1990 when it completely rewrote Section 112. It included a lengthy list of HAPs in the statute and directed EPA to set a large number of standards commonly known as "maximum achievable control technology" (MACT) standards within 10 years.[23] EPA was required to set the standards at least as stringent as the best performing facilities in the industry; only after developing this "floor level" could it consider costs (in determining whether the standards should be more stringent).[24]

Congress did not abandon the health-based approach, however. Within 8 years after EPA promulgates a MACT standard for an industry category, EPA is required to determine whether remaining emissions from sources in the category pose an unacceptable risk to human health. If EPA finds that the risks from HAP emissions *after application of MACT standards* still exceed certain levels, further emission reductions are required. This "residual risk" review is governed by the same health-based language found in the pre-1990 CAA: the technology-based standards and the potential residual risk standards must protect public health with "an ample margin of safety."[25] With regard to HAPs, the post-1990 CAA therefore still provides the public with a right to air quality levels considered protective of human health.

THE RIGHT OF CITIZENS TO SUE

States and EPA are the primary enforcers of the CAA, including regulations and standards issued under the Act. However, CAA Section 304[26] also provides citizens with the right to bring a lawsuit in federal court against EPA for a failure to carry out a nondiscretionary duty (such as the required issuance of regulations or standards). Moreover, if EPA or a state is not diligently prosecuting an alleged violation by a company, a citizen can sue the company for an alleged violation of (a) an emission standard or limitation under the Act, (b) an EPA or state order concerning an emission standard or limitation, or (c) the obligation to obtain certain types of permits.

This "citizen suit" provision is powerful. EPA frequently delays in issuing regulations and standards, and an environmental group often will bring a lawsuit that results in EPA agreeing to issue the rules or standard by a specified deadline. Before 1990, citizen suits against companies were relatively rare. However, with much better access to emissions monitoring reports (and clearer identification of standards to which companies are subject) as a result of the 1990 amendments to the Act, citizen enforcement of emission standards has increased. Thus, in addition to providing rights to clean air, the CAA empowers citizens to enforce their rights.

CONCLUSION

Although the federal Constitution does not provide a public right to clean air, certain provisions of the CAA essentially do. The rights-based approach of these provisions has led to significantly improved air quality since passage of the Act in 1970, even though much needs to be done before many areas attain ambient air quality standards for certain pollutants. Furthermore, citizens have the right to enforce EPA's nondiscretionary duties under the CAA, as well as emission standards for facilities.

Thus, in important ways, the Act can be viewed as providing the public with a right to be protected from adverse health effects resulting from air pollution.

REFERENCES

Belden, R. S. (2001). *The clean air act*. Chicago: American Bar Association.

Clean Air Act, 42 U.S.C. § 7401 *et. seq.* (Note: Although not cited in this chapter, the regulations implementing the Clean Air Act are found in volume 40 of the Code of Federal Regulations [C.F.R.])

Cusack, M. F. (1993). Judicial interpretation of state constitutional rights to a healthful environment. *20 Boston College Environmental Affairs Law Review, 173,* 175–176.

Ely v. Velde, 451 F.2d 1130, 1139 (4th Cir. 1971).

Environmental Protection Agency. (2008). *Six common pollutants*. Retrieved March 10, 2010, from www.epa.gov/air/airtrends/2008/report/SixCommonPollutants.pdf

Feller, J. M. (1994). Non-threshold pollutants and air quality standards. *Environmental Law, 24,* 821.

Martineau, R. J., Jr., & Novello, D. P. (2004). *The clean air act handbook* (2nd ed.). Chicago: American Bar Association.

Meltz, R. (1999, February 23). Right to a clean environment provisions in state constitutions, and arguments as to a federal counterpart. *CRS Report for Congress.* Retrieved March 10, 2010, from http://ncseonline.org/nle/crsreports/risk/rsk-15.cfm

Natural Resources Defense Council v. EPA, 529 F.3d 1077 (D.C. Cir. 2008).

Novello, D. P. (2004). The air toxics program at the crossroads: From MACT to residual risk. *Natural Resources & Environment, 18,* 57.

Pedersen, W. F., Jr. (1981) Why the clean air act works badly. *University of Pennsylvania Law Review, 129,* 1059–1109.

S. Rep. No. 91-1196 (1970). (Report of Senate Environment and Public Works, on the Senate's Clean Air Act bill)

Schoenbrod, D. (1983). Goals statutes or rules statutes: The case of the clean air act. *University of California at Los Angeles Law Review, 30,* 740–828.

Whitman v. American Trucking Associations, 531 U.S. 457 (2001).

NOTES

[1]See for example, Ely v. Velde, 451 F.2d 1130, 1139 (4th Cir. 1971). See also Meltz, R. (1999). Right to a Clean Environment Provisions in State Constitutions, and Arguments as to A Federal Counterpart, *CRS Report for Congress.* Retrieved March 10, 2010, from http://ncseonline.org/nle/crsreports/risk/rsk-15.cfm

[2]See Meltz, R. (1999). Right to a Clean Environment Provisions in State Constitutions, and Arguments as to A Federal Counterpart, *CRS Report for Congress*. Retrieved March 10, 2010, from http://ncseonline.org/nle/crsreports/risk/rsk-15.cfm for a discussion of these calls to amend the U.S. Constitution.

[3]See Meltz, R. (1999). Right to a Clean Environment Provisions in State Constitutions, and Arguments as to A Federal Counterpart, *CRS Report for Congress*. Retrieved March 10, 2010, from http://ncseonline.org/nle/crsreports/risk/rsk-15.cfm. See also Cusack, M. F. (1993). Judicial interpretation of state constitutional rights to a healthful environment. *20 Boston College Environmental Affairs Law Review, 173*, 175–176.

[4]U.S. Clean Air Act, section 101(b)(1), 42 U.S.C. § 7401(b)(1).

[5]U.S. Clean Air Act, section 111(a)(1), 42 U.S.C. § 7411(a)(1).

[6]CAA section 202, 42 U.S.C. § 7521 governs car and truck standards. Other sections of CAA Title II provide for regulation of aircraft, railroad engines, "nonroad" engines, and other sources known as "mobile sources." CAA section 211, 42 U.S.C. § 7545, provides for regulation of fuels; the composition of fuels has a major effect on emissions from engines.

[7]U.S. Clean Air Act, sections 109 and 110, 42 U.S.C. §§ 7409 and 7410.

[8]U.S. Clean Air Act, section 109(b)(1), 42 U.S.C. § 7409(b)(1). The World Health Organization issues similar advisory ambient "guidelines" for protecting health, for particulate matter, ozone, nitrogen dioxide, and sulfur dioxide. See World Health Organization. Retrieved March 10, 2010, from www.who.int/phe/health_topics/outdoorair_aqg/en

[9]U.S. Clean Air Act, section 109(b)(2), 42 U.S.C. § 7409(b)(2).

[10]U.S. Clean Air Act, section 109(d)(1), 42 U.S.C. § 7409(d)(1).

[11]See, for example, Schoenbrod, D. (1983). Goals statutes or rules statutes: The case of the Clean Air Act. *University of California at Los Angeles Law Review, 30*, 740. Schoenbrod notes that "[t]he Act ordains that its environmental goals must be achieved" (p. 742), and that it "conferred on everyone an absolute right to healthy air in the 1970s" (p. 748). However, he then goes on to criticize Congress' command that "[t]he public shall be protected from every harm" (p. 756) as unrealistic and naïve.

[12]Whitman v. American Trucking Associations, 531 U.S. 457 (2001).

[13]S. Rep. No. 91-1196 at 9–10 (1970).

[14]75 Fed. Reg. 2938, 2940–2941 (Jan. 19, 2010; proposed NAAQS for ozone).

[15]S. Rep. No. 91-1196 at 9–10 (1970).

[16]For trends in ambient levels of the criteria pollutants since 1990, see U.S. Environmental Protection Agency Web site. Retrieved March 10, 2010, from www.epa.gov/air/airtrends/2008/report/SixCommonPollutants.pdf

[17]For areas that are attaining a NAAQS, the principal SIP requirements are found in CAA section 110, 42 U.S.C. § 7410. Title I, Part D of the Act states additional requirements for areas that are exceeding a standard. 42 U.S.C. §§ 7501–7515. For a general description of the basic mechanics and problems of the SIP system (at least as it existed years ago), see Pedersen, W. F. (1981). Why the Clean Air Act Works Badly. *129 The University of Pennsylvania Law Review*, 1059.

[18]See Schoenbrod, D. (1983). Goals statutes or rules statutes: The case of the Clean Air Act. *University of California at Los Angeles Law Review, 30*, 740.

[19]U.S. Clean Air Act, 42 U.S.C. § 7410(a)(2)(A).

[20]U.S. Clean Air Act, 42 U.S.C. §§ 7501–7515.

[21]U.S. Clean Air Act, 42 U.S.C. § 7412.

[22]For a discussion of EPA's problems in issuing hazardous air pollutant standards during the 1970s and 1980s, see Feller, J. (1994). Air quality standards and non-threshold pollutants, 24 *Environmental Law*, 821.

[23]U.S. Clean Air Act, §§ 112(b)–(e), 42 U.S.C. §§ 7412(b)–(e).

[24]U.S. Clean Air Act, § 112(d)(2)–(3), 42 U.S.C. § 7412(d)(2)–(3).

[25]U.S. Clean Air Act, § 112(f)(2), 42 U.S.C. § 7412(f)(2). For a discussion of the MACT and residual risk process for hazardous air pollutants, see Novello, D. P. (2004). The air toxics program at the crossroads: From MACT to residual risk. 18 *Natural Resources & Environment*, 57. For a discussion of what "an ample margin of safety" means for carcinogens, see Natural Resources Defense Council v. EPA, 529 F.3d 1077 (D.C. Cir. 2008) (reviewing the residual risk standard for organic chemical manufacturing facilities).

[26]U.S. Clean Air Act, 42 U.S.C. § 7607.

CHAPTER 18

Peer Education in Prison: A Rights-Based Approach

Kathy Boudin and Corey Weinstein

Prisoners are condemned to imprisonment for their crimes; they should not be condemned to HIV and AIDS. There is no doubt that governments have a moral and legal responsibility to prevent the spread of HIV among prisoners and prison staff and to care for those infected. They also have a responsibility to prevent the spread of HIV among communities. Prisoners are the community. They come from the community, they return to it. Protection of prisoners is protection of our communities.[1]

"Each one, teach one," that was one of the best results of our peer ed groups at every prison I was at. Women who began the sessions not knowing anything about the immune system or how their bodies work learned the basics and were then both capable of and excited about teaching others what they had learned. The core of our work is the process of empowerment that accompanies peer education on health issues.[2]

INTRODUCTION

Medical care in prison is a public health matter: It concerns the health of those who are incarcerated as well as the health of communities to which incarcerated persons return. Medical intervention depends on health education and prevention services as a critical factor in communicable diseases such as human immunodeficiency virus (HIV) or hepatitis C virus (HCV). Peer education in prison—education carried out by incarcerated people who work with others who are incarcerated—is a cornerstone of HIV and HCV prevention. Educators are members of the affected community whether they are living with the disease or not. The educators become a source of focus and information and generally function as teachers and as advocates empowering the community to learn and act on its own behalf. Studies of HIV/AIDS prevention in prison demonstrate that peer education has had a strong positive influence on behaviors and intentions.[3] In addition, no country has sufficient resources to provide comprehensive primary prevention programs behind bars. Thus, there is a significant value to using peer educators who themselves are incarcerated, because of both the high potential for effectiveness and the very low costs.

This chapter will examine issues of health and human rights as they pertain to the incarcerated. It will then discuss rates of HIV and HCV among incarcerated populations. Finally, it will examine the origins of the AIDS Counseling and Education (ACE) Program and other prison-based peer education programs.

HUMAN RIGHT STANDARDS AND THE RIGHTS OF THE INCARCERATED

All persons have a human right to "the highest available standards of health care" and access to information. The enjoyment of the highest attainable standard of health conducive to living a life in dignity is a well-codified human right.[4] People who are incarcerated also have a right to health care. Article 10 of the International Covenant on Civil and Political Rights (ICCPR) imposes a positive obligation on states to ban inhumane or degrading treatment and freedom from any hardship or constraint other than that resulting from the deprivation of liberty while incarcerated.[5] Alternatively, as one who is in prison might put it, "we are in prison as punishment, not for punishment." Article 10 details that no prison system should be only retributory; it should also essentially seek the reformation and social rehabilitation of the prisoner.[6]

The U.S. Constitution, as interpreted by the U.S. Supreme Court in *Estelle v. Gamble*,[7] contains a guarantee that health care will be provided to people in prison. The constitutional standard is a prohibition against deliberate indifference to serious medical needs. *Deliberate indifference* means that if a prison system and its agents are aware of a risk of harm, they have an affirmative duty to prevent deterioration in function, pain, death, or risk to the public health.[8] The right of incarcerated persons to become educated and to become peer educators is a human right precisely because of the central role of peers in health care prevention in prison. Article 19 of the ICCPR guarantees the right to receive and impart information, whereas Article 2 prohibits discrimination of any kind that impinges on the rights guaranteed therein.

HIV AND HEPATITIS C VIRUS AMONG INCARCERATED POPULATIONS

The rates of HIV and HCV infection among incarcerated populations worldwide are much higher than in the general population. In the United States, the rate of confirmed AIDS illness behind bars in 2004 was triple that of the noninstitutionalized population.[9] It is astounding that about 1.4 million HCV-infected people pass through various U.S. penal institutions each year, accounting for as many as 33% of the total U.S. population infected with HCV.[10] In 1996, 17% of the estimated 229,000 persons living with AIDS, 35% of the total of population with active tuberculosis (TB), and 12–15% of all individuals in the United States with chronic or current hepatitis B infection spent time in a correctional facility.[11] In 2005, 19% of men and 10% of women entering the New York Department of Correctional Services (DOCS) were hepatitis C seropositive.[12]

HIV and HCV are most commonly transmitted through sharing needles while injecting intravenous drugs and during unprotected sex. Poverty has contributed to the high rate of HIV and HCV among those in prison in the United States, as has public policy: the U.S. National Commission on AIDS in its 1991 report stated, "by choosing mass imprisonment as the federal and state governments' response to the use of drugs, we have created a de facto policy of incarcerating more and more individuals with HIV infection."[13]

The provision of health care includes preventive care and prevention services. Preventing people from becoming infected with communicable illnesses, such as HIV/AIDS, sexually transmitted diseases, TB, and viral hepatitis B and C, is the central strategy for stemming the health epidemics relating to these illnesses; prevention work is particularly important to carry out in prison for several reasons. First, the high prevalence of HIV and other communicable diseases among people in prison, the reality of sexual activity, drug use, and tattooing and the widespread correctional policy of denying condoms or sterile syringes place people in prison at risk for infection. Second, more than 90% of all those incarcerated are released back into society. Prevention education before release is important to encourage safe behavior at home, thus limiting future infections.[14] Finally, prevention is critical as a public health issue. Peer-educated people are not only less likely to infect others, but they can also play a role in educating and protecting the communities to which they return.[15]

As distressing as the criminalization of the public health problem of drug addiction may be, the high rate of serious chronic viral infections in the incarcerated population presents an important public health opportunity. Prevention education in prisons succeeds because there is literally a "captive audience," and time is more available for people to think about health and illness, prevention, and safe behaviors compared to life outside prison where enormous pressures often result in placing health care low on the priority lists of people returning from prison. Without peer involvement, this prevention education will neither reach the numbers it needs nor reach people as effectively.

The Early HIV/AIDS Crisis

By the end of the 1980s HIV/AIDS became a crisis in the United States as the HIV/AIDS epidemic spread in poor and Black and Latino communities through injection drug use and heterosexual sex. Although the rates varied among prisons and jails depending on location, in New York State in 1989 according to a blind study, 18.8% of consecutive inmates entering through Bedford Hills Correctional Facility tested positive for HIV.[16] A study done on men entering Downstate Correctional Facility showed that 17.4% of the men tested positive for HIV.[17] The crisis was multilayered:

- It forced prison authorities to provide HIV/AIDS treatment and to find methods to prevent the spread of infection within the prison.
- People in prison themselves had to contend with the psychological pressure of wanting to know, but fearing to know, their own status.
- Those known to be HIV-positive were forced to cope with public shame and isolation, as well as the dread of their own deaths and deaths of loved ones outside.

The Response From Prison Administrators

The response from administrators of prisons and jails was varied. In one extreme example in Alabama, an HIV-positive prisoner had to wear a gown, gloves, and mask, and squirt disinfectant over each step every time there is a need to leave the cell.[18] More common was the practice of isolating of inmates who tested positive. There were also institutions where educational sessions were carried out by nurses, doctors, or health educators. There were few prisons that allowed the incarcerated to become educators themselves.[19] The vast majority of prison systems at that time and today did not and do not use inmate representatives to deliver AIDS education and instead rely on civilian social workers and medical experts.[20] Although in many instances, these individuals provide real relief and supportive services to prisons, when the experts are the ones doing the work they do not train and enable prisoners to do it. Experts cannot generate the kind of peer-to-peer engagement, self-initiative, and community involvement that is possible from a grassroots effort.

THE AIDS COUNSELING AND EDUCATION PROGRAM

In early 1988, a proposal was made by women at Bedford Hills Correctional Facility to create an AIDS/HIV program among women in the prison to become educated, to address the stigma, to care for those who were dying, and to try and prevent transmission inside the prison and back home.

The women were responding in part to the inadequacy of existing efforts to meet their needs: experts from the New York State Department of Health and other agencies came and did live presentations, usually supplemented by videos and written materials. Although the presentations were usually accurate and well-meaning, the audience was too large and the time was too short. Many of those who were incarcerated did not trust the presenters because they were state officials. The women were also responding to the inspirational models of community empowerment in health care outside prison; for example, the women's self-care health movement begun in the 1970s and exemplified in the publications of *Our Bodies Ourselves.*[21] Another model was the gay men's HIV/AIDS movement.

The superintendent of Bedford Hills Correctional Facility was probably alone at that time in her willingness to allow prisoners to become educated and to tackle the issues of prevention, care, and stigma. What became known as the ACE Program gained momentum and was soon funded by the New York Department of Health AIDS Institute. Dr. Robert Greifinger, then chief medical officer of the New York State Department of Corrections, determined that peer education programs were the best approach to coping with the AIDS epidemic, and Prisoners for AIDS Counseling and Education Program (PACE) programs modeled after ACE were funded throughout New York State empowering men and women to become peer educators to meet the growing crisis. He said recently, reflecting on his decision to support the development of peer education and prevention programs throughout the New York State prison system:

> I came into what was the largest HIV population of the world, 7,000 people at least with no testing and no treatment until six months before I left. So as we learned more about the modes of transmission and the ineffectiveness of existing treatments, we were looking for creative modes of prevention including among other things working with women who are known to be infected to at the least to prevent them from transmitting their virus to their partners. It was also an opportunity to work with people before they go home so that they wouldn't get infected.[22]

Following the development of ACE and similar programs in New York State, peer education efforts developed in other state systems and in some federal prisons. Also in the early 1990s, a peer education program began at Pleasanton, California as well as at Federal Correctional Institution in Lexington, Kentucky, the largest of the three main federal correctional facilities for women.

KEY CONCEPTS OF PRISON-BASED PEER EDUCATION PROGRAMS

Peer education programs are premised on several core ideas:

- People in prison have a stake in helping one another because prison is where they live and because the people they are helping are themselves. Thus commitment and caring characterize the work.
- Prisoners have greater trust, generally, with others who are also incarcerated. Prisoners can talk freely about issues of sex and drugs, which are forbidden in prison. Otherwise harm reduction approaches are generally not permitted, so having real discussions about sex and drugs are difficult with the prison professional staff.
- Prisoners have constant access to peers in the living units, in the yard, in the mess hall, and in the school, so ongoing support and education is much more available.
- Peer educators are role models for others who are incarcerated. They inspire, encourage, and support others in prison to believe that they too can grow into creating active and important roles.
- Peer education programs lead to the development of marketable skills and knowledge, serving as a basis for jobs when peer educators reenter the community.

• Peer education programs create new community leaders in the area of HIV/AIDS who subsequently serve the communities they came from.

Prevention literature shows that knowledge is necessary but not sufficient for behavior change. The theoretical underpinnings of the strength of peer education are social learning theory: the importance of attitudes, norms, role models, and context. It is in these areas that peers can play a unique role. When a supportive environment was developed through the efforts of people living with AIDS (PWAs), those who were incarcerated began to challenge the stigma and show support. People who were living with the virus could step forward and be public about their status. Their courage, their life stories, and their passion played a leading role in education and prevention work.

In the ACE program, the peers developed role plays and problem situations that they would use in classrooms as part of prerelease programs, in which women would work with real-life situations relating to drug use, sex, and disclosure. The humor, tragedy, and real-life problems, all led to a prevention approach that engaged people. At Lexington, the motto, "each one teach one," became the driving force. Women who began sessions not knowing anything about the immune system and how their bodies worked learned the basics and became capable of and excited about teaching others what they had learned. Community mobilizations sometimes accompanied the more formal educational work led by peer educators. In some prisons, the peers organized health fairs. At others, they held a walkathon where people walked around the prison yard raising money to support outside AIDS programs. Outside organizations and activists connected with those inside. Peers were allowed to accompany another person into his or her medical appointment or help the person prepare for the appointment by writing down questions and concerns to communicate to the doctor. After the visit, peers help the patient to remember or absorb the information given by the doctor. In almost all the prisons, the peer educators led in creating World AIDS Day events as a chance for the people in prison to come together and remember all whom they had known who died of AIDS, talk about the existing challenges, and connect to the outside world.

LACK OF SUPPORT FOR PRISON-BASED PEER EDUCATION PROGRAMS

Despite these activities, most American correctional facilities have not implemented or maintained HIV prison-based peer education programs. One study[23] carried out on the prevalence of HIV prison-based peer programs in U.S. correctional facilities showed that out of 1,280 facilities and 1,427,279 inmates only 18 states had an HIV prison-based peer program. Although peer programs are successful, most facilities are not using them for educational or rehabilitative purposes.

One reason for the lack of support is the disconnect between the goals of incarceration and the goals of peer education programs. The primary objectives of incarceration are control, punishment, and deterrence through social isolation.[24] Peer education health programs require initiative, self-efficacy, collective activity, and empowerment of people in prison and collaboration between the peers with administration and health officials. However, these very qualities create a contradiction with the command-and-control organizational model that dominates prison. In particular, discussions about AIDS and other infectious diseases often raise the issues of sex and drugs, yet prison administrators usually do not want to acknowledge that such activities take place, let alone provide the means to pursue sex or use drugs safely. Hence, most prison administrators rely on outside experts or civilian workers to provide the education.

Another reason for the lack of support for prison-based peer education programs is their reliance on the harm reduction model. Harm reduction strategies encourage but do not insist on abstinence from unsafe sex and drug use; any decrease in unsafe behavior is seen as a step in a positive direction.

Harm reduction in prison must take into account the fact that injectable drug use, tattooing, and sexual activity are part of daily life for numerous prisoners. Certainly, these behaviors are illegal in prison. As a result, peer educators are frequently barred from discussing proven techniques for reducing harm. For any peer education program to be successful and respected in a prison, setting the realities of the everyday must be dealt with. Peer educators in prison deal with the restrictions in creative ways. For example, they can teach about the general philosophy of harm reduction and then create role plays about real situations requiring harm reduction techniques that take place outside of prison. However, materials such as condoms or clean syringes are rarely, if ever, permitted; people who are incarcerated may be forced to invent means of preventing transmission using accessible materials building on the peer educators' information about harm reduction.

CONCLUSION

International human rights standards clarify that prisoners have a right to education and access to information. Global strategies include harm reduction for HIV and HCV, which include voluntary testing and counseling, bleach, needle exchange and opiate substitution, and condoms/dental dams.[25] International studies of harm reduction in prison find that syringe exchange programs have been successfully implemented in a diverse range of prison settings. The exchange programs reduce HIV and HCV risk and prevent disease transmission, increase referrals to substance abuse treatment, and neither result in increased drug use nor pose problems with security or violence.[26] However, these programs do not exist in almost any U.S. penal institutions. The U.S. peer education programs would be even stronger if the international human rights standards about harm reduction were applied in the United States in prison. The Joint United Nations Programme on HIV/AIDS states the importance of attention to human rights in this way:

> The risk of HIV infection and its impact feeds on violations of human rights, including discrimination against women and marginalized groups such as sex workers, people who inject drugs and men who have sex with men. HIV also frequently begets human rights violations such as further discrimination and violence. Over the past decade the critical need for strengthening human rights to effectively respond to the epidemic and deal with its effects has become ever-more clear. Protecting human rights and promoting public health are mutually reinforcing.[27]

Incarcerated people who are engaged in effective action on their own behalf can better overcome the prison pressures toward passivity, dependence, and lack of self-reliance, characteristics that are so effective in undermining the self-determination and confidence required for successful integration back into the community.[28] In California, peer education activities by the prisoners began during their difficult battle for better medical care. During that time and after when the program was formalized as a prison-supported activity, the educators played multiple roles as teachers, organizers, and advocates. They had written on the wall in their office: "We speak for women who can't speak for themselves."[29]

When men and women in prison are involved in a peer education program, they become activists and are role models for others within their community who strengthen the health of the population building skills and hope. Within this framework, prison-based peer education is fulfilling the human rights vision of education and participation, health care and prevention, and an engaged rights-based approach to dignity and well-being.

NOTES

[1]United Nations Commission on Human Rights. (1996). Fifty-second session, item 8 of the agenda. HIV/AIDS in Prisons - Statement by the Joint United Nations Programme on HIV/AIDS (UNAIDS), Geneva, Switzerland, April 1996.

[2]Personal conversation with a formerly incarcerated peer educator (January 15, 2009).

[3]Bryan, A., Robbins, R. N., Ruiz, M. S., O'Neill, D. (2006). Effectiveness of an HIV prevention intervention in prison among African Americans, Hispanics, and Caucasians. *Health Education and Behavior, 33*(2), 154–177.

[4]International Network for Economic, Social and Cultural Rights. (2000). General Comment 14 on Article 12 of the International Covenant on Economic, Social and Cultural Rights, adopted 5/11/2000.

[5]Office of the High Commissioner for Human Rights. (1992). General Comment 21 on Article 10 of the International Covenant of Civil and Political Rights.

[6]Office of the High Commissioner for Human Rights. (1992). General Comment 21 on Article 10 of the International Covenant of Civil and Political Rights.

[7]Estelle v. Gamble, 429 U.S. 97 (1976).

[8]Greifinger, R. B. (2006). Health care quality through care management. In M. Puisis (Ed.), *Clinical practice in correctional medicine* (2nd ed., p. 512). St. Louis, MO: Mosby.

[9]Murischak, L. M. (2006). HIV in Prisons, 2004. *Bureau of Justice Statistics Bulletin,* [revised 3/1/07], NJC 213897.

[10]Boutwell, A. E., Allen, S. A, Rich, J. D. (2005). Opportunities to address the hepatitis C epidemic in the correctional setting. *Clinical Infectious Diseases, 40*(Suppl. 5) S367–S372.

[11]National Commission on Correctional Healthcare. (2002). *The health status of soon-to-be-released inmates.* Report to Congress. Retrieved October 24, 2007, from http://www.ncchc.org/stbr/Volume1/Health%20Status%20(vol%20l).pdf

[12]Birkhead, G., & Wright, L. (2007, January). *Prison and jail health.* Paper presented at the University of Albany School of Public Health. Albany, NY. Retrieved from http://www.albany.edu/sph/coned/t2b2jail.htm

[13]US National Commission on AIDS. (1991). *Report: HIV disease in correctional facilities.* Washington, DC: The Commision.

[14]Bureau of Justice Statistics Correctional Surveys. (1996). *Correctional populations in the United States.* U.S. Department of Justice.

[15]Zack, B. (2007). HIV prevention: Behavioral interventions in correctional settings. In R B. Greifinger (Ed),. *Public health behind bars: From prisons to communities.* Secaucus, NJ: Springer Verlag.

[16]New York Department of Public Health. (1989). AIDS in New York State (26). Albany, NY: New York Department of Public Health.

[17]New York Department of Public Health. (1989). AIDS in New York State (28). Albany, NY: New York Department of Public Health.

[18]Conversation with John Hale, spokesman for the Alabama Department of Corrections, Winter 1995. Cited in ACE. (1998). In K. Boudin (Ed.), *Breaking the walls of silence: AIDS and women in a New York State maximum-security prison* (p. 202). Woodstock, NY: Overlook Press.

[19]Hammet, T., Moini, S. (1988). *AIDS in correctional facilities: Issues and options* (3rd ed., pp. 39–50). Washington, DC: National Institute of Justice.

[20]Collica, K. (2006, October 31). *The prevalence of HIV prison-based peer programming in American correctional facilities: Another opportunity wasted.* Paper presented at the annual meeting of the American Society of Criminology (ASC), Los Angeles Convention Center, Los Angeles, CA. Retrieved February 2, 2009, from http://www.allacademic.com/meta/p125535_index.html

[21]Collica, K. (2006, October 31). *The prevalence of HIV prison-based peer programming in American correctional facilities: Another opportunity wasted.* Paper presented at the annual meeting of the American Society of Criminology (ASC), Los Angeles Convention Center, Los Angeles, CA. Retrieved February 2, 2009, from http://www.allacademic.com/meta/p125535_index.html

[22]Private communication to author, Dr. Kathy Boudin.

[23]Collica, K. (2007, October). The prevalence of HIV prison-based peer programming in American prisons: An opportunity wasted. *J. Correct. Health Care, 13*(4), 277–278.

[24]Sullivan, L. E. (1990). *The Prison Reform Movement: Forlorn Hope.* Boston: Twaye.

[25]Jurgens, R. (2005). Prisoners who inject drugs: Public health and human rights imperatives. *Health and Human Rights, 8*(2), 46–74.

[26]Harm Reduction Coalition. (2007). Syringe exchange in prisons: The international experience. Retrieved from www.harmreduction.org/article.php?id=418&printsafe=1

[27]Joint United Nations Programme on HIV/AIDS. Human Rights and HIV. Retrieved from http://www.unaids.org/en/PolicyAndPractice/HumanRights/

[28]Irwin, J. (2005). *The warehouse prison.* Los Angeles: Roxbury Publishing Company.

[29]Interviews with Seven Prison HIV Peer Educators at Central California Women's Facility, December 2008.

CHAPTER 19

Rights-Based Approaches to Community Development: A Case Study of the Lower Ninth Ward, New Orleans

Ann Yoachim and Charles Allen III

With the support of good people and the resilience of brave people, it seems like anything can be accomplished. Sustain the nine!

Pam Dashiell, founder, Center for Sustainable
Engagement and Development (1948–2009)[1]

INTRODUCTION

As discussed in previous chapters in this volume, rights-based approaches (RBAs) to development are grounded in international human rights principles that focus on states as the primary duty bearers to fulfill the rights of individuals with a focus on strengthening accountability, promoting equality and nondiscrimination, and supporting participation and empowerment in decision-making process.[2] This is an inherently political process and requires dealing with imbalances of power.[3]

The immediate response and current rebuilding efforts related to Hurricane Katrina in New Orleans highlight the impact of these imbalances of power and disenfranchisement. These efforts can serve as a case study for how RBAs provide the opportunity to address historical and long-standing socioeconomic, racial, and regional inequality; lack of transparency and coordination at the local, state, and federal level; and limited civic engagement in postdisaster community recovery and development. The formal use of RBAs for social and economic development in the United States is relatively new and is largely the result of the adoption of these approaches by international nongovernmental organizations for development efforts. For this reason, this case study does not highlight a specific program but instead focuses a rights-based lens on recovery efforts.

HISTORY AND DEVELOPMENT OF NEW ORLEANS

Any attempt to use a rights-based lens on the current recovery and rebuilding efforts in New Orleans must begin with the physical and cultural landscapes of the city and the Lower Ninth Ward. These are the landscapes and the resulting relationship between people and the environment that have served as the foundation for the city's culture and economy. Prior to its founding in 1718 by Frenchman Jean-Baptiste Le Moyne on the relatively high ground of the natural levees of the Mississippi River, the area served as a trading route for Native Americans. Through the 18th century, colonial rule shifted between the French and the Spanish until the Louisiana Purchase in 1803, when the strategic port city came under American rule.

In the 19th and in to the early 20th century, settlement continued to hug the banks and the historic ridges and follow the natural curve of the Mississippi River, creating the "Crescent" City.[4] In 1850, New Orleans was the most diverse city in the United States when defined by the number and size of ethnic groups represented. Residents of the city faced threats from seasonal flooding, hurricanes, waterborne illnesses such as yellow fever, and ongoing sewage and drainage issues.[5] The city expanded off the banks and ridges of the Mississippi River with the invention of the wood screw pump in 1913, which allowed swampy areas once off limits to be drained and settled.[6] These areas and those that were largely settled after 1878 were the areas that flooded during Hurricane Katrina.[7]

Founded because of its location in the Mississippi River delta, for much of its existence, New Orleans has been protected by a complex coastal wetland ecosystem created as the Mississippi River shifted channels and deposited sediment along the Gulf Coast over the last 7,000 years. Following the Flood of 1927, the worst river flood in U.S. history, a decision was made to federalize the already existing levees along the length of the Mississippi River.[8] Coupled with natural subsidence, sea level rise, impacts of introduced species, and canals for oil and gas exploration, the leveeing of the Mississippi River starved southern Louisiana of sediment and has resulted in nearly 1,900 sq mi (1.2 million acres) of coastal land loss since 1930.[9] Today, 30% of the United States' coastal wetlands are located in southern Louisiana, but the region experiences 90% of the annual loss in the 48 contiguous states.[10] Although difficult to quantify, these remaining wetlands serve as buffers reducing storm surge and damage to important infrastructure.[11] Past and present, decisions on how to manage the Mississippi River for economic benefit and ecosystem protection and in turn current conversations around coastal restoration are inherently political and the complexity of the policy and legal landscape often reinforce existing imbalances of power and lack of accountability.

THE LOWER NINTH WARD

The interplay between land and culture and the city's relationship with water is dramatically apparent in the Lower Ninth Ward. The area is composed of two distinct neighborhoods, Holy Cross and the Lower Ninth. Holy Cross, settled in the early 1800s, hugs the banks of the Mississippi River. The fertile soil of the natural levees of the Mississippi River was a logical place for plantations to serve the city proper. In the mid-to-late 1800s, Holy Cross reflected the ethnic diversity that existed in the city: free people of color, freed slaves, and immigrants from Ireland, Italy, and Germany built homes in the area.[12] Predominately "shotgun" homes, they were built in harmony with the physical landscape. Built 3 ft off the ground, constructed of barge board and cypress, with high ceilings and windows that allowed air to travel through the house and create a cross-breeze for the hot, humid temperatures of summer in New Orleans, these shotgun homes were, in today's terminology, "built green."

Settlement of what is the Lower Ninth neighborhood began with the placement of surface canal drainage systems in the early 1900s and the construction of the Inner Harbor Navigation Canal, also referred to as the Industrial Canal, which was completed in 1923. Prior to the completion of the construction of the canal, the entire Lower Ninth Ward was contiguous with the rest of the city. As a deep water shipping channel connecting the Mississippi River to the Lake Pontchartrain, the Industrial Canal created jobs and resulted in a desire for housing even with drainage problems and lack of sewage system in the Lower Ninth Ward. In the mid-20th century, another bridge was added providing a second link between the Lower Ninth Ward and the rest of the city furthering development in the northern boundaries of the neighborhood.[13] Today, the Lower Ninth Ward is bounded on three sides by water, the Industrial Canal to the west, the Florida Avenue Canal to the north, and the Mississippi River to the south.

Immediately prior to Hurricane Katrina, the Lower Ninth Ward was predominately African American with a population less than 20,000.[14] The neighborhood had a high percentage of homeowners, and many of these homes had been passed down from previous generations. The Lower Ninth faced challenges common to many urban areas prior to the devastation wrought by the hurricane. Changes in the shipping industry and the collapse of the oil economy led to a lack of jobs and shift toward dependence on service industry jobs and resulting lower wages.[15] This, along with a failing public education system, disinvestment, lack of adequate public transportation, and population loss, fed into the high percentage of blighted properties and high crime rates. However, with these challenges or perhaps because of them, the Lower Ninth had not lost its social aid clubs or churches and was home to artists such as Fats Domino. Like many neighborhoods in New Orleans, the percentage of residents who were native to Louisiana was high and extended families often lived in the same block or on neighboring streets.[16]

THE IMPACT OF HURRICANES KATRINA AND RITA

It was on this physical and cultural landscape Hurricane Katrina made landfall in Louisiana on April 29, 2005 as a Category 3 storm on the Saffir Simpson Scale, with winds of 125 mph (205 km/h). Hurricane-force winds extended outward more than 120 mi (190 km) from the center of the storm and the area impacted by the storm was more than 90,000 sq mi (233,100 sq km), an area larger than the size of Great Britain. Coastal communities along the Gulf Coast of Mississippi and Louisiana were decimated by storm surges of 20–29 ft, the latter being the highest ever recorded in the United States.[17] Levee overtopping and breaches resulted in the flooding of 80% of New Orleans.[18] Homes remained in standing water until the city was completely emptied of water on September 17, excluding the Lower Ninth Ward and New Orleans East, which flooded again as a result of Hurricane Rita. A total of 1.4 million people were displaced.[19]

The impact of Hurricane Katrina and resulting levee failures in the Lower Ninth Ward was catastrophic. Storm surge funneled water from the Gulf Intracoastal Waterway (GIWW) and the Mississippi River Gulf

Outlet (MRGO) into the Industrial Canal. Rebounding off the Industrial Canal Lock, this extreme water movement was one of the factors that caused the Industrial Canal to breach.[20–22] Walls of water moving at approximately 5 ft/s and as high as 15 ft pushed homes off their foundations and moved the homes blocks away. Earthen levees of the MRGO were overtopped allowing water to pour in from the northern side of the neighborhood. Flooding was so severe that homes located in Holy Cross on the natural levee of the Mississippi River took more than 4 ft of water. Of the approximately 1,600 people who died directly because of Hurricane Katrina in Louisiana, more than 150 of them perished in the small neighborhood of the Lower Ninth Ward.[23] On September 23, sections of the Lower Ninth Ward flooded again as a result of Hurricane Rita.

AFTER THE STORM

The importance of two key features of RBAs to community development—the empowerment of individuals to "engage in the decision-making processes that affect their lives" and "building of synergies and alliances" across and among different actors in shaping return, rebuilding, and recovery—became apparent in the early months after Hurricane Katrina.[24] In late November of 2005, the Holy Cross Neighborhood Association (HCNA) began meeting weekly in a nonflooded section of the city. The importance of the neighborhood association's existence, engagement with nonprofit organizations, strong leadership, and involvement in environmental justice battles prior to the storm cannot be underestimated. At a time when residents were not allowed to stay overnight in the Lower Ninth Ward, the meetings provided opportunity for the limited number of returned residents to connect with each other, to locate displaced residents, and to connect with technical support.[25] This coordinated effort placed it ahead of other neighborhoods that had been severely damaged, and it was in these meetings that the groundwork for the neighborhood's "Sustainable Restoration Plan" was forged.[26] At the same time, the neighborhood's moderate damage relative to the rest of the Lower Ninth, its historic designation, and its location on the natural levee of the Mississippi River resulted in it being designated as an "immediate opportunity area" by the Bring New Orleans Back Commission.

The Sustainable Restoration Plan, based on a 3-day "facilitated design workshop" in April 2006, laid out a framework for a healthy and vibrant community built on sustainability, carbon neutrality, and increased safety and prosperity with recommendations placed under four themes: urban design and the built environment, quality of life, environment, and economics.[27] At the time of this initial planning process, returned residents were still unable to spend the night in their homes in the Lower Ninth Ward, and many residents remained displaced. Even with these limitations, the coordinated effort served as a catalyst for philanthropic investment in the Lower Ninth Ward around broad issues of sustainability and health, highlighted the neighborhoods' commitment to return and rebuild better, and served as a foundation for incorporating this new framework and vision focused on a healthy environment and community into the citywide Unified New Orleans Plan.[28]

The visionary nature of the plan, vocal leadership, and a diverse coalition of stakeholders has placed the neighborhood at the forefront of local, state, and national discussions at the intersections of urban planning, green building, historic preservation, and environmental justice.[29] Learning from and building on the experiences of "Greening the Ghetto" in the South Bronx and the national "Green for All" effort, the Lower Ninth Ward's vision for a "healthy environment" and "healthy community" has pushed and continues to push national organizations to expand their view of "green" building to include deconstruction, historical preservation, and hazard mitigation.[30] This broad vision is reflected in construction, policy advocacy, volunteer, and outreach efforts taking place in the Lower Ninth Ward. Ongoing home construction efforts by Make It Right will create the "largest and greenest community of single-family homes in the world."[31] Global Green continues the construction of five single-family residences and an 18-unit apartment building.[32] The Preservation Resources Center in conjunction with the U.S. Green Building Council and the National Trust for Historic Preservation is transforming a historic home in Holy Cross into a LEED Platinum community center.[33]

The synergies among academia, private entities, international and local nongovernmental organizations, community-based organizations, and residents have resulted in policy change. The Lower Ninth Ward's efforts focused on energy efficiency, and renewable energy led the New Orleans Historic District Landmarks Commission, the entity served with ensuring renovation in historic districts, to grant permits for the installation of the first solar panel systems on any homes within a local and national historic district in New Orleans.[34] With the Alliance for Affordable Energy, a local nonprofit organization, the HCNA, and later, the Lower Ninth Ward Center for Sustainable Engagement and Development, a program, which continues to bulk purchase radiant barrier insulation and support residents in installation, was developed. This program and neighborhood residents played a key role in the passage of Energy Smart New Orleans, the first citywide energy efficiency program.[35] The founding of Lower Ninth Ward Center for Sustainable Engagement and Development, a community-based nonprofit organization, has created another vehicle to support residents in their efforts to rebuild a safer and more sustainable future, to provide space for dialogue between local, state, and federal entities and for residents to know, claim, and realize their rights, especially regarding environmental issues, and to allow information exchange between Gulf Coast communities seeking to rebuild sustainability.

In laying a framework for recovery, the Sustainable Restoration Plan highlights the connections between the urban and built environment that reflect New Orleans' connection to its physical and cultural landscapes. The Sustainable Restoration Plan calls for ecosystem restoration, passive stormwater management, and other hazard mitigation measures as means not only to reduce the neighborhood's vulnerability to flooding but also to provide economic and educational opportunities. Plans to restore the Bayou Bienvenue Triangle, a degraded cypress marsh adjacent to the north side of the neighborhood, have gained momentum, garnered the attention of local, state, and federal agencies, and become feasible with the closure of the MRGO.[36] The neighborhood continues to develop their visions and calls for this restoration that would offer storm protection, provide ecotourism and green job opportunities in the form of wetland restoration, serve as a recreation and environmental education site, and enhance food security. Faced with ongoing drainage challenges and inadequate infrastructure, the neighborhood, with the support of local and national nonprofit organizations, continues to adopt passive stormwater management techniques including the installation of rain gardens in medians of major streets and on individual property and the development of the city's first permeable street.

Broadly identified in the Sustainable Restoration Plan as quality of life issues, almost 5 years after the storm, the challenges of safety and security, reliable public transportation, food security and access, and medical care remain. Collaborative efforts of local and national nonprofit organizations, community-based organizations, academia, and public–private partnerships continue to address these requisites for a healthy and "carbon-neutral" community.[37,38] Groups including the Lower Ninth Ward Urban Farming Coalition, Common Ground, the School at Blair Grocery, and the Guerrilla Garden project of the HCNA are promoting backyard gardens and urban agriculture while other organizations work with the support of local academic institutions to access federal funding and private investment to support the opening of a "green" grocery store in the neighborhood.[39] The Neighborhood Empowerment Network Association (NENA) provides "services and implements sustainable programs in community outreach, case management, design and construction administration, home and school rebuilding, and economic development."[40] The monthly Sankofa Market brings together food vendors and health screening providers, serves as a recycling drop-off, and celebrates the arts. In addition to the existing Martin Luther King (MLK) Charter School, residents continue to work for the opening of a public high school in the neighborhood. As envisioned, the school would build on the wetland-based curriculum of the MLK Charter School and serve as a hub for creating a "green" economy and job training in the Lower Ninth Ward. With the broad base of new community organizations in the Lower Ninth Ward, the neighborhoods have developed Lower 9th Ward Stakeholders Coalition to support the coordination of efforts.

CONCLUSION

This is just one snapshot into recovery of the Lower Ninth Ward. The article excludes many important facets of recovery, specifically an in-depth the discussion of the multitude of planning processes and the "right to return" and rebuild. However, highlighted in this narrow window focused on efforts around environment and sustainability are benefits of RBAs in community development that have been reflected in projects around the world: asset accumulation, capacity building, linkages among actors, and reduction of vulnerability [41] It was the devastation wrought by Hurricane Katrina that highlighted the structural causes of vulnerability and provided a valuable entry point for communities and the "state" to begin and build capacity to address imbalances of power and to enhance accountability.[42,43] The impact of the storm also forced residents to reconnect to the physical landscape of the city and recognize and deepen their understanding of the legal and policy frameworks, political decisions, and actors that have shaped this landscape. This case study also highlights the importance of going beyond traditional human rights-based frameworks that focus on the role of the state as "duty bearer." The power relationships that exist among individuals, community-based organizations, nongovernmental organizations, private entities, and the academy cannot be ignored as rights-based programs and practices are developed.

The case study also highlights challenges of implementing RBA's in the context of community redevelopment and environmental sustainability. Many of the efforts described focused on meeting "bricks and mortar" and social service needs and only indirectly used RBA's in implementation. Finding funding for long term community recovery programs specifically in post-disaster settings which incorporate or primarily use RBA's remains challenging. Sustained investment is often required to address long-standing structural inequalities and environmental degradation. At the same time, there are often limited resources available to meet "immediate" and short term relief needs. In addition, the development of strategies to use RBA's to address issues of natural resources management and climate change impacts continue to evolve.

On the ground, it is important to note that challenges remain. Population estimates suggest that only 4,000–5,000 residents currently live in the area; empty lots and blighted houses signal that displaced residents continue to struggle to return and the area remains vulnerable to flooding. Persistent worries over security and safety and a lack of access to public transportation, health services, and fresh products remain barriers to redevelopment.[44,45]

At the same time, the Lower Ninth Ward's vision focused on integrating climate change adaptation and mitigation; ecosystem services and human health; and the built environment continues to shape and support the development of innovative non-profit programming, community-based academic research, and state, federal, and local policies.

NOTES

[1]Schmit, W. D. (2009, December 7). Retrieved February 17, 2007, from http://bestof neworleans.com/gyrobase/Content?oid=oid%3A65844

[2]Foresti, M., Ludi, E., & Griffiths, R. (2007, November). *Human rights and livelihood approaches to poverty.* Retrieved April 17, 2010, from http://www.odi.org.uk/resources/download/1548.pdf

[3]Foresti, M., Ludi, E., & Griffiths, R. (2007, November). *Human rights and livelihood approaches to poverty.* Retrieved April 17, 2010, from http://www.odi.org.uk/resources/download/1548.pdf

[4]For a comprehensive physical, cultural, social, ethnic, and historical geography of New Orleans: Campanella, R. (2006). *Geographies of New Orleans: Urban fabrics before the storm.* Center for Louisiana Studies, University of Louisiana Lafayette.

[5]Campanella, R. (2006). *Geographies of New Orleans: Urban fabrics before the storm.* Center for Louisiana Studies, University of Louisiana Lafayette.

[6]For understanding of settlement patterns: Colten, C. (2005). *An unnatural metropolis: Wrestling New Orleans from nature.* Baton Rouge, LA: Louisiana State University Press.

[7]The Times Picayune. Retrieved February 21, 2010, http://www.nola.com/katrina/pages/110305/1103A01.pdf

[8]For greater understanding of this decision: Barry, J. (1998). *Rising tide: The Great Mississippi Flood of 1927 and How It Changed America*. Simon & Schuster.

[9]U.S. Geological Survey National Wetlands Research Center. 100+ Years of Land Change for Coastal Louisiana, Retrieved from http://www.nwrc.usgs.gov/upload/landloss8X11.pdf

[10]Louisiana Department of Natural Resources. (2009). Louisiana Coastal Facts. Retrieved March 5, 2010 from http://dnr.louisiana.gov/crm/coastalfacts.asp

[11]Day, J., Shaffer, G. P., Britsch, L. D., Reed, D. J., Hawes, S. R., & Cahoon, D. Pattern and process of land loss in Mississippi Delta: A spatial and temporal analysis of wetland habitat change. *Estuaries*, 23(4), 425–438.

[12]Greater New Orleans Community Data Center. Planning District 8. Retrieved February 23, 2010–March 1, 2010, from http://www.gnocdc.org/orleans/8/index.html

[13]H3 Studio Inc, Williams Architects, Facilitative Leadership Team/UNOP. (2006). Unified New Orleans Plan: District 8. Retrieved December 10, 2009, from http://unifiedneworleansplan.com/home3/districts/8/plans/

[14]Greater New Orleans Community Data Center. Planning District 8. Retrieved February 23, 2010- March 1, 2010, from http://www.gnocdc.org/orleans/8/index.html

[15]H3 Studio Inc, Williams Architects, Facilitative Leadership Team/UNOP. (2006). Unified New Orleans Plan: District 8. Retrieved December 10, 2009, from http://unifiedneworleansplan.com/home3/districts/8/plans/

[16]Greater New Orleans Community Data Center. Planning District 8. Retrieved February 23, 2010- March 1, 2010, from http://www.gnocdc.org/orleans/8/index.html

[17]Campanella, R. (2006). *Geographies of New Orleans: Urban fabrics before the storm*. Center for Louisiana Studies, University of Louisiana Lafayette.

[18]For details of impact, relief, recovery, and rebuilding: The Times Picayune, Katrina Archive. Retrieved January 2010, from http://www.nola.com/katrina/

[19]New York Times. Katrina's Diaspora. Retrieved February 18, 2010, from www.nytimes.com/imagepages/2005/10/.../20051002diaspora_graphic.htm

[20]The Times Picayune. Retrieved February 1, 2010, from http://www.timespicayune.com/

[21]For history of MR GO, see Freudenberg, W., Gramling, R., Laska, S. & Erikson, K. (2009). *Catastrophe in the making: The engineering of Katrina and disasters of tomorrow*, Washington, DC: Sheerwater Publishing.

[22]For description of storm, see Schlefstein, M. (2006). *Path of destruction: The devastation of New Orleans and the coming age of superstorms*. New York: Little Brown.

[23]The Times Picayune. Retrieved February 7, 2010, from http://www.nola.com/katrina/graphics/wide.ssf?/katrina/pdf/katrina_dead_122005.pdf?600

[24]Foresti, M., Ludi, E., & Griffiths, R. (2007). *Human Rights and Livelihood Approaches to Poverty*. Retrieved April 17, 2010, from Poverty-wellbing.net

[25]Neighborhood attendance records.

[26]Personal conversations.

[27]Personal conversations.

[28]Personal conversations.

[29]For connections between environmental justice and climate change: Park, A. (2009). *Everybody's movement: Environmental justice and climate change*, Washington, DC: Environmental Support Center.

[30]For description of Greening the Ghetto: Sustainable South Bronx. Retrieved from http://www.ssbx.org/; TED: Ideas Worth Spreading. Retrieved from http://www

.ted.com/talks/majora_carter_s_tale_of_urban_renewal.html; For Green For All. Retrieved from http://www.greenforall.org/

[31]U.S. Green Building Council. Retrieved February 13, 2010, from http://www.usgbc .org/Docs/News/CGI%200909.pdf

[32]Global Green. Retrieved March 5, 2010, http://www.globalgreen.org/neworleans/

[33]Preservation Resource Center. Retrieved March 4, 2010, from http://www.prcno.org/ programs/operationcomeback/preserving-green.php

[34]Personal conversation with author.

[35]Mowbray, R. (2009, September 11). Energy smart plan passes key New Orleans city council committee. Retrieved March 5, 2010, from http://www.nola.com/business/ index.ssf/2009/09/energy_smart_passes_key_counci.html

[36]Nelson Institute of Environmental Studies. (2009). *The Bayou Bienvenue Wetland Triangle: Issues affecting the restoration of a former cypress-tupelo swamp Lower Ninth Ward, New Orleans.* Water Resources Management Practicum, University of Wisconsin Madison.

[37]Help Holy Cross. Retrieved March 6, 2010, from http://www.helpholycross.org/

[38]Economic Empowerment and Global Learning Project. (2010, January). Lafayette College "Carbon Model: Lower 9th Ward, New Orleans" Draft Report.

[39]Our School at Blair Grocery. Retrieved from http://schoolatblairgrocery.blogspot.com/; Help Holy Cross: Lower Nine's Guerilla Garden Project. Retrieved from http://www .helpholycross.org/2009/09/guerilla-garden-project.html; Bringing Fresh Food to the Lower 9th Ward. Retrieved March 4, 2010) http://www.enterprisecommunity.org/ local_work/documents/chase_st_claude_ave.pdf

[40]People Home . . . Business Strong: Lower 9th Ward neighborhood Empowerment Network Association. Retrieved April 17, 2010, from http://www.9thwardnena.org/

[41]Foresti, M., Ludi, E., & Griffiths, R. (2007, November). *Human Rights and Livelihood Approaches to Poverty.* Retrieved April 17, 2010, from Poverty-wellbing.net

[42]Schlefstein, M (2009, November 19). *Corps' operation of MR-GO doomed homes in St. Bernard, Lower 9th Ward, judge rules.* Retrieved April 25, 2010, from http://www .nola.com/hurricane/index.ssf/2009/11/post_16.html

[43]For landmark decision to for IAHCR to take jurisdiction over a long-standing environmental racism in the United States. See http://www.ehumanrights.org/docs/ IACHR_Ruling-Mossville_petition_admissible.pdf (Accessed April 26, 2010.)

[44]Greater New Orleans Data Center. Retrieved March 7, 2010, from http://www.gnocdc .org/RecoveryByNeighborhood/index.html

[45]Needs Assessments from numerous planning assessments and community meetings.

CHAPTER 20

Rights-Based Approaches in Conflict Settings: Examples From Nepal and Israel/Palestine

Neil Arya, Judy Kitts, and Khagendra Dahal

INTRODUCTION

The term *rights* elicits a sense of obligation; a sense that someone, somewhere must be held accountable for the denial of basic human rights. In the preamble of the United Nations' Universal Declaration of Human Rights, members pledged to achieve the promotion of universal respect for, and observance of, human rights and fundamental freedoms, but how does this play out in conflict-affected countries? Who protects? Who promotes? Who provides?

Echoing the values of the United Nations' Declaration of Human Rights, the rights-based approach (RBA) starts from the ethical position that all people are entitled to a certain standard of living. It recognizes individuals as active rights holders and removes aspects of charity from the realm of development by emphasizing rights and responsibilities. A right is a basic entitlement or claim, in which an individual can assert and call on another person or institution to uphold that right.

As defined by the United Nations Commission on Human Rights, RBA focuses on raising levels of accountability by identifying rights holders and the corresponding duty bearers. In examining the role of duty bearers, RBA highlights not only our negative obligations—to abstain from violations—but also our positive obligations—to protect, promote, and provide. These three Ps are central to duty bearers, whether they be the state, the community, or nongovernmental organizations (NGOs). However, many players continue to dismiss their role, preferring to turn a blind eye instead of taking direct action. This sense of duty is what a RBA seeks to create. In using the language of rights, it automatically raises the question of accountability.

In this chapter, we examine two examples of conflict-affected countries where health organizations are committed to working for human rights in the absence of government action: Nepal and Israel/Palestine.

NEPAL PHYSICIANS FOR SOCIAL RESPONSIBILITY

Nepal, a landlocked country situated between India and China, has, until recently, been a Hindu hereditary monarchy. A 10-year armed insurgency waged by an underground Maoist Communist Party of Nepal (CPN) ended following a peace agreement between the democratic political parties and the Maoists and the resultant elected Constituent Assembly voted, by a whopping majority, to oust the monarchy and establish a federal republic system of governance in Nepal.

The new republic inherited a health system that failed to deliver the people's basic health care needs. Nepal's health indicators are among the poorest in the world. The infant mortality rate (IMR) is 46 per 1,000 live births, life expectancy of 63 years at birth, and an adult literacy rate of 55.2 per 100 (United Nations Development Programme [UNDP], 2007/2008). According to the same sources, the United States has an IMR of 6.3 per 1,000, life expectancy of 78 years at birth, and an adult literacy rate of 99 per 100. People in general have been deprived of minimal basic health care with inadequate health care facilities and meager resources (Maskey, 2004). Some reasons underlying the poor health indicators in Nepal include inequitable distribution of available resources, rampant corruption, and the bloody insurgency that has disrupted the tenuous health care infrastructure in Nepal (Singh, Dahal, & Mills, 2005).

History of Physician Involvement With Human Rights in Nepal

The documented and substantial involvement of Nepali physicians in defending human rights and helping to establish democracy dates back to 1991 (Maskey, 2004). That year, physicians and other health professionals, under the leadership of prominent physicians affiliated with Physicians for Social Responsibility, Nepal (PSRN; including Professor Mathura Shrestha, Dr. Mahesh Maskey, Dr. Arun Sayemi, and Dr. Bharat Pradhan) worked to build the movement to oust the partyless Panchayat system, which was developed and supported by the monarchy, and replace it with a multiparty democracy (Ogura, 2001). Thus, from the planning phase, physicians were involved (Adams, 1998).

Nepal's record of human rights deteriorated when the Maoist CPN launched a war against the existing establishment and the latter retaliated (Singh, Dahal, & Mills, 2005). When political demonstrations were outlawed and the government employed dumdum bullets as "nonlethal means to disperse the crowds," the doctors' critique assisted in forcing the government to withdraw the bullets from use (Adams, 1998). They organized a network of clinics and hospitals in the hideouts of the capital, Kathmandu, to provide treatment to a large number of wounded demonstrators (Maskey, 2004). The medical community of Nepal also was an integral part of Professional Alliance for Peace and Democracy (PAPAD) that coordinated the activities of civil societies in the country to defend the rights of the people and their respective professions.

When the democratic movement emerged in 2006, physicians were part of the civil society response, playing a decisive role in establishing peace and republican system in Nepal (Dahal & Singh, 2008). This movement was supported by the then-underground CPN, which was waging a violent war that had already killed more than 13,000 people and left more than 100,000 injured and displaced (Gautam, 2007). Besides supporting the movement and issuing press releases protesting the government's suppression of peaceful demonstrations, the physicians were involved in the immediate treatment of the injured, likely decreasing the number of casualties (Dahal & Singh, 2008). They defended the right to freedom, the right to peaceful assembly, the right to medical treatment, the right to walk freely, and the right to expression and opinion.

The Nepal Medical Association (NMA), an umbrella organization of Nepali physicians, coordinated the movement throughout the country through their branches in different zones of Nepal (Dahal & Singh, 2008). When communication was not possible because of the disruption of mobile phone services by the government and the imposition of daytime curfews in major cities of Nepal, activities were organized at the local level, where the communication was easier and well planned.

The Role of Outsiders

Substantial support from international health and human rights groups and other participating individuals in the movement was critical. When leaders of the movement were arrested, PSRN and allied physicians mobilized an international network to pressure the government diplomatically. Dr. Sonal Singh, a United States–based physician of Nepali extraction, helped design an e-petition, which was later signed by almost 3,000 international doctors, medical students, other health professionals, and human rights defenders (Pandey, 2006), to help release the Nepali physicians and medical students detained during the peaceful demonstrations. Singh also authored an open letter to the *Lancet* demanding the safe and immediate release of the Nepali colleagues (Singh, Arya, Mills, Holtz & Westberg, 2006). The International Physicians for the Prevention of Nuclear War (IPPNW), the federation of the physicians working to abolish nuclear weapons, supported its Nepali affiliate by writing letters to Nepalese diplomatic representatives throughout the world (Dahal & Singh, 2008).

Nepal After the "Victory"

After the signing of the comprehensive peace accord between the Maoists and the government in 2006, the 10-year Maoists' insurgency stopped and a consensus government formed to include the Maoists and other democratic parties. The Constituent Assembly to draft the constitution is inclusive, including around one-third representation of females as well as representation of people from all walks of life. The goal is to ensure that their rights are upheld and to prove that "ballots are more powerful than the bullets." This movement has set an example for the groups and rebels waging violent wars in different parts of the world, reflecting that if they work peacefully, people may support them and help them move into the political mainstream.

Because of their commitment and participation in the movement to establish democracy and rule of law, the Nepali physicians were lauded as "doctors for democracy" (Adams, 1998). They have worked to enshrine "health as a human right" in the Interim Constitution of Nepal 2007 (Dahal & Singh, 2008), "every citizen shall have the right to get basic health service free of cost from the State as provided for in the law" (Interim Constitution of Nepal 2007, part 3, art. 16 (2)). The meaning of this, however, is yet to be actualized.

In the evolving scenario, the role of physicians in Nepal has changed. Now, they work in government positions drafting new policies, advising ministers, and making and implementing plans to improve the health status of the Nepali people. The first elected president of Nepal, Dr. Ram Baran Yadav is a physician and a democratic intellectual from a "backward community" in the marginalized Terai region. With several physicians in the decision-making positions, people can be hopeful that they can work for what they have long been advocating for, to ensure the implementation of "health as a human right" in Nepal.

The Connection Between Peace, Health, and Human Rights

The doctors' participation in the movements to establish peace and democracy can be seen as occurring beyond their professional mandate. They identified the root causes of war and conflict, which in Nepal's case were lack of democracy and rule of law. They correctly identified that the lack of equal rights to the indigenous and "backward" communities, negligence of the state toward equal access to the state's resources for all citizens, and rampant corruption, which were the main causes behind the escalation of conflict and worked well before it manifested (Dahal & Singh, 2008).

Physicians in Nepal have worked to defend various forms of human rights of the people and established health as a human right, applying the principle of the collective benefit, without losing health as a basic individual human right. It is important to understand that they think strategically by creating a structure, advocating for their patients, mobilizing the community, and developing international support, they were able to achieve their goals through nonviolent political means.

Opposing the corrupt and undemocratic regime, making people aware of their rights, speaking out against the government atrocities and violations of international human rights law, and working to safeguard the physicians' right to treat people irrespective of their race, religion, and political belief were central to the Nepali doctors' efforts.

In "Peace Through Health" terms, this may be seen as primary prevention of violence and even of poor health, because corruption and lack of democratic rights are considered as root or enabling causes of structural violence, the growing disparities and dividing gaps between haves and have-nots, and the substandard health situation of the country (Adams, 1998). Doctors feel that with peace established, substantial changes can be brought to improve the health of the people through the formulation and effective implementation of right and people-oriented policies (Dahal & Singh, 2008). As the conflict comes to the end, more resources can be allocated to education, health care, and development projects. In the postconflict situation, the donor agencies are willing to invest more in rehabilitation process and development projects that engage people in sustaining peace. Thus, reciprocally in Nepal's case, peace may have been achieved through health and health may be achieved through peace.

Physicians in Nepal operated under a system, whereby a gap in the provision of health services led them to assume the rights and responsibilities typically reserved for the state. This meant that physicians undertook traditionally state-controlled roles as they served to protect the rights of Nepali citizens, promoted their security, and provided for their health needs.

PHYSICIANS FOR HUMAN RIGHTS-ISRAEL

In the occupied Palestinian territories (oPt), the health situation has deteriorated to unprecedented levels and the lack of state action has created a similar occurrence to that of Nepal, whereby physicians have found themselves not only providing health care, but also protecting and promoting the right to health.

The World Health Organization reports that in the oPt, the under-5 mortality rate is 25.3 per 1,000 (higher in the Gaza Strip than the West Bank—28.8 and 22.9 per 1,000 live births, respectively) and the maternal mortality rate is 6.2 per 100,000 births, much better than Nepal, but significantly worse than in Israel (World Health Organization, 2008). In fact, since the beginning of 2000, 68 women in labor were delayed at checkpoints or were refused permission to reach medical facilities (United Nations Population Fund, 2007). In addition, the fear of such hardships has led a significant number of Palestinian women to give birth at home, with an increase by 8.2% in home deliveries (United Nations Economic and Social Commission for Western Asia, 2007). To complicate this matter, in the oPt, there are only 1.6 physicians and 1.3 hospital beds per 1,000 people (Palestinian Central Bureau of Statistics [PCBS], 2009).

The social determinants of health in the oPt are equally dismal. Poverty in the Gaza Strip has risen to an unprecedented level, affecting 80% of households; unemployment in the Gaza Strip rose from 30% in 2005 to 38% in the third quarter of 2007 (World Health Organization, 2008). Rising poverty and unemployment has had a devastating effect on school attendance across the oPt. In the 2005–2006 school year, the number of students whose families could not afford the NIS 50 ($11) school fee doubled from 29,000–56,000 (Palestine Monitor, 2008).

In addition, the extensive system of checkpoints and barriers with arbitrary closure, the construction of the security fence, and random destruction and seizure of property, also serve to limit the right of Palestinians to shelter, mobility, health, and safety.

Unfortunately, this bleak picture is not exclusive to Palestinians in the oPt; similar conditions exist among other marginalized populations within Israel. Two of the authors (Judy Kitts and Neil Arya) have studied the social determinants of health within Israel, exploring the complete physical, mental, and social well-being of Bedouin Arabs, migrant workers, refugees and asylum seekers, Ethiopian Jews, Sephardic Jews, and ultra-Orthodox Jews. Findings suggest that other marginalized populations within Israel are experiencing similar disparities in care. For example, Bedouin Arabs in the unrecognized villages of the Negev are not connected to the national water grid, and many inhabitants are forced to obtain their drinking water from water access points located several kilometers from their villages via improvised plastic hose connections or by transporting the water in unhygienic metal containers by vehicle or donkey (Negev Coexistence Forum for Civil Equality [NCFCE], 2006).

Historical Background

From the start of the Israeli occupation in 1967, the Israeli authorities assumed responsibility for the provision of basic health, education, and other municipal services. In 1993, with the implementation of the Oslo Accords, these responsibilities were handed over to the Palestinian Authority, which is now on the brink of collapsing as it struggles with a lack of resources and a divided Palestinian population. Given Israel's retention of control over the territories— its borders and land—and many aspects of the lives of its inhabitants, according to international law, it must remain responsible for the health in the oPt. According to the Geneva Conventions, an occupying force has a duty to ensure the food and medical supplies of the population, as well as maintain hospitals and other medical services, "to the fullest extent of the means available to it" (International Committee of the Red Cross, 2005, arts. 55 & 56).

Medical ethics, as epitomized by the Hippocratic Oath, places an obligation to treat those in need at an individual level, impartially. However, in reaction to such blatant violations of health and human rights, not just at an individual but general, systemic population health level, two simple questions remain—Who *is* accountable? Who *should* respond? For physicians, there is a corollary question—when the state fails to act, is there a responsibility, as duty bearers, to provide medical or health services and to act to change the situation?

With Israel denying its responsibilities and the Palestinian Authority unraveling, the right to health including the availability, accessibility, and quality of health facilities, services, and goods in the oPt is deteriorating. The failure to meet these basic human rights has resulted in a precarious impact on the health status of people living in the oPt, and the responsibility to provide, promote, and protect the rights of Palestinians has fallen in the hands of civil society, including Physicians for Human Rights-Israel (PHR-I), as a proliferation of international donors and NGOs struggle to fill the gap in the provision of health services.

How Physicians for Human Rights-Israel Works

Established in 1988, PHR-I is composed of Israeli and Palestinian physicians and human rights activists. In the absence of government action, PHR-I works to *protect* the rights of Palestinians living in the oPt by fighting the injustices at the Israeli Supreme Court of Justice, works to *promote* their rights in Israel and around the world through the discovery and dissemination of facts, and works to *provide* immediate health care services through its mobile health clinics and training and educational services. Not surprisingly, PHR-I is recognized as a model of the RBA not only for its programs that highlight its role as a duty bearer but also by drawing attention to the lack of state accountability.

PHR-I recognizes that the medical community has a clear obligation to advocate for the realization of every person's universal right to health, medical treatment, and proper living conditions (PHR-I, 2007); however, it also maintains that Israel has effective control over the oPt.

Although the state is ultimately accountable for the provision of rights,[1] including the right to health, in recent years, the role of local NGOs has significantly increased as Israel has shirked its responsibility in the face of international law.[2]

PHR-I is one of the many actors working to combat the systemic harm inflicted on the lives of Palestinians by improving accessibility to health care, yet members of PHR-I state that their involvement with the organization has less to do with its success[3] and more to do with obligation. One member explains, "We do this work because we can't do otherwise, not because there is an evidence base . . . We do it because we are politically and morally obliged" (J. Kitts, personal communication).

It is evident that members of PHR-I recognize their role as duty bearers, yet they also question whether or not their work is directly or indirectly supplementing the responsibilities of the state, thereby allowing the government to shirk its responsibilities under international humanitarian law. International and local organizations must then consider whether they do more harm than good when working in sensitive conflict situations Collaborative for Development Action).

For example, in June 2005, 20 Palestinian organizations called for a boycott against cooperation with Israeli institutions and NGOs that were complicit with the occupation (Union of Health Workers et al., 2005). The call put forth the argument that it was not enough for Israeli organizations to promote dialogue and collaboration between Palestinians and Israelis, rather they:

> may want to consider becoming actively involved in Israeli or joint Israeli–Palestinian activities aimed at ending Israeli military occupation of Palestinian land, the removal of closures, checkpoints, siege and the Apartheid Wall, among other manifestations of the root cause of ill health: the occupation. (Union of Health Workers, 2005)

The Role of Outsiders

Outsiders who seek to use health as a connector in conflict situations must be cautious. Though their voices shedding light on the situation for the outside world is often invaluable, when they strive to protect, promote, and provide, they may become party to the conflict, being perceived as unwelcome by many, particularly if they act in what they consider solidarity with those they see as oppressed. This can have legal consequences for them and sometimes endanger the very people they seek to protect.

What happens when outsiders try to be above politics? The Canada International Scientific Exchange Program (CISEPO; Skinner et al., 2005) works from a Peace Through Health perspective, trying to be above the politics of the Middle East. As such, in developing and implementing health sector cooperative activities in the Middle East between Arabs and Israelis, CISEPO has been criticized for focusing solely on individual human relations and failing to recognize the social and political realities of the conflict (Jabbour, 2003). CISEPO, and other like-minded initiatives, may help to create and enhance opportunities for cooperation, but their failure to address the systemic inequality of conditions or justice issues may have the opposite effect (Arya, 2004). A middle ground might be seen in Healing Across the Divides, an American nonprofit organization, which uses a health RBA to peace building by increasing awareness on the part of policy makers regarding the obstacles hindering the improvement in health of both Israelis and Palestinians (Healing Across the Divides, 2009).

Physicians for Human Rights-Israel and Rights-Based Approaches

PHR-I's activities demonstrate the organization's commitment to extending altruism to "out groups" as it pushes "beyond traditional in-group identities, challenging and extending the boundaries of health care" (MacQueen & Santa Barbara, 2000, p. 294), yet members of PHR-I continue to remind themselves and others that "their work is not a substitute for a proper community-based medical system that is planned and funded by the governing authority" (PHR-I, 2010, General Information section, para. 5). How then should duty bearers respond to a state's inaction?

PHR-I has responded by moving beyond the provision of immediate health services to identifying, uncovering, and addressing the root causes of these health inequities. PHR-I's political activism, representing Palestinians before the Israeli Supreme Court, writing petitions, writing reports (in English, Arabic, and Hebrew), organizing demonstrations, and maintaining contact with the almost completely cutoff Gaza to try to advocate for their rights, is what allows the organization to gain credibility to work closely with Palestinian partners. As the president and founder, Ruchama Marton states:

> I think that everyone, including doctors, need to be politicized. Otherwise, it is a kind of mild, blind, non-affective activity. Even though a person can come home at night and tell himself how wonderful he was today, it is not very helpful to the dynamics of the whole thing. The organization and each and everyone in the organization must be outside the consensus, which is not an easy place to be. (J. Kitts, personal communication)

Central to RBA is the premise that people have inalienable and indivisible rights that cannot be addressed with quick fixes, rather it requires slow tactical steps that go beyond surface problems, taking up deep-rooted questions and challenging all parties for answers. PHR-I recognizes this inextricable link between health and politics and has likened to the realization of health to the end of the occupation:

> Our vision is to end the occupation . . . It won't help even if we bring 500 people out of Gaza for medical treatment in Israeli hospitals. It won't help them afterward. It is just a band-aid. The system in [the oPt] will remain the same. (J. Kitts, personal communication, November, 2007)

The fact that the basic health rights of Israeli citizens are also overlooked may actually serve to create a sense of solidarity as Palestinians and Israelis alike come to recognize that the state of Israel has an obligation to provide basic health rights.

CONCLUSION

The capacities of health professionals to act when states abdicate their responsibilities differ in the contexts of Israel/Palestine and Nepal. However, in both countries, physicians continue to document and speak out against injustices, engage in diplomacy with political leaders, write petitions on behalf of marginalized populations, and treat patients impartially; they have done this all while accepting the severe consequences of these actions.

RBA proposes that a right is a basic entitlement, in which an individual can assert and call on another person or institution to uphold that right. Although we continue to struggle with the questions, who protects, who promotes, and who provides, we find duty bearers taking various shapes from everyday citizens who actively participate in human rights organizations to physicians who uphold the Hippocratic Oath as a framework for service. These duty bearers recognize that although international humanitarian law holds states accountable for the provision of human rights, inaction cannot be met with further inaction, or it will only serve to legitimate the system that continues to place obstacles in the way of human rights, whether it is concrete walls of separation or economic and social barriers.

Could such approaches work in other contexts? Would this help in the case of genocide as in Rwanda, or unaccountable regimes with great power as in Burma (Myanmar) today? This is less certain. As such, this would become the responsibility of the international community to act to protect vulnerable populations.

Systemic issues are often the main cause of intractable conflicts, and central to minimizing conflict is the ability of duty bearers to transform the structures and dynamics that create the foundation for such injustice, and being above, but not beyond, politics unites the doctors of Israel/Palestine and Nepal.

REFERENCES

Adams, V. (1998). *Doctors for democracy: Health professionals in the Nepal Revolution*. Cambridge, UK: Cambridge University Press.

Arya, N. (2004) Peace Through Health I: Development and use of a working model. *Medicine, Conflict, and Survival, 20*(3), 242–257.

Collaborative for Development Action. *Do no harm: Development assistance and humanitarian aid in conflict*. Retrieved September 4, 2010, from http://www.cdainc.com/cdawww/project_profile.php?pid=DNH&pname=Do No Harm

Dahal, K., & Singh, S. (2008). *Role of health professionals in the Peace Through Health movement in Nepal*. Unpublished report, PHRI-PtH Program of McMaster University–Canada.

Gautam, B. (2007). *Maoist struggle: A period of insurgency*. Nepal: Martin Chautari.

Healing Across the Divides. (2009). *Healing across the divides*. Retrieved September 10, 2010, from http://www.healingdivides.org/

Interim Constitution of Nepal. (2007). Fundamental Rights, Part 3, Article 16 (2).

International Committee of the Red Cross. (2005). International humanitarian law - Treaties & documents. *Fourth Geneva Convention*, Articles 55 and 56. Retrieved September 10, 2010, from http://www.icrc.org/ihl.nsf/FULL/380?OpenDocument

Jabbour, S. (2003). Health and development in the Arab world: Which way forward? *British Medical Journal, 326*(7399), 1141–1143.

MacQueen, G., & Santa Barbara, J. (2000). Peace building through health initiatives. *British Medical Journal, 321*(7256), 293–296.

Maskey, M. (2004). Practicing politics as medicine writ large in Nepal. *Development*, 47(2), 122–130.

Negev Coexistence Forum for Civil Equality. (2006). *The Arab-Bedouins of the Naqab-Negev Desert in Israel*. Retrieved September 10, 2010, from http://www2.ohchr.org/english/bodies/cerd/docs/ngos/NCf-IsraelShadowReport.pdf

Ogura, K. (2001). *Kathmandu springs: A narrative of the people's movement in 1991*. Nepal: Himal Books.

Palestine Monitor. (2008). Palestine monitor factsheet: Children. Retrieved September 10, 2010, from http://www.palestinemonitor.org/spip/spip.php?article11

Palestinian Central Bureau of Statistics. (2009) *Special report on the 61th anniversary of the Nakba*. May 13, 2009. Retrieved September 10, 2010, from http://www.pcbs.gov.ps/Portals/_pcbs/PressRelease/nakba_61E.pdf

Pandey, K. (2006). Doctors in Nepal take part in democracy protests. *British Medical Journal*, 332(7547), 931.

PHR-I. (2010). About the mobile clinic. General information. Retrieved September 10, 2010, from http://www.phr.org.il/default.asp?PageID=136

Physicians for Human Rights-Israel. (2007). Information Booklet. Tel Aviv, Israel: Physicians for Human Rights.

Singh, S., Dahal, K., & Mills, E. (2005). Nepal's war on human rights: A summit higher than Everest. *International Journal for Equity in Health*, 4(9), 1186–1193.

Singh, S., Arya, N., Mills, E., Holtz, T., & Westberg, G. (2006). Free doctors and medical students detained in Nepal. *Lancet*, 367(9524), 1730.

Skinner, H., Abdeen, Z., Abdeen, H., Aber, P., Al-Masri, M., Attias, J., et al. (2005). Promoting Arab and Israeli cooperation: Peacebuilding through health initiatives. *Lancet*, 365(9466), 1274–1277.

Union of Health Work Committees, Union of Palestinian Medical Relief Committees, Central National Committee for Rehabilitation, Health Development Information Policy Institute, General Union of Palestinian Workers, General Union of Palestinian Charitable Societies, et al. (2005). [An open letter to the Palestinian and international community]. *Occupation Magazine*.

United Nations Development Programme. 2007/2008

United Nations Economic and Social Commission for Western Asia. (2007). Social and economic situation of Palestinian women. *Economic and Social Commission for Western Asia (ESCWA)*. Retrieved September 10, 2010, from http://www.escwa.un.org/information/publications/edit/upload/ecw-07-tp1-e.pdf

United Nations Population Fund. (2007). Checkpoints confound the risk of childbirth for palestinian women. May 15, 2007. Retrieved September 10, 2010, from http://www.unfpa.org/public/site/global/News/pid/310

World Health Organization. (2008, May 13). *Health conditions in the occupied Palestinian territory, including east Jerusalem, and in the occupied Syrian Golan*. Retrieved September 10, 2010, from http://www.reliefweb.int/rw/RWB.NSF/db900SID/EGUA-7EUNGW?OpenDocument

OTHER RESOURCES

Arya, N. (2007). Peace Through Health? In C. Webel & J. Galtung (Ed.), *Handbook of peace and conflict studies* (pp. 367–394). London: Routledge.

United Nations International Children's Emergency Fund. (2006). *Nepal statistics.* Retrieved from http://www.unicef.org/infobycountry/nepal_nepal_statistics.html

Yusuf, S., Anand, S., & MacQueen, G. (1998). Can medicine prevent war? Imaginative thinking shows that it might. *British Medical Journal, 317*(7174), 1669–1670. Retrieved September 10, 2010, from http://bmj.com/cgi/content/full/317/7174/1669

NOTES

[1] Under the International Covenant on Economic, Social and Cultural Rights, states are required to take immediate steps for the progressive realization of the rights concerned, thus a failure to take the necessary steps, or any retrogression, will flag a breach of the state's duties. Under the International Covenant on Civil and Political Rights, states are bound to respect the rights concerned, to ensure respect for them, and to take the necessary steps to put them into effect.

[2] The Israeli government maintains that it does not regard the fourth Geneva Convention as legally applicable to the West Bank and Gaza Strip. The Fourth Geneva Convention prescribes rules for an occupying power in relation to the inhabitants, who are described as "protected persons." Among other things, the rules prohibit the occupying power from willfully killing, ill-treating, or deporting protected persons. It also prohibits it from transferring its own civilian population into the territory and from carrying out reprisals or collective punishments.

[3] PHR-I has influenced the lives of thousands of Palestinians (in 2007, PHR-I's mobile health clinics treated 10,676 patients, of which 2,591 were children), but still struggles to have an effect on Israel's discriminatory policies.

CHAPTER 21

Rights-Based Approaches to Essential Medicines

Elvira Beracochea and David Lee

INTRODUCTION

On a hot and rainy afternoon, an illiterate mother in her midteens brings her firstborn, a 7-to-8-month-old girl, to a rural health center in an African country. After waiting for several hours, she gets to see the center's only nurse. This baby is the nurse's 76th patient that day. The mother says the baby has been hot for 2 days. The nurse would like to take the baby's temperature but she cannot because she does not have a thermometer. She touches the baby and confirms that the baby's skin is hot. Without doing a blood test, the nurse tells the mother that the baby probably has malaria and gives her a prescription. The mother takes her crying baby to the center's pharmacy. Through a narrow crack in the pharmacy window, the pharmacy dispenser tells her the center has run out of malaria medicines and suggests that she go to a private pharmacy. The mother asks how much it would cost, but the pharmacy dispenser has already closed the window to prevent the escape of the air conditioning and does not hear her question. The mother leaves.

No one will ever know whether the mother knew how to read, understood what was written on the prescription, went to the private pharmacy, was able to afford the treatment, actually bought it, or was able to give her baby the medicine in the correct dose and frequency. Did this baby girl survive or did she become another infant mortality statistic?

The Universal Declaration of Human Rights and the United Nations Convention on the Rights of the Child state that this infant's right to access health care. However, these rights cannot be fulfilled if medicines are not available or are used incorrectly.

THE RIGHT TO MEDICINE AS A COMPONENT OF THE RIGHT TO HEALTH

Access to safe, effective, affordable, and quality medicines is a fundamental element of the right to health. General Comment 14 on Article 12 of the International Covenant on Economic, Social and Cultural Rights states that the right to health includes access to facilities, goods, and services (see Figure 21.1) and that acts of omission, such as failure to offer vital medicines or prevent unsafe medicines from being marketed, constitute a violation of the right to health.

In many developing countries, seeing a health worker would seem enough to fulfill the government's responsibility to respect, protect, and fulfill the right to health of its people. However, as shown in the story earlier, the fact that neither the nurse nor the dispenser explained the treatment or helped the mother figure out a way to obtain the medicine are acts of omission that voided the entire interaction, put a baby's life at risk, and wasted the mother's and nurse's time. In addition, the government (the duty bearer) made an investment in facilities and staff that do not have the willingness and/or the

FIGURE 21.1 Article 12 of General Comment 14 of the International Covenant of Economics, Social and Cultural Rights: The right to the highest attainable standard of health.

Article 12.2 (d). The right to health facilities, goods and services (General Comment 14, United Nations, 2000)

17. "The creation of conditions which would assure to all medical service and medical attention in the event of sickness" (art. 12.2 [d]), both physical and mental, includes the provision of equal and timely access to basic preventive, curative, rehabilitative health services and health education; regular screening programmes; appropriate treatment of prevalent diseases, illnesses, injuries and disabilities, preferably at community level; **the provision of essential drugs**; and appropriate mental health treatment and care. A further important aspect is the improvement and furtherance of participation of the population in the provision of preventive and curative health services, such as the organization of the health sector, the insurance system and, in particular, participation in political decisions relating to the right to health taken at both the community and national levels.

---

equipment to diagnose or treat according to quality standards. Unfortunately, this futile patient encounter occurs every day in many health centers around the world, and it is up to us as public health professionals to change it.

In the United States, the picture may be a bit different but the outcome sometimes is the same: poor quality of care and health deterioration. Consider the following scenarios: An uninsured newly diagnosed patient with diabetes wonders how he will afford his medication for the rest of his life; an asthmatic child, whose single parent has just been laid off, has an attack and is taken to the emergency room because the family cannot afford his chronic treatment; and a woman recently diagnosed with lupus is forced to stop her treatment after her insurance company informs her that it will no longer cover her medicines because the lupus was a preexisting condition.

This chapter will discuss three main concepts for implementing a rights-based approach to improve the supply of medicines: the need for essential medicines; the need for an effective supply system; and the rational use of medicine.

ESSENTIAL MEDICINES

Since 1977, the World Health Organization (WHO) has disseminated an essential medicine list (EML)—a list of scientifically proven medicines that are selected by an expert committee. Now in its 16th edition, the EML uses generic medicine names only and is available worldwide. WHO has developed guidelines so that expert committees can be formed at the country level; thus the WHO model is adapted and updated by individual countries based on their unique epidemiological needs. WHO evaluates not only the scientific evidence for the medicines, but also the pharmacoeconomic criteria to ensure that selected medications offer the best value for the money, which is equally important (Flynn, Hollis, & Palmedo, 2009). A children's EML started to be disseminated in 2007, which is especially fortunate because medicines for children are particularly scarce (Robertson, Forte, & Trapsida, 2009). Also an interagency list of essential medicines for reproductive health is available.

EFFECTIVE SUPPLY SYSTEM

An effective supply system includes the selection, procurement, distribution, and use of medication. Care should be provided by trained, accredited, and efficient providers. Sustainable financing strategies are needed to fund all these activities. Prescribers and dispensers need to work as a team with their patients and must be empowered to suggest and oversee improvements of each function in the supply system to achieve the best health outcomes.

Using a rights-based approach, various stakeholders play important roles in the implementation of these functions. They include the following:

- The *right holder* is the patient (or, if a minor, his or her guardian) and is the ultimate user of the medicine. Ideally, the patient should be informed, aware of his or her rights, and willing and able to ask questions about whether the medicine is required, its effects, how to best take it, and for how long.

- The *provider* includes the public or private prescriber (usually a doctor or nurse) and the dispenser (a pharmacist or pharmacy assistant in developed countries, or a trained dispenser in most developing countries). Providers may represent the government; if so, they play the duty bearer's role. Alternately, they may be intermediaries who advise and educate the patient about the best treatment choices. In such cases, they are *intermediary users* because they decide what medicine the patient (the final user) needs.

- The *duty bearer* is the government that has the responsibility of respecting, protecting, and fulfilling the right to health of all its citizens. Governments usually appoint an agency that is in charge of ensuring the safety, efficacy, and (in some cases) efficiency of medicines. In the United States, the Food and Drug Administration (FDA) fulfills this duty. City and county governments are usually in charge of procuring medicines for their public clinics. Selection of approved medicines usually follow well-defined criteria in developed countries. In Australia, for instance, states have formulary committees that approve medicines based on their cost-effectiveness (Walkom, Robertson, Newby, & Pillay, 2006). Many developing countries now have medicine regulatory agencies. In addition, developed country donors sometimes share in the responsibility of ensuring medicine safety quality and availability for developing countries. For example, the United States Agency for International Development (USAID) provides antimalarials, antiretrovirals, and contraceptives to millions of people in developing countries every year.

- *Drug manufacturers* have the duty to follow government regulations and good manufacturing practices (GMP) to ensure the safety and efficacy and quality of their products. Enforcement of this duty is in the hands of *procurement agencies* that must inspect manufacturing plants and assure the quality of the products they purchase;

and regulatory agencies that have the responsibility to monitor product quality in the market place.

- The task of financing medicines may be handled by employers (who pay insurance premiums), insurance companies, and governments (as in the case of Medicare and Medicaid in the United States and the national health systems in the United Kingdom). It may also be managed by parastatal agencies (such as, for example, the Philippine Health Insurance Corporation). In developed countries, insurance companies and government agencies have increased negotiating power and can obtain medicines at considerably lower prices than retail. In most developing countries, on the other hand, patients are left to their own resources; and have to pay proportionally higher retail prices than patients in developed ones. For many patients in developing countries, unregulated medicine prices result in catastrophic out-of-pocket expenditures. Community insurance schemes and revolving medicine funds have emerged to help reduce this risk to poor patients.

General Comment 14 lists four interrelated essential elements to be applied to ensure the right to health and that are relevant to the supply of medicines: availability, accessibility, acceptability, and quality (see Figure 21.2.). In addition, the progressive improvement of a supply system using a rights-based approach requires ownership, accountability, and efficiency and affordability. We will examine each of these concepts over the following pages.

Availability: An effective supply system requires several processes to ensure that medicines are available to patients, including registration and selection of medicines, procurement of essential medicines in appropriate quantities according to epidemiologically defined disease patterns, distribution to health facilities, proper storage to ensure medicines do not get damaged, correct diagnosis and prescription,

FIGURE 21.2 Elements of a RBA in Supply Management

- *Availability*
- *Accessibility*
- *Acceptability*
- *Quality*
- *Ownership*
- *Accountability*
- *Efficiency and affordability*

and informed dispensing. Trained, deployed, and supervised managers and providers also need to be available to ensure the smooth functioning of each step in the process. For example, medicines need to be stored at the right temperature in a clean warehouse free from pests and rodents, secure to prevent break-ins, and inventoried and distributed according to date of expiry (First in–First out). The continuous and smooth operation of the supply system is what ensures the sustained availability of medicines. This is even more important for medications used in the management of lifelong chronic conditions such as AIDS and diabetes (Mendis et al., 2007).

Accessibility: The international legal framework of the right to health ensures the access to medicines, which can be even enforceable by courts (Hogerzeil, Samson, Casanovas, & Rahmani-Ocora, 2006). In the United States, having insurance increases access to medicines; many uninsured are left to their own resources if they do not meet Medicare criteria. In developing countries, revolving medicine funds such as the Bamako initiative have proven effective—even conflict settings such Sudan (Mohamed Ali, 2009).

Lack of unbiased medicine information makes it hard for prescribers to assess the benefits of new medications and therapies. For this reason, the role of professional organizations such as the American Society of Health Systems Pharmacists is essential to ensure access to proper treatment. However, access to medicines alone is not enough in chronic conditions such as diabetes. In such conditions, medications are only one part of a comprehensive primary care system that ensures the patient's best outcome by applying evidence-based case management (Beran, McCabe, & Yudkin, 2008).

Acceptability: Duty bearers need to ensure that patients can access their medicines independent of their ability to pay, race, gender, or other forms of discrimination.

Quality: The supply system needs to include processes to ensure that only medicines produced by registered manufacturers with acceptable and safe practices are marketed. Visits to manufacturing plants by trained inspectors or potential buyers are necessary to verify the information before awarding registration or tenders.

Ownership: It is essential that the supply system remain in the hands of those that ultimately have the responsibility to manage it every day and that supply processes are as simple as possible. In developing countries, duplication of efforts managed by multiple donors and the creation of parallel systems to support various programs make improvements unsustainable and waste resources. In developing and developed countries, ownership also means ensuring that the prescriber, dispenser, and patient all work within a system that empowers them to find the best treatment for the patient's condition. Informed treatment decisions should be made by the patient and medical providers according to scientific evidence, not by insurance companies or financial interests.

Accountability: Accounting for failures to finance, prescribe, or supply the right medicine to those that need it should be part of the country's surveillance or health information system. This is the only way to learn how to reduce the number of such negative events. Accountability for negative medicine side effects is also ensured through reporting and surveillance systems. Duty bearers and providers have a duty to report potential undesirable medicine effects to their patients. Knowledge of legal implications has demonstrated that also strengthens accountability to the patient for administering the right medicine and respect for the patient's right to self-determination (Griffith & Davies, 2003).

Efficiency and affordability: There are ways of ensuring the efficient supply of medicines and that essential medicines are affordable in every country. What is the use of having several brand names of acetaminophen? They all are the same. Having various brands in the market creates price competition that can lead to increased purchase savings. However, this benefit is lost if a hospital is required to purchase several brands of the same medicine. The use of generic medicines ensures that the lowest price is paid for medicines, independent of the brand, and that treatments remain affordable for all. Pharmacoeconomics is a growing field that assesses the cost of introducing a new medicine and avoids the waste "me too" brand names. Mendis et al. (2007) also suggest that prices are reduced by improving purchasing efficiency, eliminating taxes, and regulating markups. Pooled procurement also known as group purchasing programs that pool the purchasing power of several hospitals, provinces, and small island nations have demonstrated considerable savings of more than 30 and 40% (Huff-Rousselle & Burnett, 1996; Tordoff, Norris, & Reith, 2005).

RATIONAL USE OF MEDICINE

Medicines must need to be prescribed, dispensed, and used according to standard evidence-based treatment guidelines. Having access to the medicines is half of the solution; having the information to use medicine rationally is the other half. Many professional publications and online resources, include treatment guidelines; in addition, many countries have developed their own treatment guidelines for various levels of care. U.S. hospitals use diagnosis-related groups, which determine not only the most effective treatment but also how much hospitals will be paid for their services. In general, continuing education and use of job aids are essential to ensure that medicines are used correctly to minimize side effects and complications.

STRATEGIES FOR PROGRESSIVE IMPROVEMENT

Duty bearers need to implement a minimum of nine strategies to progressively develop and strengthen the supply systems and protect and serve right holders (Figure 21.3) and thus ensure the availability and rational use of medicines.

Ensuring the Availability of Medicines

The National Regulatory Agency and Good Manufacturing Practices and Quality Assurance

There are some functions that only governments can regulate and enforce. Ensuring that all medicines are registered and that manufactures meet GMP are two such regulatory functions. Duty bearers need to ensure that manufacturers (both public and private owned) are responsible and accountable for the consequences of the medicines they produce. A GMP certificate

FIGURE 21.3 Selected Proven and Effective Pharmaceutical Management Practices to Ensure the Right to Health

Ensure Access and Availability:
1. National regulatory agency and good manufacturing practices
2. The Essential Medicine List
3. Global Alliance for Vaccines and Immunisation (GAVI)
4. Green Light Committee
5. The Global Fund
Ensure Rational Use:
6. Therapeutic committees
7. Children's doses and presentations
8. Pharmacies and prescriptions
9. Standard treatment guidelines to prevent antimicrobial resistance

asserts that a manufacturer does not produce counterfeit or substandard medicines. Counterfeit medicines are still a widespread problem that duty bearers need to address (Caudron et al., 2008). Those in charge of procurement need to request a certificate of registration and of having met GMP.

Regulatory agencies also need to share information about undesirable side effects; these are compiled in a list of medicines that have been banned, restricted, or not approved. The WHO[1] publishes this list and governments should ensure that medicines used in their countries are not included in the list. (As an aside, one of the medicines on this list is metamizole [Dipyrone], an analgesic that has been demonstrated to cause agranulocytosis, a blood disorder. However, the authors have personal experience that this medicine is still used for the treatment of fever in many countries, even in children.)

Weak medicine regulatory agencies may cost lives. To address this problem, WHO is promoting regional harmonized efforts (Azatyan, 2008) to disseminate technical requirements, establish a common framework for joint medicine evaluations, and develop a shared information system that would strengthen regulatory capacity and oversight by developing nations.

The Essential Medicine List

The infant who did not get its malaria treatment at the beginning of this chapter is the result of a long sequence of unfortunate events that started when the country's government did not anticipate the needs of its citizens and did not procure the right quantities of the right medicines and/or did not distribute them in a timely manner to the health facilities. Not procuring the right medicines may be partly caused by not having a prioritized and updated list of essential medicines. An EML is essential to a rights-based approach in medicine supply (Hogerzeil, 2006). Many developing and developed countries use an EML to prioritize procurement of medicines and to determine levels of use (e.g., which medicines can only be used by specialists or hospital care providers). Australia's cost–benefit criteria for medicine selection is another example of using the EML to avoid offering multiple medicines that have the same effect and therefore no additional benefit.

There is a significant gap between the access to medicines on one hand and the pharmaceutical companies' concerns over their intellectual property on the other. Galvao (2005) describes how in Brazil, the government's concern for AIDS patients led to the first universal policy of free access to antiretrovirals as an inspiration for other governments to follow. Progress toward narrowing the gap between the right to access to medicines and intellectual property rights is still slow. Academic institutions involved in pharmaceutical research can ameliorate the gap (Sampat, 2009).

Benchmarking win–win solutions that allow for incentives in research and development while protecting the right to health need to be developed (Musungu, 2006).

In the United States, there is no national EML or generic medicine name policy unfortunately. To improve availability and access, the health care reform bill of 2010 included three main cost-containment measures that are hoped to promote the access to medicines and reduce over medication:

- Medicare beneficiaries in the Part D prescription medicine coverage will receive 50% discounts on all brand-name medicines.
- Over-the-counter (OTC) medicines not prescribed by a doctor will no longer be reimbursable through flexible spending arrangements or health savings/medical savings accounts.
- An annual, nondeductible fee will be imposed on pharmaceuticals and importers' branded medicines, based on market share.

Unfortunately, the creation of a rational effective supply system that leverages public and private recourses seems to still be far in the future, and the protection of the rights of Americans to essential medicines is still in the hands of human rights advocates and consumer's rights activists and not the U.S. government.

Vaccines. The Global Alliance for Vaccines and Immunisation (GAVI),[2] helps 72 countries and civil society organizations purchase vaccines through the GAVI fund. Developing countries need to access the fund to ensure the continuous supply of vaccines and support that the alliance provides; this protects infants and children against several preventable infections such as polio, TB, measles, and so forth and helps meet the targets of the fourth Millennium Development Goal (MDG) of reducing infant mortality.

Green Light Committee.[3] Established in 2000, the Green Light Committee (GLC) is another fund countries can use to finance medications for their citizens. The GLC provides expensive second-line TB medicines for cases of multidrug resistance and helps countries protect and fulfill the rights of TB patients to an effective treatment. The GLC is essential to the achievement of TB reduction target of MDG 6.

Global Fund.[4] Since its creation in 2002, many developing countries have used the Global Fund (GF) to purchase mosquito nets, lab supplies, and medicines for their TB, AIDS, and malaria programs through performance-based grants. In addition, through the Joint United Nations Programme on HIV/AIDS (UNAIDS), USAID, and other donors, countries access assistance to strengthen their procurement and supply systems. By December 2009, the GF has disbursed more than $19 billion to 144 countries and saved almost 5 million lives since its foundation (GF, 2010). The current financial crisis has affected the revenue that the GF gets from its investments and reduced the commitments made by the G8 donors that contribute to fund and reduced.

Ensuring Rational Use

Therapeutic Committees

Governments are duty bearers, but they are not solely responsible for every aspect of effective supply systems. Health workers need to make correct diagnoses and prescribe the right medicines. In addition, medicines need to be dispensed correctly, and patients and/or caregivers must understand how to use them properly.

Expert committees that review and research the use of medicines need to develop standard treatment guidelines and monitor adherence to these guidelines. All hospitals must have a rational use committees (also known as medicine and therapeutic committees) that ensure the right medicines are selected, procured, and used according to standard treatment guidelines. At national and provincial levels, many countries have developed these committees to ensure the rational use of medicines and quality of care. Internationally, case management guidelines such as the Integrated Management of Childhood Illnesses (IMCI) have demonstrated improvements in the use of medicines (Zhang, Dai, & Zhang, 2007).

Children's Doses and Presentations

Children have special concerns when it comes to medication issues. Many developing countries do not have suspension formulations or pills in the doses and quantities required for small children (Robertson et al., 2009). Childproof packaging and other safety measures to prevent intoxications are still not widespread in developing countries. A rights-based approach would consider children's needs in the development, procurement, and supply of effective medications.

Pharmacies and Prescriptions

Patients obtain their medicines in government-funded or private-run pharmacies or medicine shops. Pharmacies face many challenges such as high medicine prices, lack of trained staff, inadequate medicine administration procedures, and poor monitoring and information systems (Doloresco & Vermeulen, 2009). A way of addressing some of these problems is to ensure the dispensation of medicines only by prescription. In most countries, a prescription is required for most medicines, except those that have been approved by government agencies to be sold OTC. Prescribers are usually physicians; however, in developing countries, nurses may also prescribe medications for a majority of primary care level conditions. There are legal issues that need to be addressed when nurses are allowed to prescribe (Miles, Seitio, & McGilvray, 2006).

A prescription is an important medical document that can protect populations from the negative consequences of irrational use of medicines, such as antibiotic resistance, medicine overdose, and/or overmedication. A prescription also prevents the inappropriate use of products. For example, in Papua New Guinea, where diarrhea kills hundreds of children because of contaminated bottles, baby bottles cannot be purchased without a prescription. Along with the prescription, the prescriber can provide the mother with information about bottle hygiene and other infant nutrition practices.

Standard Treatment Guidelines and Antimicrobial Resistance

After intentional or unintentional overdose, antimicrobial resistance (AR) is the most common negative result of the sale of antibiotics without a prescription by the informal sector in developing countries and the irrational use of medicines. In addition, inadequate case management and the unnecessary prescription of antibiotics for viral conditions such as diarrheas, colds, and upper respiratory conditions has rendered many first line antibiotics useless and created "superbugs" that kill patients all over the world and increase the cost of health care. In developing countries, AR has caused TB to become a major killer again, particularly in patients who are HIV positive. In the United States, the Federal Interagency Task Force on Antimicrobial Resistance, along with the Department of Health and Human Services and the Centers for Disease Control and Prevention (CDC), have research, surveillance, and education programs to prevent and control AR. The FDA is also conducting research to prolong the "life" of antibiotics and the search for new products.

CONCLUSION

Public health professionals, whether they are acting as duty bearers, advocates, or health providers, need to be aware of the issues in ensuring the right to essential medicines and medical supplies to progressively contribute to improve access, availability and rational use. We envision that this will be a role that will grow for public health professionals worldwide.

REFERENCES

Attawell, K., & Mundy, J. (2003). *Provision of antiretroviral therapy in resource-limited settings: A review of experience up to August 2003.* London, England: Health Systems Resource Centre, Department of International Development. Retrieved April 20, 2010, from http://www.who.int/3by5/publications/documents/en/ARTpaper_DFID_WHO.pdf

Azatyan, S. (2008). African Medicines Regulatory Harmonization Initiative (AMRHI): A WHO concept paper. *WHO Drug Information, 22*(3).

Beran, D., McCabe, A., & Yudkin, J. (2008). Access to medicines versus access to treatment: The case of diabetes. *Bulletin of the World Health Organization, 86*(8), 648–659.

Bird, R. (2009). Developing nations and the compulsory license: Maximizing access to essential medicines while minimizing investment side effects. *Journal of Law, Medicine & Ethics Pharmaceutical Regulations,* 209–221.

Caudron, J., Ford, N., Henkens, M., Mace, C., Kiddle-Monroe, R., & Pinel, J. (2008). Substandard medicines in resource-poor settings: A problem that can no longer be ignored. *Tropical Medicine and International Health, 13*(8), 1062–1072.

Doloresco, F., & Vermeulen, L. (2009). Global survey of hospital pharmacy practice. *American Journal Health-System Pharmacy, 66*(Suppl. 3),S13–S19.

Flynn, S., Hollis, A., & Palmedo, M. (2009). An economic justification for open access to essential medicine patents in developing countries. *Journal of Law, Medicine & Ethics, 37*(2), 184–208.

Galvao, J. (2005). Brazil and access to HIV/AIDS drugs: A question of human rights and public health. *American Journal Public Health, 95,* 1110–1116.

Global Fund. (2010). The Global Fund 2010–Innovation and impact. Replenishment Report. Retrieved May 10, 2010, from http://www.theglobalfund.org/documents/replenishment/2010/Global_Fund_2010_Innovation_and_Impact_en.pdf

Griffith, R., & Davies, R. (2003). Accountability and drug administration in community care. *British Journal of Community Nursing, 8*(2), 65–69.

Hogerzeil, H. (2006). Essential medicines and human rights: What can they learn from each other? *Bulletin of the World Health Organization, 84,* 371–375.

Hogerzeil, H., Samson, M., Casanovas, V., & Rahmani-Ocora, L. (2006). Is access to essential medicines as part of the fulfillment of the right to health enforceable through the courts? *Lancet, 368,* 305–311.

Huff-Rousselle, M., & Burnett, F. (1996). Cost containment through pharmaceutical procurement: A Caribbean case study. *The International Journal of Health Planning and Management, 11*(2), 135–157.

Mendis, S., Fukino, K., Cameron, A., Laing, R., Filipe, A, Jr., Khatib, O., et al. (2007). The availability and affordability of selected essential medicines for chronic diseases in six low- and middle-income countries. *Bull World Health Organization, 85,* 279–288.

Miles, K., Seitio, O., & McGilvray, M. (2006). Nurse prescribing in low-resource settings: Professional considerations. *International Nursing Review, 53,* 290–296.

Milstien, J., & Kaddar, M. (2006). Managing the effect of TRIPS on availability of priority vaccines. *Bulletin of the World Health Organization, 84,* 360–365.

Mohamed Ali, G. (2009). How to establish a successful revolving drug fund: The experience of Khartoum state in the Sudan. *Bulletin of the World Health Organization, 87,* 139–142.

Musungu, S. (2006). Benchmarking progress in tackling the challenges of intellectual property, and access to medicines in developing countries. *Bulletin of the World Health Organization, 84,* 366–370.

Oliveira, M., Zepeda, J., Costa, G., & Velásquez, G. (2004). Has the implementation of the TRIPS Agreement in Latin America and the Caribbean produced intellectual property legislation that favours public health? *Bulletin of the World Health Organization, 82,* 815–821.

Robertson, J., Forte, G., & Trapsida, J., Hill, S. (2009). What essential medicines for children are on the shelf? *Bulletin of the World Health Organization, 87,* 231–237. Retrieved September 15, 2010, from http://apps.who.int/medicinedocs/documents/ s14099e/s14099e.pdf

Sampat, B. (2009) Academic patents and access to medicines in developing countries. *American Journal of Public Health, 99,* 9–17.

Seuba, X. (2006). A human rights approach to the WHO model list of essential medicines. *Bulletin of the World Health Organization, 84,* 405–411.

Shaffer, E. R, & Brenner, J. E. (2009). A trade agreement's impact on access to generic drugs. *Health Affairs, 28*(5), w957–w968.

Tordoff, J., Norris, P., & Reith, D. (2005). Managing prices for hospital pharmaceuticals: A successful strategy for New Zealand? *Value in Health, 8*(3), 201–208.

United Nations. (2000). The right to the highest attainable standard of health. General Comment 14. Retrieved March 4, 2010, from http://www.unhchr.ch/tbs/doc.nsf/(Symbol)/40d009901358b0e2c1256915005090be?Opendocument

Walkom, E., Robertson, J., Newby, D., & Pillay, T. (2006). The role of pharmacoeconomics in formulary decision making. *Formulary, 41*(8), 374–386. Retrieved April 28, 2010, from http://formularyjournal.modernmedicine.com/formulary/article/articleDetail.jsp?id=364692

WHO. (2006). The interagency list of essential medicines for reproductive health. Retrieved September 15, 2010, from http://apps.who.int/medicinedocs/documents/s14099e/s14099e.pdf

Zhang, Y., Dai, Y., & Zhang, S. (2007). Impact of implementation of Integrated Management of Childhood Illness on improvement of health system in China. *Journal of Paediatrics and Child Health, 43,* 681–685.

NOTES

[1] World Health Organization. Consolidated List of Products whose Consumption and/ or Sale have been Banned, Withdrawn, Severely Restricted or Not Approved by Governments. Retrieved from http://www.who.int/medicines/areas/quality_safety/ safety_efficacy/who_emp_qsm2008.3.pdf

[2] The Global Alliance for Vaccines and Immunisation. Retrieved from http://www .gavialliance.org

[3] World Health Organization. Retrieved from http://www.who.int/tb/challenges/mdr/ greenlightcommittee/en/

[4] The Global Fund to Fight AIDS, TB and Malaria. Retrieved from http://www.theglobal fund.org/en/

Conclusion: Rights-Based Approaches in Public Health

Elvira Beracochea, Dabney P. Evans, and Corey Weinstein

Throughout this volume, we have explored how rights-based approaches (RBAs) in analysis, planning, program development, and evaluation can infuse any public health activity. The chapters demonstrate various ways in which public health practitioners are exploring and shaping the contours of the road map toward the right to health. Here, we summarize some of the key findings of this volume and offer suggestions to public health professionals, who are in a unique position to investigate and implement RBAs in their work.

THE LINKS BETWEEN RIGHTS-BASED APPROACHES AND PUBLIC HEALTH

The International Covenant on Economic, Social and Cultural Rights (ICESCR), as introduced in chapter 1, makes it clear how the concerns of a human rights approach parallels those of public health. The ICESCR outlines the activities required for the realization of the right to health, including attention to maternal and child health, to environmental and industrial hygiene, to the prevention of epidemic, endemic, and occupational disease, and to the availability of accessible medical care. These concerns could also be the focus of any public health department.

The use of a human rights paradigm highlights the concern of the public health community with social justice and can move the field from a welfare or needs-based approach to a RBA. The needs-based approach identifies and assists people who most require goods and services to help mitigate adverse health outcomes. In such an approach, the obligation of the State to intervene comes out of an interest in decency, fairness, or the desire to subvert dissent. Needs-based approaches tend to be analyzed within a given particular system and can create dependency on service agencies.

RBAs, on the other hand, are based on participation and empowerment. They recognize the right of all people to assert their claims, and they make clear what obligations the duty bearers must fulfill. RBAs look past a particular health system or service. As a result, vulnerable groups strengthen their abilities to address the root causes of poverty, marginalization, and health disparities and to lay claim to the civil, political, social, and economic resources to meet their needs.

As outlined in the United Nations Development Program 2003 Human Rights Approach Statement of Common Understanding, individuals are key actors in their own development, not passive recipients; participation is both a means and a goal. UN programs focus on marginalized, disadvantaged, and excluded groups to reduce disparities. Vulnerable populations are a preoccupation of public health because of its emphasis on population-based health as opposed to individual health. However, individual and group demographics such as sex, race, and disease status are often the exact criteria that place individuals at risk of unequal access or disparate treatment (see chapters 10 and 12). An emphasis on vulnerability from a human rights perspective allows public health professionals to maintain their population-based focus while addressing the needs of those who require the most attention. Clearly, health care reform that removes economic barriers to accessible care is needed (see chapter 4). However, any rights-based change requires that the delivery system be rationalized to meet the needs of the rights holders-not just the financial interests of insurers and providers.

THE ROLE OF THE STATE IN FULFILLING
THE RIGHT TO HEALTH

There are great challenges in fulfilling the right to health of disaffected and marginalized populations, such as the poor, women, substance users, immigrants, persons with mental illness, prisoners, and others. States have the obligations to respect these vulnerable groups while protecting them and fulfilling their right to health. These requirements—to respect, to protect, and to fulfill—are the core State responsibilities.

States implement these responsibilities in various ways. They can formulate laws in accordance with human rights doctrine. They can also implement administrative regulations that make the protection and fulfillment of the right to health a compulsory part of the daily work of government agencies. Finally, States, along with other organizations (such as the American Public Health Association and the Association of Schools of Public Health) are encouraged to increase human rights education for public health professionals and all health science students.

Rights-based public health approaches assert that any given population has the right to organize to demand improvements in the quality of life as part of its right to health. For example, as the duty bearer, States have a responsibility to work toward food safety, clean air and water, accessible efficient transit, and other aspects of communal life that bear on the health of the population. This includes issues of violence at all levels. From a rights-based perspective, violence is seen as a symptom of inequalities and despair. Violence control then becomes a matter of community development within a human rights framework. Although the issue of violence becomes more complex on an international scale, rights-based analysis can be used to clarify causes and solutions to civil war and cross-border interventions. Chapters 13 and 20 offer some examples of rights-based health programs that are being used in high-conflict areas.

GLOBAL RESPONSIBILITIES AND THE RIGHT TO HEALTH

On a global scale, life on our planet needs to start to be fairer for the billions whose right to health is not fulfilled. A baby born in Kenya to an HIV-positive mother has the same rights as a baby born to a healthy mother in the United States or Europe. Postponing a child's or his or her mother's right to health is unacceptable in a world where the knowledge and technology to protect the baby and the mother exist, and under the international law and public health practice, it must be made illegal.

Making the right to health a reality is a continuous process. It requires global responsibility and leadership to ensure that the right to health is truly universal (see chapter 5). We need a global plan (see chapter 6) to ensure that our investments in health offer a strong return in the numbers of people served and lives saved. We also need new forms of partnership between developed and developing nations that empower the developing nations to take ownership of their own development process. The new way is an RBA in which developed and developing states fulfill their respective duties as stated in the Millennium Declaration (see chapter 5).

As with other human rights, our understanding of the right to health is constantly evolving. Great progress in this area has been made in recent years. The complexities of the right to health have been explored by various national and international bodies. Courts have heard cases on the topic, demonstrating that economic, social, and cultural rights are just as justifiable and enforceable as civil and political rights. However, States vary widely in terms of how well they respect and enforce human rights. Monitoring of compliance with human rights treaties is left largely to the states themselves—and none of the findings of the UN monitoring committees is legally binding in any case. In this murky world of accountability, some clarity can be developed through institutions of public health.

PUBLIC HEALTH PROFESSIONALS
AS ADVOCATES OF HUMAN RIGHTS

The correspondence between human rights principles and the basic tenets of public health means that the public health community has a special role in asserting these rights in society. Our educational programs, research agendas, preventive programs, and health care services can all serve to realize basic human rights, monitor state compliance, and protect vulnerable populations. Thereby public health institutions can directly advocate for the State. Public health can help guide governments in setting priorities and adopting policies that improve the lives of people using human rights principles.

On an individual level, how public health practitioners approach their work has human rights implications. For example, as discussed in chapter 16, Doctors for Global Health only works in areas where they have been invited, and they ensure that the community is an active participant in every step of the process, from defining its health needs to delivering care. As a result, the community not only benefits from the health services provided but also builds its own infrastructure capable of sustaining any development achieved. In this new paradigm, members of the public health program staff work as facilitators as much as providers of care.

Public health professionals should have only one loyalty: to the citizens and communities we serve. Our work respects and protects those rights (see chapter 7). The right to health includes creating policies, regulations, programs, services, and other public health mechanisms and instruments to ensure access to timely and quality care to all. In an RBA, our imagination and creativity are the only limit to find better and more effective ways to serve.

Protecting the right to health of poor illiterate women, children, intravenous (IV) drug users, prisoners, and those affected by conflicts is and will be a responsibility for public health professionals worldwide (see Part 3). We must unite, work in real and virtual networks that share information, and account for those we serve.

Throughout Part 4, this book offers examples of how organizations and individuals have implemented RBAs in various settings and geographic locations. Many have shared their tools so that you can join the work of rights-based public health professionals. Perhaps, the impact of embracing an RBA is best summarized by Ariel Frisancho, Jay Goulden, and Helene D. Gayle (see chapter 15) when they state,

> our global experiences shows that a rights-based approach to health makes a difference, not only in how you approach the work you do but also in what you do, who you do it with, and, with increasing surety, the nature and quality of the impacts achieved. p. 287.

RBAs do contribute to the fulfillment of our mission as public health professionals. Now it is your turn to adopt the human rights principles and take public health practice to a new level, to the level of universal access to health and justice. It is time. It is our time.

Appendix: List of Acronyms

AIDS	acquired immunodeficiency syndrome
CAA	U.S. Clean Air Act
CAFTA	Central American Free Trade Agreement
CAIPES	*El Centro de Atención Integral para la Prevención y Educación en Salud* [The Center for Integrated Care for Prevention and Education in Health]
CAT	Convention Against Torture and Other Cruel, Inhuman or Degrading Treatment or Punishment
CEDAW	Convention on the Elimination of All Forms of Discrimination Against Women
CERD	Convention on the Elimination of All Forms of Racial Discrimination
CESCR	UN Committee on Economic, Social and Cultural Rights
CHW	community health worker
CIDI	*Centros de Integración Desarrollo Infantil* [Centers for Integrated Child Development]
CISEPO	Canada International Scientific Exchange Program
CISOMOZ	Committee for Health in Southeast Morazán
COBRA	Consolidated Omnibus Budget Reconciliation Act
COPC	Community-Oriented Primary Care
CPN	Communist Party of Nepal
CRC	Convention on the Rights of the Child
CSO	civil society organization
DAC	Development Assistance Committee
DFID	U.K. Department for International Development
DGH	Doctors for Global Health
ECHUI	Ending Child Hunger and Undernutrition Initiative
EMTALA	Emergency Medical Treatment and Active Labor Act

EMR	electronic medical record
EPA	U.S. Environmental Protection Agency
ERISA	Employee Retirement Income Security Act of 1974
FAO	Food and Agriculture Organization
FBO	faith-based organization
FDA	Food and Drug Administration
GAVI	Global Alliance for Vaccines and Immunisation
GC	general comment
GDP	gross domestic product
HAP	hazardous air pollutant
HHRE	Health and Human Rights Education
HIPAA	Health Insurance Portability and Accountability Act
HIV	human immunodeficiency virus
IADB	Inter-American Development Bank
ICCPR	International Covenant on Civil and Political Rights
ICESCR	International Covenant on Economic, Social and Cultural Rights
IMR	infant mortality rate
IPPNW	International Physicians for the Prevention of Nuclear War
MACT	maximum achievable control technology
MD	Millennium Declaration
MDGs	Millennium Development Goals
MNC	multinational corporation
MoH	Ministry of Health
NAAQS	National Ambient Air Quality Standards
NBA	needs-based approach
NGO	nongovernmental organization
NIS	new Israeli shekel
NMA	Nepal Medical Association
NSPS	new source performance standards
OECD	Organisation for Economic Co-operation and Development
OHCHR	United Nations Office of the High Commissioner for Human Rights
oPt	occupied Palestinian territories
PAHO	Pan American Health Organization
PAPAD	Professional Alliance for Peace and Democracy
PD	Paris Declaration
PHR-I	Physicians for Human Rights-Israel
PMTCT	prevention of mother-to-child transmission
PSRN	Physicians for Social Responsibility, Nepal
RBA	rights-based approach

SIP   state implementation plan
SOA   School of the Americas
SR   special rapporteur
STD   sexually transmitted disease
SUDs   substance use disorders
TB   tuberculosis
TNC   transnational corporation
UDHR   Universal Declaration of Human Rights
UN   United Nations
UNDP   United Nations Development Programme
UNFPA   United Nations Population Fund
UNHCR   United Nations High Commissioner for Refugees
UNICEF   United Nations International Children's Emergency Fund
USAID   United States Agency for International Development
WFP   World Food Programme
WHA   World Health Assembly
WHINSEC   Western Hemisphere Institute for Security and Cooperation
WHO   World Health Organization
WIC   Women, Infants, and Children program

Index

Note: Page numbers followed by f indicate figures, and t indicate tables.